Understanding pain for better clinical practice

DEDICATION

To my mother, Doris Melton Linton,
my father, the late Michael Linton
for teaching me
just about everything
and
to Gabriel, life is a sport

**PAIN RESEARCH AND
CLINICAL MANAGEMENT**

Understanding pain for better clinical practice

A psychological perspective

Steven James Linton PhD

Professor of Psychology
Department of Occupational and Environmental Medicine
Örebro University Hospital
    and
Department of Behavioral, Social and Legal Sciences – Psychology
Örebro University
Örebro, Sweden

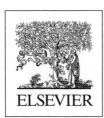

ELSEVIER

EDINBURGH   LONDON   NEW YORK   OXFORD   PHILADELPHIA   ST LOUIS   SYDNEY   TORONTO   2005

ELSEVIER

First published 2005

ISBN 0444515917

British Library Cataloguing in Publication Data
A catalogue record for this book is available from the British Library

Library of Congress Cataloging in Publication Data
A catalog record for this book is available from the Library of Congress

Notice
Knowledge and best practice in this field are constantly changing. As new research
and experience broaden our knowledge, changes in practice, treatment and drug
therapy may become necessary or appropriate. Readers are advised to check the most
current information provided (i) on procedures featured or (ii) by the manufacturer
of each product to be administered, to verify the recommended dose or formula, the
method and duration of administration, and contraindications. It is the responsibility
of the practitioner, relying on their own experience and knowledge of the patient,
to make diagnoses, to determine dosages and the best treatment for each individual
patient, and to take all appropriate safety precautions. To the fullest extent of the law,
neither the publisher nor the author assume any liability for any injury and/or damage
to persons or property arising out of or relating to any use of the material contained in
this book.

The Publisher

Working together to grow
libraries in developing countries

www.elsevier.com | www.bookaid.org | www.sabre.org

ELSEVIER   BOOK AID International   Sabre Foundation

**your source for books,
journals and multimedia
in the health sciences**
www.elsevierhealth.com

Printed in China

Commissioning Editors: Elly Tjoa, Mary Law
Development Editor: Hannah Kenner
Project Manager: Anne Dickie
Designer: Judith Wright

The
publisher's
policy is to use
**paper manufactured
from sustainable forests**

Preface

This is a book about how putting psychological aspects of pain perception into clinical practice can affect you and the patients you care for. It is the story of how psychological factors work to influence the thoughts, feelings and behaviors we have when in pain. By understanding pain from a psychological perspective, you will be better equipped to comprehend the reactions patients have to pain as well as to how you can best care for them. During the past 20 years, my students, colleagues and I, as well as a host of internationally renowned scientists, have explored the exciting nature of psychological processes and pain. This book is an attempt to put this knowledge into a workable format for the student and clinician.

Pain is an ever-present experience, but despite its common occurrence it is nevertheless difficult to grasp and explain. Some might even say it is baffling. Yet a good knowledge of pain is essential for understanding patients and providing optimal healthcare. To facilitate a modern, scientific appreciation of pain, this book poses intriguing questions about how we perceive pain and why we react to it in certain ways. New inroads in research have broadened our view of pain and provide insights that simply were not previously possible. Even though many descriptions of pain dissect it into small fragments, a modern view underscores how integrated our pain perception system actually is. In fact, it is an amazing arrangement that includes biological and psychological processes that clearly help us to deal effectively with our environment.

I have written this book for individuals interested in pain and psychology, and in particular for those in the healthcare professions. My aim is to help healthcare professionals comprehend the psychology of pain so that they may provide better care for their patients. My hope is that others will also find the book interesting and useful. In this endeavor I have chosen to use musculoskeletal pain problems, like back and neck pain, as the main examples. In part this is because I work with these problems and thus have better insight into them than other pain problems; however, this is also because back and neck pain are such common problems that most readers will be able to relate to these examples. But let there be no confusion, the principles illustrated apply to pain perception in general and not just back or neck pain.

The book integrates a theoretical model and clinical practice and therefore it has two parts. In the first half of the book, we examine pain from a psychological perspective. Here we delve into the depths of pain perception and explore how attention, cognitions, beliefs and behaviors influence our pain. Indeed, the intriguing role of psychological processes is underscored and I maintain that psychology is crucial for pain perception. Although these processes are intricate and complicated, I have developed a relatively simple model of pain perception that will aid in remembering the basic concepts. Further, a typical patient with a pain problem, "Hank", is provided as a case study to help illustrate the main points in an actual case. This case is built upon in each chapter to show how pain problems develop. A good comprehension of the psychology of pain is highlighted and sets the stage for application.

In the second half of the book, we turn to utilizing the psychological perspective in clinical situations. Most books on treatment start with a full-fledged pain patient typically already suffering a chronic pain problem: the focus is on relieving chronic pain. Instead of this, I have concentrated on prevention and start with the first contact with the patient. Our case study, "Hank", is ever present and used to illustrate the application techniques. Consequently, the second section starts with why seemingly normal acute pain may become chronic and this information is used for the early identification of patients who risk developing persistent pain and disability. Because communication with the patient is so crucial for successful intervention, an entire chapter is given to applying psychological principles for enhancing contact with the patient and arriving at relevant goals for treatment. Further, we examine basic methods, from a psychological perspective, for dealing with patients at the very first consultation. Although excellent medical care is a prerequisite,

it is quite surprising how important and powerful a psychological approach can be. This is clearly documented in the chapters concerning a cognitive-behavioral approach to early treatment. Here a program has been carefully established to help patients, at an early point in time, more effectively cope with their pain problem. You will learn how this treatment is actually conducted in the clinic. The results of the cognitive-behavioral treatment as an intervention to prevent persistent disability has been impressive. Indeed, in several studies the risk of developing long-term work disability has been reduced quite significantly.

This book has been stimulated by enormous amounts of information that I have had the benefit of accessing through the scientific literature, but also through endless hours of discussion, research and clinical practice. I am indebted to the countless people who have helped me along the way with information, feedback, ideas, reports and so on. Some are acknowledged through the references, while others are not mainly because the support has taken the form of a discussion. This ranges from patients to students, colleagues, teachers and mentors. It would be impossible to name them all, but let me sincerely thank each and every one of them anonymously.

Finally, it is my hope that you will enjoy reading this book. I will delight in every laugh, every question, every surprise, every insight, and even every opposition you have! My goal is to stimulate your thought and curiosity about pain. My conviction is that by putting this knowledge into practice you will become a better practitioner and provide outstanding pain management. May the satisfaction of excellent pain care be with you, your patients, and your loved ones.

Steven James Linton
Fingerboda, Sweden

Contents

Part 1:

The psychology of pain perception and behavior

1

The need to understand the psychology of pain

The thing worse than death is the pain.

—Terminally ill pain patient

Never before has there been such an urgent need to understand the psychology of pain. We are at a unique junction where understanding and applying information on the psychology of pain could have a major impact on how we deal with pain problems as diverse as ordinary back pain to life-threatening cancer pain. This could have an enormous impact on how we care for patients in pain. Moreover, since pain is as ubiquitous as any emotion, there is a need to study the mysteries of pain perception and behavior.

Pain truly presents a number of mystifying experiences that are difficult to understand without a proper knowledge of the psychology of pain. Take, for example, the development of a chronic disabling backache. While it is widely recognized that acute pain serves as an important "warning signal", it is difficult to understand any biological value in chronic pain. The pain does not easily resolve and it results in great suffering and numerous functional problems. In fact, having persistent pain would seem to reduce our biological ability to survive and therefore might be a disservice rather than a service to us. Why, then, does chronic pain develop?

Another mystery is the relationship between the degree of tissue damage and the pain experience. A simple, Cartesian model would postulate a direct link: the more damage, the more pain. This would appear to be biologically "correct" in that appropriate action could then be taken that would directly reflect the seriousness of the tissue damage. However, healthcare professionals and lay people alike are acutely aware that there are numerous instances when tissue damage is not directly related to the amount of pain experienced. One of the first modern researchers to develop this theme was Beecher, who served as a surgeon for the Allies in World War II. Beecher observed that soldiers with severe injuries ordinarily required few painkillers as compared to his surgical patients at home in civilian settings. An enticing explanation put forward by Beecher was that the situation in which the injury occurs exerts influence on pain perception. While patients view a surgery as a threat to their normally good health, Beecher's soldiers were overjoyed to have survived the battle and to be on their way home. Other examples abound. I have personally witnessed a man stick a rusty nail through his arm without the slightest complaint or flinch, while as a child I experienced a simple injection as excruciating.

Still another example is the tremendous variation in the effects of painkillers and placebos. The effects of the so-called placebo are so well known that scientists around the world require that new drugs be tested against them. In short, simply taking a tablet or injection that is believed to contain an active ingredient produces some benefits such as pain relief even when the true ingredient is neutral. The question is why. Today scientists look to the role of learning and especially to the role of "expectations" in explaining the placebo effect. Moreover, rather than viewing the placebo as a problem, attention is now turning to how this effect might best be utilized clinically.

If pain were a highly mechanical operation it would be simple to circumvent it; but interestingly we are equipped with a wide variety of coping strategies to help us deal with pain. Why do we need to cope with pain rather than simply to discover and remove the source of it? Moreover, why isn't one particular coping strategy universal, that is, why isn't there one strategy that is always superior to others?

All these mysteries demonstrate that a simple, mechanical view of pain does not explain human pain perception and thus underscore the role of other factors. The list of the seeming mysteries of pain could fill this whole book, but the point is that many aspects of pain cannot be fully understood without considering pain from a psychological perspective. Pain is truly a multidimensional phenomenon where biological and psychological processes are extremely well integrated.

PAIN IS A PREVALENT PREDICAMENT

Another cogent reason for studying the psychology of pain is the fact that pain problems are so common (Crombie et al., 1999). Pain is a natural perception and nearly everyone has a pain problem at some point. This is not only normal, but extremely important for survival as pain curbs our behaviors so that we do not injure ourselves; it helps us to deal efficiently with the problem and thereby increases our ability to survive. The few people born without pain sensations demonstrate this advantage as they have a truly difficult time surviving. But while we are aware of the basic need to be able to feel pain, we are also equipped with mechanisms to decrease, escape or avoid pain as best we can.

Pain is common regardless of age, color or culture. While we might expect pain to be prevalent in the elderly, it is an experience that affects humans from birth. Research shows that infants react to pain even though their nervous system is not fully developed. Moreover, children may suffer from chronic pain problems ranging from headaches (estimated prevalence of up to 37%), knee, back, cancer and abdominal

pain (McGrath, 1996). Chronic pain problems are more prevalent for older people (Helme and Gibson, 1999). The elderly suffer a variety of persistent pain problems dominated by pain in the joints, back, legs and feet. And although cultural factors influence how we experience and cope with pain, the associated suffering appears to be universal (Moore and Brödsgaard, 1999).

It is not surprising then that pain is the main reason that people in developed countries seek healthcare. In the United States, pain is said to account for over 80% of all visits to the doctor (Gatchel and Turk, 1996). But pain also results in numerous other healthcare visits to other professionals such as physical therapists, nurses, medical technicians, psychologists or occupational therapists. Often medical assessments include laboratory, imaging or other advanced techniques. Actual treatment may include a variety of methods and needs to be followed over long periods of time. Thus, treatment costs alone amount to more than $5 billion dollars annually in the United States. Moreover, so-called complementary medicine such as massage, chiropractics, baths, etc., are a fast-growing alternative that attracts numerous patients. In fact, in our studies of musculoskeletal pain problems, patients sought alternative forms of care as often as they sought help from a physical therapist or general practitioner (Linton et al., 1998).

In fact, healthcare expenditures, of which pain is an important part, now consume a noteworthy part of the Gross Domestic Product in many countries. A study using 1995 values (Table 1.1) showed that countries spent up to 14% of their GDP on healthcare (Waddell and Nordlund, 2000).

In addition to healthcare, people purchase gigantic amounts of pain medications, remedies and other paraphernalia in the hope of relieving their pain. Although the advances in pharmacological methods have dramatically increased our ability to manage pain, it also reflects on the number of people suffering. Health economists point to the considerable costs that patients and their families incur because of pain (Goossens and Evers, 1997; Goossens, 2002). These include out-of-pocket costs for managing the pain, but

Table 1.1 Healthcare expenditures as % of Gross Domestic Product, 1995.

Germany	7.7%
The Netherlands	8.8%
United Kingdom	8.2%
United States	14.2%

Based on data in Waddell and Nordlund, 2000.

also costs for accommodating the person in pain at home, e.g. particular chairs, beds, stairs or equipment in cars. In addition, people in pain incur expenses in the form of paid and unpaid help in the home as well as for travel. Historically, the Food and Drug Administration came about as an authority to oversee the literally hundreds of remedies that were devised in the United States and elsewhere in the late 1800s and early 1900s designed mainly to relieve pain.

Pain is also a leading cause of functional problems and work disability. Pain from the back, neck and upper extremities is the single most common reason for being off work sick in many countries. Undeniably, this may represent the "treatment failures" that we want to avoid in our practices. In a wide range of painful illnesses, there is a real risk that the condition develops into a chronic problem. Estimates of the prevalence of chronic pain, for example, range from 7% to 40% (Crombie and Davies, 1999). In one study, as an illustration, it was determined that as many as 10% of the population may suffer from widespread chronic pain (McBeth and Macfarlane, 2002). A general survey in Sweden showed that for adults about 12% of the population reported chronic neck or back pain (Nachemson and Jonsson, 2000). Other estimates of chronic back pain are as high as 45% of adults (Nachemson and Jonsson, 2000)! And the development of long-term pain problems is not uncommon after a variety of illnesses including headache, stroke, surgery, stomach disorders and most forms of musculoskeletal disorders (Crombie et al., 1999). In fact, back and neck pain are by far the most common sources of pain in persistent problems (McBeth and Macfarlane, 2002) and this is one reason that this book puts spinal pain in the spotlight as an example of how chronic pain may develop.

Pain also results in extensive work loss. In fact, pain-related illness is involved in the majority of work loss due to ill-health. As an example, consider that a national health survey in the United States showed that 17.6% of American workers lost an estimated 149 million days of work as a result of back pain alone (Guo et al., 1995). And the rate of work loss may be rising. Figures from Sweden show that the percentage of employees off work for back pain rose by eight times between 1970 and 1992 (Nachemson and Jonsson, 2000). Add to these figures work loss due to other painful disorders such as cancer, rheumatic diseases, cardiovascular conditions and the like and the numbers become overwhelming.

The total economic burden that the individual and society bear for pain is staggering. Indeed, in the United States, the costs of healthcare, disability and lost productivity due to pain was estimated at over

Table 1.2 The direct costs of back pain in Sweden in 1987 as compared to 1995 as calculated in 1995 price levels.

Type of expenditure	1987 (cost in millions of Swedish crowns)	1995 (cost in millions of Swedish crowns)
Inpatient care	419	415
Outpatient care	1,082	1,869
Drugs	167	152
Total costs	1,668	2,436

Based on Nordlund and Waddell (2000).

$100 billion dollars in 1990 (Bonica, 1990). Costs have skyrocketed since 1990. A recent national study conducted in Sweden underscored the costs of medical care for back pain. As Table 1.2 illustrates, the total cost for care was calculated using 1995 currency and price rates. It shows a substantial increase of about 36% between 1987 and 1995.

However, the costs for treatment are but a small portion of the total costs. The largest cost is for compensating people who are unable to work because of their pain. Table 1.3 provides an overview of the breakdown of how societal resources are spent on back pain in Sweden. The numbers are shocking as the vast majority of the resources are spent on various forms of compensation for lost work such as sick days and early retirements. This appears to be true in several developed countries (van Tulder et al., 1995; Goossens, 2002). Moreover, of the money spent on healthcare, only a small portion appears to be focused on early preventive interventions or comprehensive pain rehabilitation services.

What are the total costs for back pain and how do they vary from country to country? Some analyses have

Table 1.3 An overview of the costs for back pain.

Type of expenditure	% of total expenditure
Indirect costs, e.g. compensation, early retirement	92
Direct costs	8
Physician visits	26
Physical therapy	36
Drugs	8
Other interventions	30

Based on data from Nachemson and Jonsson (2000).

Table 1.4 A comparison of costs for back pain in various countries. The cost is calculated in US dollars (1991 value) and is the cost per inhabitant.

Country	Direct costs	Indirect costs	Total costs per inhabitant
United Kingdom	7	113	120
The Netherlands	24	299	323
Sweden	24	266	290

Based on data from Nordlund and Waddell (2000).

been attempted and one is summarized in Table 1.4. Here the direct medical costs as well as the indirect costs such as for compensation have been determined. Subsequently, the total cost has been calculated on a per capita basis so that the total cost of back pain per inhabitant (and per year) may be used as a basis for comparison. As may be seen, the cost is enormous and ranges from $120 per inhabitant and year in the United Kingdom to $323 per inhabitant and year in the Netherlands. We may truly wonder if we are getting good value for our expenditures. A thesis is that early preventive interventions that truly employ a psychological perspective will be more cost-effective because they address the problem more adequately.

MULTIDIMENSIONAL VIEW OPENS NEW ROADS FOR CARE

The real value of the multidimensional view of pain where psychological and other factors are weighed in is the new avenues for care it presents. To be sure, applying psychological principles can enhance pain treatments and provide insights into how uncomfortable, disabling pain might be prevented.

The biological–psychological interface shows that these factors are highly integrated. As such, changes in one therefore influence changes in the other. The biology of pain shows a magnificent system that is dynamic and well tuned. To optimally serve its purpose, it is, however, integrated into a psychological system in order to react to the demands the environment places on us. Thus psychological processes influence the biological system. For example, a pinprick does not represent a large trauma and ordinarily is short-lived and not particularly intense. However, if the person is frightened or anticipates that the healthcare professional is not competent and may "jab" the patient, then the same pinprick may be experienced as an ordeal that is quite painful and traumatic. By understanding the psychological mechanisms, it is possible to develop methods for reducing the pain and trauma even though the pinprick will still do the same biological "damage" as before.

Often psychological methods are the best or the only methods available for relieving the pain. At other times, they are helpful in enhancing the effects of other methods. Certainly, psychological methods may be used on their own. Still, most often these techniques are used in conjunction with other methods to enhance results. Importantly, psychological methods are helpful in assisting the patient to deal with the entire pain situation. The experience of pain may be overwhelming and influence everyday life in a variety of ways. Psychological methods can be of help in dealing with these changes, even in cases where it is not possible to influence the pain intensity. Moreover, while some methods may require long training such as in a psychology program, others are most powerful when used by other professionals like doctors, nurses or physical therapists.

AIMS OF THE BOOK

This book aims to elucidate the psychology of pain for healthcare providers. By incorporating the latest scientific knowledge available, a basic overview of the psychology of pain will enhance your understanding of the experience of pain. We will follow a typical case in order to illustrate the main points in the text. A central goal is to provide a model that may be applied to a wide variety of illnesses, pain patients and settings. To provide clear examples, we will focus on musculoskeletal (neck, back, muscles, etc.) pain. Yet the information provided can be applied to virtually all situations where people experience pain.

In Part I, the focus is on developing a model of pain that illustrates our current knowledge and that will serve as a heuristic aid. Each chapter develops a particular, basic aspect of the psychology of pain to provide an in-depth understanding of the model. These chapters underscore the psychological processes involved in attending to painful stimuli and interpreting their meaning. Further, the beliefs and cognitions we have about pain are examined with an emphasis on how these influence our coping strategies for pain. Learning is a central aspect as the environment in which the pain occurs shapes our perception of pain and our response to it.

After "picking apart" the basic biological and psychological elements, they will then be put back together again so as to highlight a model that underscores how biological, emotional, cognitive and behavioral factors are integrated. A major theme is that this integrated system underlies the "normal" psychology of pain. This system is highly developed and helps us efficiently deal with injury and pain and increases our ability to survive. On occasion this "normal" psychology nonetheless leads to problems such as the development of persistent pain or inefficient coping strategies. The model will help us to understand when and why this tends to happen.

In Part II, the implications of the psychology of pain are explored to enhance application. Rather than starting with rehabilitation, as most textbooks do, we start with early interventions. Thus, the first chapter in Part II deals with why chronic pain develops. We then proceed to the implications this has for how the very first healthcare visit might better help patients with pain. The continuing chapters proceed with a focus on how early interventions might prevent the development of a full-fledged chronic pain problem.

The aim of Part II is to explore the consequences of applying the psychology of pain in healthcare settings. We will work on how applying psychological knowledge may help us develop our clinical skills to best serve our patients. For example, we will explore how we might actually identify very early on those patients who risk developing chronic pain and disability. Moreover, as psychological processes may play an important role in a given pain problem, we will delve into how interventions might best reflect this. As a result, designing treatment to meet the psychological needs of the patient can greatly enhance outcome, and methods for achieving this are provided. Prevention is an ultimate goal and the final chapters provide detailed information on psychologically oriented secondary prevention methods that help avert the development of disabling chronic pain problems. Armed with this knowledge, a variety of healthcare professionals will be able to apply these techniques.

My overall aspiration with this book is to open new roads for healthcare professionals in dealing with pain problems. By better understanding the mechanisms involved in acute pain and the development of persistent pain and disability, you should be in a better position to prevent, alleviate or lessen the burden of the pain. Hopefully, new paths may be opened to provide for better assessment, treatment, and the prevention of unnecessary pain, disability and suffering.

CHAPTER 2

Models of pain perception

*Our actions and
thoughts are all
steered by the
models we embrace.*

—Author unknown

LEARNING OBJECTIVES

To understand:

- historical models of pain and how they influence our view today;

- that pain is a perception characterized by several aspects, e.g. the sensory, emotional, cognitive and behavioral;

- modern views that integrate biological and psychological knowledge.

Because of its negative and ubiquitous nature, pain has demanded an explanation throughout history. Conceptual models have thus been developed to aid in comprehending pain. These have been based on various religious, philosophical, political and cultural as well as scientific considerations. In order to understand and accept the scientific models of today, we need to understand how historical models continue to exert influence on our thinking. In this chapter, a brief history of pain models will be presented and then a modern model will be outlined that sets the framework for this book. A case study will also be introduced to help us apply the models to patients and their problems. In this way we may contrast past beliefs about pain with our present knowledge about pain from a scientific perspective.

As we can see from the case study, Hank's back pain has developed into a considerable problem that affects him and his family dramatically. An important question is how we might best understand Hank's problem in order to provide the best care possible. Let us examine this by looking historically at models of pain and progressing to a modern view of pain and disability.

PAIN AND PUNISHMENT

Today pain is viewed with compassion and we seldom think about moral or religious implications that may put the sufferer to blame for his or her pain. However, in several historical models of pain, the word "pain" is related to punishment and suffering, and this is sometimes seen as a consequence of

CASE STUDY: HANK

In order to visualize the problems patients may face with pain, let us consider a particular case. This will also help us to illustrate the principles to be underscored throughout the book. This case study is based on a composite of clinical experience and would be a typical scenario for back pain patients seeking rehabilitative care.

Hank is a 44 year old who suffers from neck and back pain. He is married, the father of two boys (9 and 12) and one girl (8). The family live in their own home. They enjoy an active family life with friends and relatives and participate in several sports. Hank has a high school education and has worked in construction for 20 years. His wife is also employed part-time at a large grocery store. Although Hank basically enjoys his work, he does find it monotonous and there is often considerable pressure to finish jobs quickly. At home, Hank is an active family member. He spends considerable time participating and assisting the children in various activities and he also maintains the home and vehicles and does various household chores. When Hank is not with the family, he likes to do sports. This ranges from watching sports on TV to participating in everything from softball to hunting.

About 2 years ago Hank hurt his back. He was surprised that he could not relate the onset of the pain to a specific event. Instead, he woke up with a stiff back that got progressively worse during the day. Hank's back ached as it occasionally had done earlier such as after a sporting event. However, at inception Hank also felt a sharp pain that made him wince. It felt as though someone was sticking a knife in his back. Every movement of the back seemed to exacerbate the pain and it sometimes caused a shooting pain. Bending and twisting movements resulted in a sharp jolt. Naturally, Hank wondered what was wrong with his back. He had never felt anything like this before. He was concerned that something serious must have happened to his back. Since the pain felt like a knife and was at times shooting, he wondered if a nerve might be pinched. Moreover, as movement seemed to set off the bouts, he thought a vertebra might be damaged or chipped. He was concerned that a nerve might be severed leaving him permanently injured. With encouragement from his wife, he rested and made an appointment with his doctor.

The doctor briefly examined Hank and listened to his complaints. However, the doctor could not say exactly what the cause of the pain was although she did find tight, sore muscles in the lower back region. Instead, she said that back pain was common and he would likely recover within a few weeks. She said that this often happened to men doing manual labor and that it would be helpful to give the back a rest. Given the severity of the pain, the doctor also prescribed a painkiller and provided a certificate so that Hank could be off work for a week.

However, after a week the pain still had not subsided. Although a little better, Hank still had considerable pain. He tried to take it easy and spent some time resting every day. Hank also attempted to return to his work. However, this was not easy as his work required lifting, carrying, hammering, and bending and twisting. Hank felt handicapped and that he could not "hold his own" on the job. This put Hank in a difficult position as the company needed to complete the current building project within the next week and much was left to do. After one particularly stressful day at work, Hank's back pain increased significantly that evening. Consequently, he visited his doctor again the next day. The doctor said she would increase the painkillers and extend his sick leave another 10 days.

After resting the additional 10 days, Hank again returned to work. Fortunately, he now felt better. He tried to be careful at work so as not to strain his back and at home he rested. His wife encouraged him to take good care of his back and she and the children pitched in to do some of the chores that Hank normally took care of. Thus, a new routine was developed that Hank and his family trusted would be helpful.

However, after working a couple of weeks, Hank suffered a relapse. Once again he felt a sharp pain and his back really ached. Hank was frustrated and angry that this should happen again when he had worked so hard to avoid a new injury. When Hank returned to his doctor, she was quite concerned. As a result, she ordered images of the back to be taken, provided a stronger pain medication, and advised Hank to be careful with movements that might hurt the back. She provided an additional certificate for sick leave and provided Hank with a referral to a physical therapist. The physical therapist was to provide some pain relief as well as instruction about working in an ergonomic manner.

Unfortunately, Hank suffered more relapses. Each time he received more treatment in the form of medications, some time out from work and physical therapy. Although Hank appreciated these treatments because they made him feel better, they did not really cure his pain. Instead, Hank felt that the pain was getting progressively worse. He now had pain more or less the whole time. Furthermore, the medications and physical therapy seemed to be having less and less effect. In addition, Hank was finding it difficult to do a number of things. For example, he could no longer participate in sports and he found it hard to do several of his normal household duties. Hank also found it demanding to keep up with social activities such as visiting friends and relatives and going to sporting or cultural events.

Because the pain seems to be getting worse rather than better, Hank feels he must do something. In point of fact, he is convinced that something must be wrong that the doctor has not yet discovered. He is well aware that increases in activity normally result in an increase in pain.

He is also concerned that trying to work and attempting his usual household work might be aggravating the injury. Although the images of Hank's back did not show any clear abnormality, the doctor nevertheless decided to refer Hank to an orthopedic specialist. In addition, Hank continued with physical therapy, medications, and being on sick leave. Hank looked forward to getting to the bottom of the problem by visiting the orthopedic surgeon.

However, after being examined by the orthopedic surgeon, it was concluded that an operation was not warranted. The specialist said that there was nothing more he could do. His diagnosis was that the back pain was due to muscle spasms and soft tissue "injuries".

Hank was frustrated. Two years had now gone by, he had seen several doctors. He now realized that his life had profoundly changed because of the pain. Something needed to be done. Yet none of the health-care professionals involved could offer to cure him or even to provide a good explanation for why he had so much pain. Further, his workplace and the insurance authorities were questioning his case. Although Hank wanted to work, he could not understand how he could possibly resume his job in construction in his condition. Indeed, he was depressed by the fact that he had not been able to work for months. He felt guilty that he was not performing his usual part in the family; his wife and children were doing many of his chores. Hank wondered how he could get the right help.

"Lust and pain are like twins, they are joined and where the one appears, the other is close by" (Leonardo da Vinci).

In some cultures it is a great merit to have survived great pain. Thus, hunters, warriors and the like who have actually survived a painful ordeal are prized. This may represent hardiness, but also seems to reflect moral purity. This seems to be related to a number of rituals and ceremonies where participants self-inflict great pain in order to reach higher religious status or overcome some perceived evil. In one tribe of American Indians, warriors expose themselves to rattlesnake bites in a ceremony. Survivors are said to be pure and obtain great status in the tribe.

Historically, pain has been explained by factors ranging from magical fluids to the work of the gods (Fig. 2.1). Indeed, each culture appears to have a rather unique explanation which is also a product of the time. The Greeks attempted to develop several aspects of their model of pain. For example, Hippocrates asserted that pain was the result of imbalances in the vital fluids. Aristotle, on the other hand, asserted that pain was due to evil spirits and the gods. These entered the body via an injury. The brain was not believed to have any direct influence; for years the heart was considered to be the center for pain sensation.

sins or misbehavior. In fact, the Latin root word *poena* means punishment. Yet, to this day, the word is coupled with blame, chastisement, discipline and anguish (Morris, 1999). Almost all religions have addressed human suffering and pain. Pain is often believed to originate with the gods. In Christian writings pain has often had contradictory meanings. On the one hand it appears to be the result of sin, that is, pain is viewed as a form of divine punishment. Certainly, various painful illnesses have been viewed with a moral overtone. Morris (1999) points out, for example, that gout (a congenital form of arthritis) was once viewed with contempt much as venereal disease is today because it was associated with the lavish lifestyle of the rich and decadent. On the other hand, pain can be viewed as a trial or test of a person's faith. For example, in one notion, pain is seen as a wound that God inflicts, lovingly, to humble and to discipline the restless spirit (Morris, 1999). Similarly, just as Jesus suffered on the cross, so pain might be a trial where the victim is suffering for a cause. Remnants of these views are not only seen in models of pain, but may form the base for some of the beliefs patients hold about their pain.

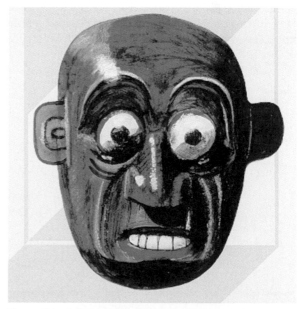

Figure 2.1 Culture influences our perception of pain and our expectations concerning treatment. This pain mask from Sri Lanka (Abutasanniya) is designed to frighten away evil pain and disease spirits. (Mask: painting by Peter Ekström.)

Descartes and the Cartesian "mind–body" model

René Descartes (1596–1650) was a philosopher whose mission was to show that humans are a mechanical body governed by a rational soul. According to Descartes, the nerves were hollow tubes through which spirits flowed in a mechanical manner. Further, the nerves were connected to the brain and the brain was the center of the senses. In order to explain pain, Descartes put forward an example as a model (Fig. 2.2). In this example, a man whose hand is being hit by a hammer serves as the injury. A hollow nerve path is also shown from the injury to the brain and this was compared to the pulling of a rope to make a bell strike on the other end. Although several aspects of the model were correct and well advanced given the scientific evidence of the time, the model also advanced a rather mechanical, dualistic view of mind and body. Indeed, pain was viewed as an injury causing a mechanical-like rope to be pulled which rang a bell in the person's mind. The body was like a machine, then, which could be explained by the laws of nature. Yet the body was governed and controlled by the rational soul.

Hurt is harm

To this day, Descartes's model of pain continues to exert influence on how people view pain. First, and most straightforward, is the assumption that there is a direct link between the amount of tissue damage and the level of pain experienced. In other words, the more damage incurred, the greater the pain. As we will see later in the book, this is a view patients frequently hold. Moreover, it appears to feed the idea that all pain

is caused by injury, so that increases in pain are interpreted as the result of additional organic damage. There is an intuitive appeal to this assumption and obviously tissue destruction is an important element in pain perception. However, as this book aims to make clear, a host of factors actually determine the experience of pain intensity.

The division of mind and body

A second assumption in the Descartes legacy is the division of mind and body where pain is consequently considered to be either strictly physical or strictly psychological. Indeed, throughout the twentieth century, doctors attempted to distinguish between true physical and psychologically derived pain. Unfortunately, when pain symptoms were difficult to treat or even understand, the question arose as to whether the pain actually was caused by a psychological condition. The implication was that the patient was mentally ill rather than physically ill. While this may have provided the medical professions with a method of dealing with some difficult cases, it does not seem to have helped patients very much. Accordingly, the distinction appears to have taken on social meaning. There still seems to be a certain amount of apprehensiveness about considering pain from a psychological perspective.

A corollary of the idea that pain is either physical or psychological is that the pain from true injury cannot be controlled or influenced by any other means than physical ones. Thus, the patient is a slave to the physical injury and is in need of physical treatment to relieve the pain. Yet psychological techniques offer additional tools in the treatment arsenal and in several situations may be the only feasible intervention available.

AN INTEGRATIVE, PSYCHOLOGICAL MODEL OF PAIN

A modern and scientifically based model has been developed over the past few years that incorporates biological, cognitive, emotional, behavioral, and to a great extent even social aspects of pain perception. Although the model involves many aspects, its focus is on psychological processes and it may be used as a heuristic aid. Let us explore an overview of the model here, before delving into the details in the coming chapters.

What is pain?

To appreciate a more psychological model of pain perception there is a need to consider what pain is and we need to attempt to define it. This is a surprisingly difficult task for a word that most of us intuitively understand. However, pain may have many meanings and the large number of words that may be used to describe pain underscores this point. One way of

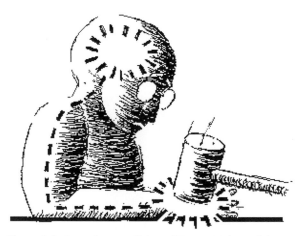

Figure 2.2 A modern rendition of Descartes's model of pain. This is a mechanistic model where injury is directly related to pain intensity. This model underscores a dualistic mind–body view that still exerts influence on us today. (Drawing by Peter Ekström.)

looking at historical models is to examine the words used in them. It is interesting to note that a distinct word(s) for pain appears to be of relatively recent origin. Moreover, as noted above, the word for pain is derived from punishment in Latin and associated with punishment in several other languages. Words are essential in developing a model as this is one of the main methods we use to communicate our pain.

Normally, we use adjectives to describe our pain ("feels like a cut, pressure, sting") rather than different synonyms (pain, hurt, ache). Adjectives help us to describe our pain from a physical and emotional standpoint. This fact was utilized in making the McGill Pain Questionnaire (Table 2.1) (Melzack, 1983). This instrument is a valuable tool in pain assessment. It employs a variety of descriptors in an

Table 2.1 Words used to describe various aspects of the pain experience from the McGill Pain Questionnaire.

Sensory words

Temporal	*Spatial*	*Punctate pressure*	*Incisive pressure*	*Constructive pressure*
1. flickering	jumping	pricking	sharp	pinching
2. quivering	flashing	boring	cutting	pressing
3. pulsing	shooting	drilling	lacerating	gnawing
4. throbbing		stabbing		cramping
5. beating		lancinating		crushing
6. pounding				
Traction pressure	*Thermal*	*Brightness*	*Dullness*	*Sensory misc.*
1. tugging	hot	tingling	dull	tender
2. pulling	burning	itchy	sore	taut
3. wrenching	scalding	smarting	hurting	rasping
	searing	stinging	aching	splitting
			heavy	

Affective words

Tension	*Autonomic*	*Fear*	*Punishment*	*Affective misc.*
1. tiring	sickening	fearful	punishing	wretched
2. exhaustive	suffocating	frightful	grueling	blinding
		terrifying	cruel	
			vicious	
			killing	

Evaluative words

1. annoying				
2. troublesome				
3. miserable				
4. intense				
5. unbearable				

Miscellaneous words

1. spreading	tight	cool	nagging
2. radiating	numb	cold	nauseating
3. penetrating	drawing	freezing	agonizing
4. piercing	squeezing		dreadful
	tearing		torturing

attempt to capture the pain the patient is experiencing. It was constructed by examining which words were actually used to describe pain in the English language. This was no small task as the researchers compiled a list based on a variety of sources such as clinicians, information from the literature and interviews with patients. Words were then grouped together by empirically studying how patients actually used the words. The final scale consisted of 20 subclasses. The sensory aspects of pain were captured with 42 words in 10 different classes. In addition, 14 words in five categories cover the affective aspects. Finally, the evaluative parts produced 5 words in one category, while various miscellaneous aspects consist of 17 words in four classes. In the clinic, patients are asked to select one word from each category that describes their pain.

Since pain may be described in so many different ways, with so many different words, it appears difficult to define and measure. We speak of pain when describing a wide variety of things such as a cut, a toothache, a muscle ache, or even when we have been disappointed ("it really hurt when I realized I was wrong") or at the loss of a loved one. How can all of these seemingly different things still be called pain?

Fortunately, an international organization has studied this problem and developed a working definition for healthcare professionals. The definition provided by the International Association for the Study of Pain is: *An unpleasant sensation and emotional experience which is associated with actual or potential tissue damage or is described in terms of such damage and which is expressed in behavior*. Thus, pain is recognized as having many facets. It includes psychological aspects as well as biological and is truly a multidimensional phenomenon. I have added the underlined words to the definition to underscore that the way we communicate pain to others and an important consequence of the pain experience is behavior.

Feeling no pain

A central goal for healthcare professionals is to relieve pain. In many healthcare situations it would seem that pain is an evil to be gotten rid of. However, even though it is rare, a few people are born with no feeling for pain. While this might seem positive from the perspective of a pain patient, it has dire consequences. The study of people who feel no pain, that is, who have congenital insensitivity to pain, has had a substantial impact on modern models of pain. To be sure, pain seems to serve the imperative role of the warning signal.

Insensitivity to pain is an ominous handicap. These people often die in childhood as a result of illnesses or injuries they have not noticed. Thus, there seems to be compelling reasons to view pain perception as having immense survival value. Pain in fact protects us from the complications of dangerous tissue damage.

Interestingly, congenital insensitivity to pain has two main forms (Nagasako et al., 2003). In the first form, congenital insensitivity to pain, patients do not perceive sensations of pain. Thus, they have a marked inability to distinguish the intensity, type or quality of the pain. This appears to be a hereditary disease where there is an abnormality in the autonomic nervous system (hereditary sensory and autonomic neuropathy: HSAN). These patients may have considerable injuries, but with no apparent experience of pain. For example, patients may have painless burns or painless mutilated or broken fingers.

The second form is congenital *indifference* to pain. As the name suggests, these people can discern the type, intensity and quality of the noxious stimulus. Thus, the ability to detect various adverse stimuli is intact, but the individual does not respond with pain behaviors. Typically, these individuals have painless injuries, but normal results on sensory and neurological examinations. One case (Landrieu et al., 1990) reported on a 5-year-old girl who had painless fractures and indifference to other injuries. While she did exhibit withdrawal reflexes and even grimaces to pinpricks and hot water stimuli, she was all the same indifferent to prolonged or repeated application of the painful stimuli. Nevertheless, she had normal neurological findings including a biopsy of the nerves and she had normal psychomotor development. Some patients even seem to lack the specific emotional aspects of a pain response. Such individuals may lack responsiveness to intense noxious stimuli such as having no withdrawal responses, no pain behavior, and sometimes even inappropriate responses suggesting pleasure.

The description of people with congenital insensitivity to pain has fascinated pain researchers and provided an impetus for the construction of models. It underscores the importance of pain in survival. Moreover, the various types of insensitivity suggest that pain perception is more than simple nerve stimulation. In fact, insensitivity to pain was one of the main bases for the distinction between sensory and affective aspects of pain in the development of modern models (Nagasako et al., 2003).

Biopsychosocial model

Scientific research has clearly shown that many factors influence our pain perception; pain is not simply a neurophysiological phenomenon. To emphasize this, consider Fig. 2.3 where selected factors that are known to influence pain perception are shown to the left.

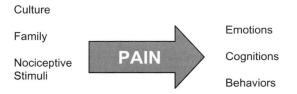

Culture

Family

Nociceptive
Stimuli

PAIN

Emotions

Cognitions

Behaviors

Environment

Figure 2.3 A large variety of factors influence our perception of pain. The experience of pain includes subjective, behavioral and physiological aspects.

The figure also underscores that pain perception involves physiological but also cognitive (subjective) and behavioral aspects. Indeed, it is important to remember that pain perception involves how we process and react to physiological stimuli.

Figure 2.3 emphasizes the so-called biopsychosocial approach to pain. The sensory stimulus associated with injury is a central input on the left-hand side. However, social and psychological aspects have also been selected for inclusion. To be sure, social aspects set the framework for how we react to pain. They determine what is acceptable as well as what is taboo in how we deal with pain. Our culture, for example, sets boundaries for how we experience and describe our pain. Several research reports highlight the fact that people from different cultural heritages respond somewhat differently to painful stimuli (Moore and Brödsgaard, 1999). There is considerable evidence, for example, of distinctive ethnic variations in the experience of pain (Moore and Brödsgaard, 1999; Morris, 1999). This includes how much pain is tolerated, but more importantly how the pain is interpreted and dealt with. Several cultural "rituals", for example, involve what we might consider to be tremendous pain, yet they are done voluntarily and with great vigor. Consider the traditional Sun Dance performed by Native Americans. In this dance, young men receive cuts in the chest area and thongs are slipped through these and then tied to a pole. The dance may continue for hours as the men tear their flesh to break free; pain is central to this ordeal and has a specific cultural meaning.

Another example of social and cultural influence is the description of our pain and what it means. Skevington (1995) points out, for example, that most patients rehearse and develop their description of their pain. In particular this is done through interactions with others. This provides social feedback that shapes our view and presentation of the pain. For example, describing some leg pain as feeling like a "gooey glob" would certainly get a different response from friends, relatives and workmates than describing it as "tender and sore".

The family also plays an important role in our experience of pain (Keefe et al., 1996; Kerns and Payne, 1996). First, parents teach their children a good deal about how one should react to pain and they serve as important models. The foundations for decisions such as the need to take a pain tablet or to see a doctor are laid here (Edwards et al., 1985). Not only do children from families where a parent has a chronic pain problem have a higher rate of pain problems, but some research suggests that these children learn inappropriate coping strategies from their parents (Turkat, 1982).

Second, the family constitutes a powerful source of feedback. Just as with social feedback in general, the family may be instrumental in shaping pain perceptions. This is true for adults as well as for children. For example, family members may encourage "sick behavior" by suggesting a course of action ("you should probably take a tablet and rest") as well as by providing feedback ("you seem to be a bit better after your rest"). This can significantly contribute to the development of sick behavior. On the other hand, family members may encourage appropriate coping strategies and be a most powerful positive help. This is why some practitioners include the family in the treatment of persistent pain (Kerns et al., 1990; Keefe et al., 1996; Kerns and Payne, 1996). One particular method is to teach spouses appropriate ways of prompting appropriate behavior as well as to provide encouragement for them.

Temporal aspects: acute, subacute, recurrent and persistent pain

Any model of pain needs to deal with the temporal aspects because the length of the suffering has far-reaching implications. Certainly, the temporal aspects of pain influence our perception as intermittent pain is clearly different from nonrelenting pain. Similarly, the length of time we have experienced the pain influences our perception. Thus, the various factors that influence pain may work differently depending on the point in time considered. These temporal aspects then have essential consequences for our understanding of the pain problem.

One basic temporal distinction is the length of suffering on the acute to persistent pain time line. Here pain is viewed on a continuum and an assumption is that the pain is experienced during the entire time period. Keep in mind that the description here is primarily focused on patients with musculoskeletal pain, although many of the attributes are true for most pain sites. *Acute pain* is generally defined as pain experienced up to about 3 or 4 weeks. It is characterized by temporary decreases in activity, reliance on medication

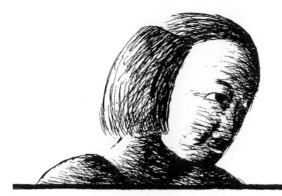

Figure 2.4 Pain may affect just about anyone. Before the onset of the pain, this person is otherwise healthy. (Drawing by Peter Ekström.)

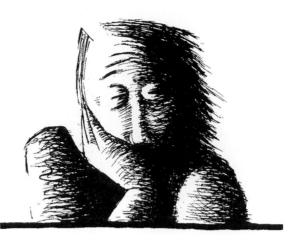

Figure 2.6 During the subacute phase the pain continues and becomes difficult for the patient to understand. It affects several aspects of the patient's life such as activities and sleep. Further, the pain may begin to spread to other areas of the body and become more or less constant. (Drawing by Peter Ekström.)

or other pain relief methods, and help seeking. It is accompanied by psychological distress, for example, anxiety, worry and feeling blue, in addition to beliefs that pain is controllable through medication and active coping. Biologically the patient may have various organic findings including soft tissue mechanisms such as muscle spasms. In the next stage, *subacute pain*, considered to be between 4 and 12 weeks, patients may exhibit altering patterns of increasing and decreasing activity and withdraw or become reliant on medication. They often attempt to continue working and use various coping styles. Pain of varying intensity is experienced and depressive symptoms may begin to develop. Patients tend to focus on the physical symptoms and these are affected by stress. Anxiety may persist and anger and frustration are common. As time passes, the likelihood of finding organic pathology decreases. In *persistent or chronic pain*, defined as more than 3 months' duration, activities may have decreased sharply, patients may "doctor shop" and

overuse medications. As these lifestyle changes become stable the person may fall into a sick role. The pain usually becomes more constant, although patients may experience "good" and "bad" periods. Depression and passive coping strategies as well as a preoccupation with symptoms are common, as are beliefs that the patient himself has no control over the pain. From a biological point of view there are few distinct findings, but the patient may suffer from chronic spasms, and decreased muscle strength and endurance.

Although the above stages of pain development underscore the time line, the assumption that pain is experienced continuously in the same way is mistaken. Instead, the experience of pain is dynamic and it is normal to experience increases as well as decreases.

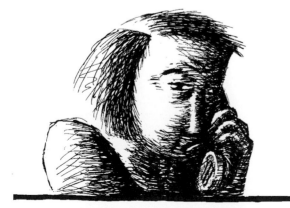

Figure 2.5 During the acute phase, the pain may be quite intense. Yet this patient is active in seeking help. (Drawing by Peter Ekström.)

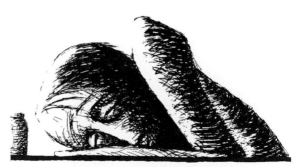

Figure 2.7 During the chronic or persistent pain phase the pain influences just about every part of the patient's life. The symptoms have often increased in number and quality of life decreases. Patients often feel depressed and uncertain of the future. (Drawing by Peter Ekström.)

It is also typical to experience periods of little or no pain followed by periods of considerable pain.

Does pain always cause disability?

Pain sometimes results in considerable disruption of our daily activities. Certainly, as seen in Chapter 1, pain is a frequent reason for not being able to work. Consequently, the patient may be considered disabled and the implication is "disabled by the pain". However, although disability is often considered to be a direct result of pain, modern research indicates that pain and function are not always closely related.

The idea of disability due to injury is a relatively old one that is based on the traditional medical model. This approach originated in Prussia during the nineteenth century and developed in parallel with the "disease model" (Waddell, 2002). In this system, symptoms and signs obtained during the examination are used to infer an underlying injury and a diagnosis is given. Based on this diagnosis, treatment is then provided aimed at alleviating the underlying injury. Once treatment is provided, the patient is expected to recover rather quickly. However, even if cured, some residual disability could be present as a result of the disease process (such as scar tissue or weakness). An extension of this system is that disease causes physical impairments that in turn result in disability. The question is whether this is absolutely true.

During the past two decades evidence has emerged suggesting that physical function, disability and pain may not be as strongly linked as previously thought. In other words, although we would expect some relationship, pain and injury may not be 100% related to function or disability. Certainly, some patients may continue to work despite considerable pain, while others may find it difficult to work even though they suffer less pain. A good deal of light has been shed on this question for low back pain. One reason that scientists began exploring the relationship was that there is frequently no medical evidence of anatomical damage (e.g. damaged nerves or bones) in patients with long-term disability (Nachemson and Jonsson, 2000; Waddell, 2002). Studies also began to be published demonstrating that pain was not crucially linked to function. For example, it has been found that for every patient off work with back pain, there are at least two with the same pain intensity and duration in the general public who are not off work (Linton et al., 1998). While there is no doubt that pain and function are related, there is a question as to the *strength* of the relationship.

Some studies showed that pain was not strongly related to work disability for back pain. The point was driven home to us in an epidemiological study we conducted aimed to elucidate back pain in nursing personnel in relation to their workplace (Linton and Buer, 1995). We examined licensed practical nurses (LPNs) and nurses at a large hospital and assessed their pain, work environment, and psychological and physical status. Interestingly, we were able to match a group of nurses all of whom reported moderate to severe pain, often or all of the time. However, some of these nurses had been off work during the preceding year (about 90 days average), while the others had not. This in itself was a surprising finding. We set out to determine which factors were related to the work disability. An examination of the work environment showed that the physical work performed by the two groups of nurses was quite similar. Further, the physical exam showed tight hamstring muscles, but these were also very similar in the two groups.

What then might explain the differences in disability? In the final analysis, we saw that psychosocial factors could explain the difference between the two groups. Those off work tended to react more emotionally toward their pain, and employed more passive coping strategies. *Thus the psychological factors were the most powerful variables for distinguishing between the groups.* An interview with the participants indicated an additional important fact. Initially we suspected that one method of coping with the pain that might differ between the groups was that those working put their effort into work, but instead were inactive at home. Conversely, we suspected that those at home had a more active home and leisure life. To our astonishment, the results of the interview indicated the opposite! Those who were working reported a more active home and leisure life *than those off work.* This seemed to be related to the beliefs the participants held about the relationship between activity and pain.

In fact, we have now begun to understand that while pain, function and disability overlap somewhat, the strength of the relationship varies greatly. Clinically, it is well known that some patients may continue to work and function well even though they suffer intense pain, while others may have great difficulties functioning with moderate pain. Waddell (2002) examined the literature on this subject and showed that pain intensity has a relatively weak relationship with time off work. Further, he asserts that pain, disability and time off work are three related but distinct concepts. That is, while there is some overlap in who is experiencing pain, or functional problems, or work incapacity, there are many people suffering only one of these. Indeed, the correlation between pain severity and disability is relatively weak. This means that having pain does not necessarily equate with functional problems or time off work. Pain is simply not the same as function!

Implications

There are two clear implications concerning the relationship between pain and function. First, we need to be very clear about terminology and the assumptions we have about these words. Pain is often used to mean pain intensity and this in turn is often assumed to be directly and strongly related to function. As noted above, pain has many qualities and is not the sole determiner of function. A second implication is that pain treatment may need to be oriented toward several variables in order to be effective. Traditionally, pain treatment has been focused on relieving the symptom. A sole measure has often been pain intensity ratings. However, the discussion here demonstrates that pain intensity may be addressed with little or no effect on function. Likewise, even if pain intensity cannot be influenced, treatment focused on other aspects such as function may have dramatic effects for the patient. Thus new roads for pain treatment may be opened.

SUMMARY

Pain has been an important experience throughout recorded history and various models of how pain functions have evolved. These continue to exert some influence in the way we view pain today. Pain may still have some moral overtones that date back to models where pain was equated with punishment. Perhaps the most influential model that continues to infiltrate is Descartes's model where the body and mind are separated. Modern research, however, demonstrates that our pain system is highly integrated and involves biological as well as psychological aspects. Thus, the definition of pain underscores not only the role of tissue damage but the psychological experience as well. While the biological and psychological processes are highly integrated, the relationships are not necessarily simple ones. For example, the relationship between pain and function is not as straightforward as previously believed. Finally, the temporal aspects of pain are an important aspect of pain. How we experience pain changes with time as do the consequences for us.

3

The biological–psychological interface: pain perception

After all these years, just looking at a potato field makes my back hurt.

—John, a potato farmer

LEARNING OBJECTIVES

To understand:

- the biological basis of pain perception;

- that pain is a sensory and emotional experience, not simply a nerve signal or tissue injury;

- the interaction between biological and psychological processes;

- that pain signals are modified within the central nervous system (CNS) before reaching the cortex and consciousness;

- that the nervous system is plastic and changes over time, and changes such as sensitization in the CNS can influence the development of pain;

- that the perception of pain involves biological, emotional, cognitive and behavioral aspects that occur in particular settings.

Pain is an amazing perception that involves an entire biological system that is regulated by the brain in reaction to environmental stimuli. Certainly all sensations, feeling, thoughts and behaviors have a biological counterpart. This seems to be nature's way of giving us an edge on survival. This interface between psychological and biological mechanisms is comparable to other perceptions like vision or hearing. By having psychological dimensions interact with biological ones we are in a much better position to adapt. In this chapter we will examine the interface between biological and psychological aspects of pain perception.

At first, the traditional medical model only considered pain to be of interest as a symptom. The description of the pain was viewed as providing clues as to what the actual cause might be. However, pain was not seen as something of interest in its own right. Consequently, for years pain was only of interest in making a diagnosis. Once the diagnosis was made, the alleviation of the disease was believed to be the cure for the pain. Several discoveries have put an end to such thinking. Some trauma, for example, occurs in regions of our body that have few pain nerves and thus major injury results in little or no pain. Likewise, some people suffer incredible pain although we cannot locate any tissue damage to explain it. It turns out, then, that pain is much more than an uncomplicated case of neurophysiology.

A further example that demonstrates the relationship between biological and psychological processes are the reactions of patients to injury. If pain was a simple neurophysiological state (as Descartes's model would suggest), then the amount of tissue damage should correspond to the intensity of the pain. However, as mentioned above, during World War II an American surgeon, Henry Beecher, made some impressive observations (Beecher, 1959). Beecher observed that soldiers with serious wounds often did not ask for painkillers. This was in considerable contrast to the patients Beecher worked with at home during peacetime. In a field study, Beecher reported that although the soldiers were not shocked or otherwise mentally unclear, only a relatively small fraction said they were in need of an analgesic. A persuasive argument was made that the pain perception was influenced by the situation in which the injury occurred. For these severely injured soldiers, the wound also meant that they would be going home. In a more formal comparison with civilian surgery where the conditions were much better and the amount of trauma much less as compared to the soldiers, Beecher found that while only 32% of the soldiers wanted painkillers, 83% of the civilian surgery patients did! Again, the explanation provided by Beecher was the context: the environment appeared to exert considerable influence over how the pain was perceived. This also raises the question of how pain stimuli are processed and integrated into pain perception and behavior.

Pain, like other perceptions, is greatly influenced by developmental and learning processes. Although we seldom consider it, vision is highly dependent on experiential learning and in fact people who have been deprived of this (such as with certain diseases) as children have difficulty "learning to see" as adults. Likewise, we learn to experience pain. Even though we ordinarily deem pain to be an automatic biological reaction, it is in fact highly influenced by our experiences. It is true that some basic pain reactions are automatic such as the reflexive withdrawal of your hand if you burn it on the stove. However, most other behaviors, feelings and cognitions concerning pain are the product of experience. Psychological factors, then, influence the biology of pain.

It is not surprising that biological pain signals also affect us psychologically. A typical reaction to intense pain is anxiety or worry. Again, this helps us to better adapt to the situation at hand as worry motivates us to check for tissue damage and to take necessary action. Persistent pain also leaves its mark on us psychologically. The constant ache of a back problem or the gnawing pain from cancer typically affects our mood and steers our thoughts. Thus there is an interaction between biological processes and psychological processes that help us to most adequately adapt to the situation at hand.

This chapter looks at the link between biological and psychological processes. We will review the physiological aspects of pain and in particular how biological and psychological processes interface. While thousands of signals are being sent to the brain, we are conscious of only a very small number. The nervous system has a complex system for processing and filtering these stimuli. We may wonder why and how this is done as well as what consequences this process has for pain perception. Indeed, as we shall see, it has considerable impact as the plastic nervous system alters and integrates signals throughout the process.

PAIN PHYSIOLOGY IN THE BIOLOGY–PSYCHOLOGY INTERFACE

Pain physiology involves a complex process rather than simply a connection between nerves. Traditionally pain has been viewed as a sensation resulting from the stimulation of a specific nerve that sends an impulse through the spinal cord up to the cortex. Like Descartes's model, this view suggests that pressing a "pain" button somewhere in the body rings a bell in the brain's cortex. In fact, pain has been considered to be a neurophysiological entity during a considerable part of the twentieth century. Unfortunately, this specific and simplistic view is a gross oversimplification that is erroneous.

Great advances in our understanding have been made during the last decade and these underscore some fundamental concepts. Basically, these conceptions draw attention to the true interface between the biological and psychological processes (Flor et al., 1990; Flor, 2000). Amazingly, pain signals are filtered and modulated continually on their journey through the nervous system. Contrary to the mechanical view, pain and emotions are closely linked in the neurophysiological processes in the brain; thus they occur and influence each other at the same time. Sensory and motor processes are also connected closely in the nervous system so that pain behavior is a basic part of the pain experience.

Nerve stimulation

Pain involves nerve stimulation where signals are first sent to the brain (ascending nerve signal). They are then processed in various areas in the brain. Subsequently, a response is sent (descending nerve signal) back to the periphery. Let us examine the process more closely to understand how the signal may be modulated during transmission.

Stimulation of nociceptors (nerves sensitive to tissue damage) creates a nerve impulse. These receptors transmit information from the skin, muscles, joints and viscera. Although it was originally believed that nerves were specific to one type of stimulation, these nerves may respond to touch as well as to other stimuli such as temperature. In fact, some nerves carry nociceptive impulses directly, while others carry impulses that affect our perception of pain, but are not nociceptors per se (Skevington, 1995; Wall and Melzack, 1999; Flor, 2000).

The impulses are transmitted by two basic types of nerves. The A fibers are myelinated nerves, that is, they are surrounded by a thick fatty sheath that allows them to transmit a signal quickly. Damage to A fibers results in sharp, immediate and often intense acute pain. On the other hand, C fibers are relatively small, unmyelinated nerves associated with slow, diffuse and aching pain. A and C fibers are the principal nerves involved in pain and they tend to overlap in terms of sensitivity.

Transmission to brain

After the nerve is stimulated the impulse is sent to the spinal cord where "gating" takes place. This occurs in the dorsal horn of the spinal cord and constitutes the first synapse, i.e. where one nerve transmits the signal to the next nerve. Melzack and Wall (1965) provided the gate control theory to explain how the nerve signals were modulated during this transmission. This theory postulates that the balance between impulses from the A and C fibers is important in the modification that occurs in the spinal cord. As sensory information arrives from the periphery to the spinal area, specifically to the dorsal horn, the balance of this activity may stimulate or inhibit the transmission to the next nerve. Thus, a sort of "gate" is formed where some nerve impulses are hurried through (stimulated, open gate) and others are inhibited (closed gate).

Several factors steer whether the "gate" is closed or open. The closing of the gate is in part regulated in the spinal cord by the activity of the nerve impulses. For example, a predominance of activity in the larger A fibers closes the gate for the smaller C fibers whereas considerable small C fiber activity facilitates an opening of the gate. This process explains how some forms of "contrastimulation" analgesia function. Contrastimulation involves stimulating nerve cells to close the gate. This may be achieved with transcutaneous nerve stimulation or massage and explains why these provide pain relief. In essence these procedures send A fiber impulses that close the gate and block the ascending nerve impulses creating analgesia.

The gating process may also be influenced by processes higher up in the nervous system. The brain, for example, may send descending nerve signals that close the gate, thus blocking transmission. One example of this is a reaction to very stressful situations. It has been noted that in extreme situations such as a war or accident, people may have severe injuries but not suffer from pain. Because attention is focused on survival, the gate is closed and pain is not experienced.

Another avenue of influence is the release of certain chemicals such as endorphins that produce analgesia. These chemicals are part of a large system and are released when certain conditions are met. While exercise may enhance the release of such chemicals, other factors like stress may inhibit them. Thus peripheral nociceptive nerve stimulation is modulated by sensory feedback and higher CNS influences.

Brain processes

There is no single "pain center" in the brain. Instead, there is a continuation of the modulation of the nerve signals that occurs in the gating process described above. Earlier it was thought that the nerves were specific to stimuli and that the brain likewise had specific areas that processed information about pain. Thus, it was thought that the location, sensory and emotional aspects of pain were processed in different, distinct areas of the brain. Today it is clear that there is not a "hard-wired" system for processing pain. What is perceived is determined by the brain abstracting a barrage of signals representing spatial, temporal and emotional aspects. Thus, it is logical that several areas of the brain might be involved.

Advances in technology have recently allowed researchers to investigate which parts of the brain are active during pain perception. This is done with magnetic resonance imaging and positron-emission tomography (PET). The results show that many parts of the brain are involved. Indeed, pain is not only a response of the whole brain, it appears to be a response of the whole being!

Pain signals are altered throughout the nervous system as they are processed and become conscious. A central control mechanism in the brainstem is an integral part of the filtering. Several parts of the brain send descending signals to the dorsal horn where gating occurs. These signals may modify or close the gate. One part of this system is located in the brainstem and it appears to be an effective modifier in the nervous system.

Once the signals reach the brain they are projected to several areas of the cerebral cortex. Here pain, emotions and pain behavior are closely integrated. Emerging data suggest that the processing of emotions, behavior and pain are closely linked. Emotional distress is a central feature of pain that is associated with fear, anxiety, anger and depression (Craig, 1999). Such processes taking place in the brain underscore the connectedness of perceptual, emotional, cognitive and behavioral aspects (Craig, 1999). This biological system is well tuned to enhance survival as we may adapt to a tremendous range of situations because of it.

Plasticity and sensitization

The central nervous system is astonishingly plastic. It adjusts, alters and changes to adapt to prevailing conditions. If an injury occurs to the nervous system, adjustments are made so that we may function normally. This may involve the rerouting of information or "secondary" nerves becoming more primary in the information they provide. This has great importance for understanding pain. Although damage to a nerve may be a relatively specific cause of pain, it is also a relatively rare cause of pain. In other words, the damaging of nerves is not a primary cause of pain. This is particularly true for aches and pains such as common low back pain. Further, the complex neurophysiology of pain and the plasticity in the system explains why surgical operations to cut pain pathways usually are unsuccessful (Waddell, 1998); the system simply adjusts via the extended interconnection within the system.

The experience of pain also appears to sensitize the nervous system over time. This involves some basic changes in the nervous system where less stimulation is required for the signal to be experienced as pain. For example, tissue damage in peripheral areas may produce sensitization so that normal stimuli begin to be perceived as pain. Similarly, central sensitization may occur in the spinal cord and brain so that the nerves are easily stimulated to send impulses. This may be likened to a path through the woods. The more times the path is tramped on, the easier it is to use the pathway as it becomes wider and more worn. Having focused on sensitization, we need to keep in mind that for the most part the pain system is highly developed and adaptive and it adjusts well to continued pain and tends to reduce sensitivity (Flor et al., 1990; Flor, 2000).

The brain exerts a regulatory influence on pain perception that attempts to maintain balance in our bodies. We try to maintain balance through homeostasis. Several states that we perceive are related to maintaining balance such as hunger, thirst or an itch. Pain seems to be no different; it involves a distinct sensation that is connected to cognitions and behavior (Craig, 2003). The connectedness of the systems, then, helps us to maintain balance by appropriately responding to the stimuli. Thus, we may seek food and eat if hungry, or seek to care for an injury if in pain. This process underscores how the neurophysiological system is plastic and the various parts connected to one another.

Behavior influences physiology

Ordinarily we concentrate on how biological processes affect our feelings and behavior, but our behavior may also influence the processing of pain perception. For example, learning to deal with a painful stimulus might alter the way it is processed. Consider the hiker who gets aches from walking. At first these may be alarming and distressing. However, after the hiker learns that these are normal and due to the extra exertion, they may become less distressful. Indeed, many pain patients learn that activity may be a helpful way of coping. Shouldn't these behaviors influence the way that our pain signals are biologically processed?

To be sure, some researchers have found that behavioral changes also result in physiological changes. For example, behavioral changes may result in the development of new patterns of reactions in the brain. As an illustration, consider that through learning experiences the expectation ("I will now administer the painful stimulus") of a painful stimulus (but in reality a nonpainful stimulus is given) actually stimulates the same areas of the brain as the actual "painful" stimulus (Bushnell et al., 2004). In other words, through learning the pattern of brain responses is influenced. Moreover, Waldenström (2004) in a series of experiments with rats found that the pain system develops physiologically through learning. Specifically, she found that even the withdrawal reflex needed learning to develop properly. Thus, the organization and processing of the nerve signals corresponds to learning the new behavior. In essence this highlights that

---

CASE STUDY: HANK

We might wonder if it would be possible to see Hank's pain in the nervous system. We might suspect that Hank has an abnormality somewhere that might be seen and perhaps even corrected. Unfortunately, there is no magic test to determine why Hank is experiencing the pain. In fact, his nervous system is functioning normally. While it would be possible to conduct PET imaging, these pictures would not be particularly helpful in diagnosing or treating Hank's problem. The PET images would show which areas of the brain are active in processing his pain, but they would not show why he is suffering. Nor would such images provide much help in knowing how to treat the pain. Other tests could help us to determine if the nerves in Hank's system are functioning properly. However, Hank has no symptoms that would suggest any such problems. Again, it appears that his nervous system is functioning properly.

One process that may affect Hank, however, is sensitization. He has now suffered pain over a longer time period. Consequently, the pathways may be well established and the nervous system may even react easily to such "pain" stimuli. This might help to explain why the pain has persisted. Still, it says little about why the pain started in the first place. Further, there is no simple treatment for sensitization either. In fact, sensitization may be seen as a physiological explanation of what is going on in the body when long-term problems develop.

Thus, in Hank's case, there is no neurological test or image that can help us to a better treatment. It is fortunate, in a sense, that Hank does not have any signs of a neurological disease.

biological and psychological processes are highly integrated. Changes in one part of the system create effects in the whole system.

SUMMARY

The biological–psychological interface provides a fantastic system for dealing with pain in an effective way. Despite previous notions of simple nerve stimulation resulting in a specific pain sensation, modern research shows that there is an integrated system that is also very plastic. This means that the system is conducive to change. The nerve signals may be modulated in every step of the processing of the signal in the nervous system. It also means that when changes take place in one part of the system, a host of effects may be seen in the system. This provides for a tremendous versatility and makes the system quite adaptive. It also underscores that pain perception involves the entire nervous system and indeed the entire body. Moreover, while we often think of biological changes causing the pain experience and pain behavior, we have also seen that learning and behavioral changes can result in physiological changes in the way we process information. Simple neurophysiology, then, cannot explain the human pain experience. Pain behavior is not a mere series of reflexes. Instead, the experience of pain involves biological, emotional, cognitive and behavioral aspects that take place in a variety of social and cultural settings. Let us now turn to how psychological processes work in the experience of pain.

Attending to pain stimuli: vigilance and distraction

The more I think about the pain, the more upset I become and the more it hurts. If I start anticipating the terrible pain when I move and the healing scabs crack, I almost get paralyzed.

—18-year-old burn patient

I waited for the injection. All my body was focused on the moment the needle would break the skin, and the jab would pierce and mutilate.

—Healthy person

LEARNING OBJECTIVES

To understand:

- attention is a critical process involving filtering and modulation of pain stimuli;

- pain demands attention and is a vital warning signal;

- attending to stimuli influences how we perceive pain: focusing attention may increase pain, while distraction may decrease pain;

- vigilance involves the continual checking of the body to discover possible evidence that a painful injury has occurred, and is associated with an increase in pain;

- attention and particularly vigilance are closely linked with emotional and cognitive processes.

Jane and her two-year-old son were driving in town one afternoon when a truck suddenly pulled out in front of them resulting in a terrible crash. Jane's first thought after the car stopped was to get to her son and make sure he was safe. She consequently got out of the car and went around to the other side where she struggled for several moments to get the smashed door open. She retrieved her son who fortunately was not injured. It was not until the ambulance arrived that she noticed that her arm was severely bruised and greatly swollen. She had felt no pain. Jane's experience is not uncommon; after such trauma, acute pain is often "blocked" and the person is unaware of injuries. This has obvious value for Jane. It is quite a different story for those suffering chronic pain. For those with persistent pain problems, attending to the pain appears to be a waste of energy since the pain persists even though no injury can be alleviated. There seems to be no advantage for survival either; the person is not able to escape or eliminate the pain. Why do we ignore the acute pain that needs treatment, but attend to chronic pain that appears to have no survival value?

Although attending to the "pain" stimulus would appear to be an unpretentious process, it is in fact an important and remarkable step in pain perception. Attention is a prerequisite for our reaction to a nociceptive stimulus, and it provides opportunities for the filtering and modulation in the central nervous system described in Chapter 3. In part this process is under the unconscious control of basic brain processes. However, it is also influenced by attention and a number of psychological factors assert control over our attention. Simply stated, the brain receives a huge number of stimuli every minute, but we only attend to a very limited number of them. In a sense, our brain operates a bit like a satellite dish: although several signals are being received by the dish, we can only tune into one station at a time.

Moreover, the relationship between attention and pain perception is a two-way street: distraction may decrease pain perception, but pain by its very nature demands attention. To be sure, we normally consider pain to be quite distracting or annoying. It grabs our attention. However, while it may be important to attend to pain, there is also an apparent need to ignore pain such as when we cannot control a headache or aching muscles. What factors, then, steer our attention to pain?

Attention serves to motivate behavior. Therefore, attention is linked to our need to take action. This ordinarily involves escaping from or avoiding the source of the pain or taking care of an injury. Since motivation is involved, the attentional process has close links with emotional and even cognitive processes (Villemure and Bushnell, 2002). Once again we see that pain involves a dynamic, interactive system. In the following sections we will examine this system more closely.

PAIN IS A WARNING SIGNAL

Pain serves the fundamental function of a warning signal. Pain alarms us to dangers so that we can appropriately deal with them in a timely manner. Consequently, it has "threat value". Without pain, we would have difficulty avoiding serious injury and death. Our central nervous system has evolved in such a way as to maximize the discovery of stimuli that are true warning signals. Amanda Williams, a pain psychologist in London, has developed a theory of the evolution of facial expressions of pain (Williams, 2002). The function of pain from an evolutionary point of view is to demand attention and prioritize escape, recovery and healing. So, pain performs an enormously useful function as an alarm.

To understand the experience of pain it is vital to keep in mind that pain is an "alarm" that begs action. Pain plays an important role in helping us deal with

injury and these tendencies are in part programmed into us through evolutionary development. Remember that, from an evolutionary point of view, we are very similar to cave dwellers as it takes thousands of years for natural selection to work. Thus, our genetic heritage is to survive acute trauma that may greatly affect our ability to endure. Let us consider a "prehistoric" man who has fallen and sustained several cuts and bruises. Interestingly, our behavior following an injury shows remarkable consistency not only across cultures but across species (Walters, 1994; Williams, 2002). In fact, Wall (1999) suggests that our nervous system is designed to synthesize pain to give priority: first, escaping the painful stimulus, then to limiting further damage, and subsequently to seeking safety and relief. From a prehistoric point of view, an injury puts one at risk of being attacked by predators or enemies. The "fight or flight" response allows this person to temporarily feel little pain through neurophysiological responses that "block" the pain signals. It is important to get to a safe haven or to prepare for an impending fight. After safety has been achieved, the man may attend to his wounds and the pain will help set limits to activities that may be harmful during healing. This pain response served this man well, just as it serves us (and Jane!) well in similar situations.

Pain is such an important warning signal that it normally demands attention. Remarkably, pain itself modifies our ability to focus attention. For example, in experiments where participants are asked to divide their attention between pain and some other sensory input such as temperature, attention to the pain dominates (Miron et al., 1989). Further, chronic pain patients have been found to have difficulties on attention tasks as compared to normals (Grisart and Plaghki, 1999), which could be explained by difficulty in attending to pain at the same time as attending to some other stimulus.

The late Patrick Wall, mentioned earlier as a founder of the gate theory of pain, described these stages when he suffered a gunshot wound. After being shot, he recalled surprisingly little pain. He was able to retreat from the situation and seek care. Upon arrival at the hospital, he still felt relatively little pain. However, after receiving first treatment and when the shock of the events subsided, the pain intensity increased dramatically. In addition, the character of the pain changed radically. The initial pain in the seconds after being shot was sharp and shooting. It fairly rapidly was transformed into a numbed but sensitive area. This was, of course, accompanied by a psychological state of being stunned. At first, energy was spent on getting oriented to what had happened. Shock followed where effort was made to find safety and treatment.

This illustrates how attention is influenced by acute pain and in particular it shows that pain is a crucial warning signal.

ATTENTION AND DISTRACTION

An obvious and often studied psychological variable that modifies our pain experience is our attentional state. To be sure, the advice to "think about something else" is probably one of the oldest treatments for annoying pain, and there seems to be evidence to support its value. Conversely, focusing on a pain stimulus often results in increases in pain. Thus attention is related to our experience of pain. In turn, a variety of factors influence our attentional state. These include how novel the stimulus is as well as personality and coping style.

Novel stimuli and warning signals

The purpose of attending to pain stimuli is to discover early on the damage that is causing the pain so that it may be prevented or treated. To function optimally, certain cues need to draw our attention to pain and heighten our awareness. This has survival value. One important example of this is that we are more likely to attend to new stimuli such as those we have never experienced before. New stimuli need to be evaluated and we learn rapidly to "ignore" common stimuli, false alarms if you will, that have little to add to our ability to adapt and survive. Novel stimuli, then, are attended to so that we may evaluate them properly.

A clever demonstration of this principle illustrates how novel pain stimuli do indeed attract attention. A group of researchers in Belgium (Crombez et al., 1994) asked healthy students to discriminate between noises of long and short duration, but to ignore visual and thermal stimuli. However, during the experiment a pain-producing heat stimulus (46°C) was nevertheless briefly applied. None of the participants had previous experience with this type of heat stimulation and so this stimulus was truly novel. Although instructed to ignore the heat stimulus, the application of the novel thermal pain resulted in large disruptions in the primary task of discriminating the long and short sounds. This shows that subtle but novel stimuli do in fact attract considerable attention as well as distract participants from ongoing tasks. This would seem to mirror the experience of patients with pain who report difficulties in concentrating and working because the pain disrupts.

The amount of threat the pain signal has appears to be related to the level of attention given to the stimulus. Consider an additional experiment in the role of pain as a signal warning of a threat (Crombez et al., 1998a). As in the experiment above, healthy students were asked to discriminate between long and short noises. At the same time, electrodes were attached to the skin so that short electric shocks could be given. One group was "threatened" that highly intense pain stimuli would at some point be applied, while the other group was not "threatened". In fact, both groups received mild, low-intensity electric shocks. The results indicated, however, that the group threatened with intensely painful shock had much larger disruption in discriminating between the short and long sounds as compared to the other group. Thus, increasing the threat value of a stimulus increased the focus of attention to that stimulus. This reinforces the idea that pain is a warning signal that plays an important role in protecting us from harm. The higher the threat the stimulus represents, the more it demands our attention and disrupts our ongoing activities.

The disrupting nature of pain is quite relevant for patients with persistent pain. Certainly, if pain solicits our attention, then those patients with high levels of pain should have more difficulty concentrating on other tasks. This idea was tested experimentally in a study that compared paitients with "high" versus "low" pain intensity reports (Eccleston et al., 1997). Each participant was asked to complete a task on the computer. These were difficult, attention-demanding tasks involving conflicting information. An example of the task was the presentation of colors where, for instance, the word "red" was printed in blue. Subjects were asked to provide the word (red) as quickly as possible. When the experiment was completed, it was found that the group with high pain intensity demonstrated a pronounced disruption of their attentional performance. The comparison group with low pain intensity was better at the task. This, then, illustrates that pain demands attention and disrupts.

Similarly, pain that is of a drastically different quality or intensity may constitute a novel stimulus and tend to get our attention. Back pain offers clear examples of the role of novel stimuli. Most people experience muscle pain regularly during their life. Fortunately, this pain is usually mild to moderate in intensity, of an aching quality, and it recedes over the course of a few days or weeks. We learn that this type of pain is not dangerous and therefore we do not pay much attention to these stimuli.

On the other hand, imagine waking up one morning with sharp pain in the lower back and numbness in your leg. You might describe the pain as "stabbing", as if someone was sticking a knife in your back. Surely, this pain stimulus would be likely to draw your attention as you have never felt anything quite like it before. The novelty of the stimulus, then, demands our attention as a warning signal.

Research into why people seek healthcare exemplifies the role of novelty and attention. Although about 75% of us have symptoms at any one time, only about a quarter seek care for a symptom (Hannay, 1979). While a third of such patients have pain, the majority appear to have pain symptoms that are definitely not serious. The question arises as to why they then seek care. The answer is related to novelty of the symptom which seems to create worry (Skevington, 1995). Indeed, in a psychosocial analysis Skevington finds that the symptoms are inconvenient (disrupt) and worry the patient, for example, concerning what the cause of the pain might be.

External versus internal orientation

Environmental factors and personality style can influence our pain perception by means of directing attention internally or externally. By focusing our attention inward we increase the likelihood of attending to a pain stimulus. Basically anything we do, consciously or unconsciously, to direct attention inward will increase the number of pain stimuli we discover. In personality research we refer to "introverts" and "extroverts" to describe the basic orientation that people may have. Those who have a personality tendency to concentrate on internal processes also have a tendency to attend to internal cues such as pain.

Environmental processes may also influence our attention, thus indirectly pointing our attention inward or outward. The more stimulation we have externally, the less likely we will attend to internal stimuli. Take for example the elderly. My grandmother at one time lived in a sterile, gray, housing unit with little to do during the day but stare at the walls. Clearly, her attention could easily be oriented to internal stimuli since there were so few external events taking place. Upon visiting her in the evening she had a long list of pain-related complaints that could take from 30 to 60 minutes to describe. Fortunately, she was able to move to a housing unit for the elderly where there were other people to visit with, planned social activities, and regular visits by personnel. In a word, there were significantly more things happening to divert her attention to the external world. While my grandmother still had pain complaints, I was impressed that they were far fewer and took no more than 5 or 10 minutes to describe. By turning attention to the outside world, that is, external events, awareness of internal stimuli decreased.

The effects of turning attention to internal stimuli can be demonstrated by doing a small experiment. Set aside a few minutes and sit in a quiet room with your eyes closed and just concentrate on what is going on inside your body. After a few moments most people begin to be aware of sensations that they normally do not feel. There may be, for example, a twitch of a muscle. Or the stomach may slightly "growl". You may feel your heart beating. Some will feel sensations such as an ache or a small spasm. If you return your attention to the external world, these sensations will subside. By focusing your attention inward, you have become aware of signals that you probably would not have felt had you been driving, listening to a lecture or cooking. At times we all have our attention focused internally or externally. Shifting our attention inward has profound effects upon discovering a "pain" stimulus.

Attentional modulation of pain: distraction

While pain demands attention and distracts us from ongoing tasks, pain is also perceived as less intense when we are distracted from it (Villemure and Bushnell, 2002). In fact, an important coping strategy is based on this fundamental principle. As a coping strategy, distraction is based on altering our attention from the painful stimuli to other, more neutral stimuli. Given that pain begs attention, it may be quite difficult to just think of something else. To be sure, distraction is related to the intensity and quality of the pain as well as to the situation in which it occurs. To enhance the effect in laboratory situations, distraction is often achieved by having the subject attend to another stimulus modality such as auditory, tactile or visual stimuli (Bushnell et al., 1999).

The effects of distraction on pain have been demonstrated in several interesting studies (Williams, 1999). Levine and associates (1982), for example, manipulated attention by having postsurgical patients rate their pain more or less often. Those who rated their pain more often also reported greater pain intensity. Indirectly, this shows that attention to the pain increases intensity, while distraction from it decreases pain intensity. Similarly, White and Sanders (1986) reported that patients who were encouraged to focus on their pain and talk about pain actually reported higher pain intensity ratings than similar patients who were encouraged to talk about nonpain topics (distraction).

Distraction seems to work best for low- or moderate-intensity pain and when the distraction is emotionally charged. Emotional aspects of pain will be described in more detail in the next chapter. At this point, however, let us begin to think about the impact of emotions on attention. An experiment sheds light on this in a very unique way (Stevens et al., 1989). Participants were asked to think about very pleasurable things (such as making love), pleasurable things (a cool breeze on a hot day), things that cause considerable anger (family conflict), and things that create low amounts of anger (a parking ticket) while at the same time undergoing an experimental pain procedure; namely, pressure was applied to produce pain. The scientists observed the amount of time the subject tolerated the pressure stimulus in relation to the emotional state. Interestingly, the emotional content seemed to steer pain tolerance. Results showed that pleasant emotions *increased* tolerance while anger *decreased* tolerance. This supports the idea that emotionally charged thoughts were related to distraction and thereby the experience of pain.

VIGILANCE

Sometimes we need to pay special attention to events that may be harmful. For example, when the weather is particularly nasty, we need to pay special attention when driving. We do not want to be taken by surprise by slippery road conditions or poor visibility. This helps us to take appropriate action to prevent an accident. In point of fact, the word "vigilance" refers to paying special attention to a particularly dangerous stimulus or situation.

Since pain is a warning signal, it poses a threat that we may need to be attuned to. Vigilance helps us to discover possible threats so that action may be taken. Vigilance is a heightened awareness to the source of the danger and involves focusing attention upon possible symptoms or signs that may warn us that the particular threat is in truth imminent. Moreover, it helps us to select the threat over other demands for our attention; we give priority to the painful, threatening stimulus. For the pain patient this translates into attention being concentrated on internal stimuli. As shown above, focusing attention inward may also increase the number of signals we experience. Thus, vigilance serves a vital function, but may also in itself increase the number of pain signals that we experience.

The emotional link

It has become clear that emotional factors are tied to vigilance and attentional processes (Eccleston and Crombez, 1999; Villemure and Bushnell, 2002). We saw above that distraction may be tied to emotions. The same is true of vigilance. High emotional "threat" value greatly influences how vigilant we are. It also may influence the focus of our vigilance.

Consider this example. Imagine being home alone late at night. It is dark and completely quiet. Some robberies have been reported in your neighborhood recently. Suddenly you hear a sound. You become frightened and believe that someone may be trying to break into your home. You listen intensely for sounds that may confirm or disconfirm that a robber is attempting to break in. Your concentration is totally on these events and you hear and sense the minutest sounds. You are emotionally charged, and extremely alert. Obviously, you will hear sounds that you normally would not hear, such as creaks from the floor, the wind, the sounds of electrical devices and so on. This demonstrates the close link between our attention and our emotional state.

Anxiety is a key to understanding how we govern our attention for painful stimuli. Psychologically speaking, the role of anxiety is to focus our attention on possible dangers. When we become anxious, we also become alert. Our senses are heightened. We focus our attention on possible threats. Anxious people begin by scanning the environment until a threat signal is detected. Attention is then "hyperfocused" narrowly and intensely on the potential threat stimulus. This results in greater perceptual sensitivity and often distortion (Rachman, 1998).

When anxiety levels increase, we typically focus our attention and become vigilant. If our anxiety or fears deal with health-related issues—as opposed to a robber—it is natural that our attention is specifically focused on internal cues. Thus, we may begin to scan our bodies for possible signs of the event we are anxious about. This is well known in the literature about heart problems. People concerned about cardiac problems may begin to focus attentions on symptoms that may confirm this process. The more attention is focused on such symptoms, the greater the likelihood that some symptoms are discovered. The person seeks to confirm their fear that something serious is happening. While this is normal, too much attention may lead to a vicious circle of increased attention toward symptoms that leads to a (false) perception of the symptom that in turn increases the anxiety even more. In the end, this process may result in a number of troubling emotions and behaviors, e.g. unnecessary healthcare seeking, suffering and emotional anxiety.

Since attention and vigilance are designed to identify threats, our attention is partly steered by our fears and concerns. If a patient is concerned that reaching for a book on the top shelf may pull a muscle in the shoulder, then attention may focus on the shoulder area. Moreover, the attention may be rather specific, focusing on signs that the muscle may be pulled. Remember that pain signals are sent through a number of nerves and modulated continually on their journey through the nervous system. This provides opportunities to discover any twitches, aches or other feelings in the shoulder. By heightening awareness to the shoulder region we increase the probability of detecting signals. Just as important, the concern that damage may have been done to a muscle focuses

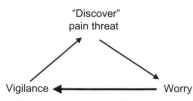

Figure 4.1 The role of attention in the maintenance of pain. Focused attention in the form of vigilance increases the likelihood of discovering a painful symptom. This symptom may constitute a threat. This in turn leads to worry which automatically increases the vigilance.

attention on *painful* or other stimuli that would coincide with such an injury.

Worry

What happens if the threat does not go away, such as is the case in persistent pain conditions? A bilateral effect occurs where pain also affects our emotions and thus attention. Recently, a group of researchers have presented a compelling model that asserts that persistent pain results in worry (Fig. 4.1) (Eccleston and Crombez, 1999; Aldrich et al., 2000). Essentially, worry is a negative emotion with a series of thoughts and images that attempt to mentally solve a problem, but where the outcome is uncertain and quite possibly negative. Worry tends to interrupt other cognitions and behavior and it may become repetitive and self-degrading. For example, chronic pain patients may ruminate about the possible causes of their pain and worry that a catastrophe may occur (Sullivan et al., 1995). Eccelston and Crombez (1999) as well as Aldrich et al. (2000) argue that worry is a dynamic view of how we try to make sense of a threat that does not seem to go away. This worry in turn maintains a heightened vigilance

CASE STUDY: HANK

Attentional factors seem to play several roles in Hank's pain problem. First, the problem demanded Hank's attention in the beginning because the symptoms were unusual. Thus, he could hardly ignore them. Second, the attention also led to disruption. Hank could not ignore the pain, but it often disrupted his thoughts or function. This made the problem difficult to tolerate and was a central factor in the decision to seek care. Third, the condition

resulted in vigilance. Hank experienced the pain as a threat to his health and well-being. Thus, he became vigilant in order to detect any early signs of danger such as the condition resulting in permanent damage. The vigilance in turn has made him more attuned to various stimuli in his body including pain. This in itself appears to have increased Hank's discomfort. Finally, Hank began to worry more about his pain. This is a natural result of pain being experienced as a "threat". Consequently, the worry results in more vigilance as seen in Fig. 4.1. A vicious circle may in fact develop that greatly influences how attuned Hank is to internal stimuli that may signal a threat.

to painful threats. Thus, a kind of vicious circle may develop where the pain heightens awareness, which in turn creates worry that also maintains the heightened awareness.

SUMMARY

Paying attention to internal stimuli is the first step in pain perception. Psychological factors steer this process. By shifting attention inward, we increase the chance of perceiving symptoms, while shifting it to the environment around us decreases this chance. Attention is such an important factor that distraction has been delineated as an important coping strategy. For sure, experiments show that paying attention to a stimulus influences perception and pain experience. Pain serves the very useful function of a warning signal. It helps us to appropriately deal with various threats to our health. However, because pain has "threat" value, it also demands attention. This demand may be conceptualized as vigilance. If a threat is suspected we become watchful and alert in anticipation of the threatened stimulus. This, however, also increases the chance that we will perceive symptoms. In a sense it may sometimes lead to the "false" perception of a pain stimulus. Moreover, if we do discover an internal stimulus that may signal pain, this results in worry. This in turn automatically leads to more vigilance. Thus, attentional factors are central in pain perception and may contribute to a vicious circle that perpetuates pain problems.

The next step in processing the information is to evaluate and interpret them, that is, to determine if the signal actually constitutes a threat. Let us turn to this in the next chapter.

CHAPTER 5

Emotions and the experience of pain

When the pain comes, it is just overwhelming. I feel like I can't breathe. It's so dis-heartening that I can't see how I can go forward.

—Chronic pain patient

I am not afraid of death but of what may happen to me before it comes. Afterward doesn't frighten me, before does.

—Vilhelm Moberg, *A Time on Earth* (1984)

LEARNING OBJECTIVES

To understand:

- pain signals are integrated in the central nervous system where connections are automatically made with the emotional systems;

- pain is experienced and expressed emotionally, that is, pain results in emotions and emotions influence the experience of pain;

- pain typically results in emotional distress;

- fear and anxiety are normal emotional reactions to acute pain;

- depressed mood may develop in conjunction with pain, especially long-term pain;

- the emotional reaction reflects previous learning and is integrated with cognitive sets;

- the interactive and bidirectional nature of these.

One of the most disruptive features of pain is the emotional distress. This emotional reaction typically includes anxiety, fear, anger and depression. Guilt, disgust and frustration are also usual. In fact, pain and emotions are so integrally related that pain is typically experienced and expressed emotionally. Accordingly, pain shapes our emotions just as our emotions influence how we experience pain.

To be sure, negative affect is a key reason why we associate pain with *suffering*. Hence, pain activates negative emotions that vary from tolerable to those that provoke misery (Craig, 2003). It is interesting, then, that clinicians focus more on the sensory aspects of pain (e.g. intensity) than on the emotional aspects. Emotional aspects play an essential part in the experience of pain and we might provide better treatment if we had better knowledge about them. Indeed, negative affect is a singular predictor of negative outcome for treatment for low back pain (Linton, 2000c) and chronic pain (Robinson and Riley, 1999).

A powerful demonstration of the effects of emotions comes from laboratory research showing that a change in emotional state results in drastic changes in pain perception. In such experiments, participants are subjected to a series of painful stimuli such as electric shocks. The shocks are of varying intensity and given in a random order. Subjects rate their pain after each trial. After establishing a baseline level, the emotional state is then altered. Watching a depressing video clip might influence mood, or reading a particular text might provoke anxiety. Then the series of shocks is repeated. In this way, the effects of an emotional alteration on pain perception can be measured. Indeed, increasing anxiety or depressing mood result in a lowering of pain thresholds and tolerance.

Negative emotions might be related to pain perception in several ways. It is not yet clear whether there is a causal link between the two, but an interaction is clear. Robinson and Riley (1999) have described four possible routes of connection. First, negative emotions might increase somatic sensitivity. As described in the previous chapter, negative emotions such as anxiety might make us more aware of somatic pain sensations. Second, negative emotions might actually cause pain. In this scenario, the emotions would have a direct link, such as neurologically, with pain stimulation. Indeed, emotions like depression share many neurophysiological entities with pain. Thus, a depressed mood might conceivably cause pain. A third method of possible influence is that negative emotions might be the result of the pain. Surely, suffering nonrelenting back pain over long periods of time might affect mood. Finally, pain and negative emotions might coexist and interact. This seems a likely scenario given the similar biological foundations. The two may simply be different ways of describing and modeling the same phenomenon. Let us turn our attention to the main emotional factors.

ANXIETY

Anxiety is closely linked to pain perception. One way of understanding anxiety is to view it as a reaction to a perceived threat. Because pain may be an imminent threat to our welfare, it is not surprising that anxiety focused upon pain is frequent (Salkovskis and Warwick, 2001). Indeed, such anxiety is frequently recorded in community and clinical studies (Salkovskis and Warwick, 2001). Those with persistent pain typically have higher rates of anxiety disorders than normal controls. As an example, Atkinson et al. (1991) found that a group of male patients with chronic low back pain had twice the rate of anxiety disorders (31% vs. 14%) than did a matched sample of pain-free men. In fact, pain patients report significantly higher levels

of anxiety as compared to normal values and a significant part of their pain reports can be explained by anxiety (Robinson and Riley, 1999). There appears to be a temporal relationship where increases in one are associated with direct increases in the other. Consider the following study. We asked chronic back pain patients to rate their pain intensity as well as their anxiety levels daily for a period of six weeks (Linton and Götestam, 1985b). The results showed that 56% of the patients in fact had a significant relationship between their ratings of anxiety and their ratings of pain over the six-week period. However, the size of the correlation was moderate at 0.59. Thus, there was a clear tendency that when their ratings of anxiety increased, so did their ratings of pain. Consequently, the relationship holds over time and daily changes in anxiety were associated with rather immediate changes in pain perception. We might wonder, though, how this relationship works.

Anxiety may influence pain perception in several ways. One mechanism might be that pain is experienced more intensely if anxiety levels are increased. For example, in a laboratory study it was found that participants with high levels of health anxiety tolerated less cold pressor pain than did those with low levels of anxiety as shown in shorter tolerance times (Gramling et al., 1996). Another mechanism might be that anxiety heightens awareness to pain signals. Thus, this focus on the pain would in essence lower pain thresholds. Anxiety may also result in physiological changes such as increases in muscle tension, blood pressure and sweating (Barlow, 2002) which in turn cause painful nociception. In particular, increased muscle tension has been linked to pain (Lundberg and Melin, 2002). As an example, Flor and colleagues (Flor et al., 1992a) found that chronic pain patients, compared to normal controls, demonstrated elevated reactivity (tension increases) when confronted with a personally relevant stressor. Not least, anxiety appears to increase distress and suffering. We all experience a wide variety of physical symptoms. Yet those with high levels of anxiety seek more care and appear to suffer more extensively (Martin et al., 2001). In reality, some research indicates that less than half of those with clear physical symptoms actually seek medical help and this may be because they are not particularly anxious about the symptom (Scambler and Scambler, 1985).

Although we may first consider anxiety to cause or exacerbate pain, the two are integrally related. While anxiety may influence pain, perceptions of pain may also affect anxiety. This interrelationship is fundamental for understanding pain perception. Reflect on an early conception of the relationship, the anxiety–muscle tension–pain model where anxiety is said to result in muscle tension which in turn leads to more

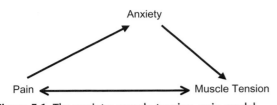

Figure 5.1 The anxiety–muscle tension–pain model. The experience of pain generates anxiety which in turn results in increases in muscle tension. This increased muscle tension subsequently results in more pain.

pain (Fig. 5.1). A vicious circle develops that once set on its way may continue even if the original injury heals (Linton, 1992; Ohrback and McCall, 1996). Although the relationship does not appear to be this simple in reality, the model nevertheless illustrates convincingly how the variables are intertwined. In fact, once such a vicious circle is started it may be impossible to know which variable "caused" what. Fortunately, the interconnections between the variables suggest that we need to understand the system rather than individual factors.

Health anxiety

One particular aspect of anxiety is the concept of *health anxiety*. Rather than regarding all forms of anxiety as in some studies mentioned above, the definition involves fears and the belief that bodily signs and symptoms indicate serious illness (Lucock and Morley, 1996). Health anxiety is linked to interpretations and misinterpretations of these signs and symptoms. Indeed, in its extreme form health anxiety results in vague but nevertheless normal bodily sensations being interpreted as serious diseases. The continuum from "normal" fears to abnormal health anxiety is determined by the degree of fear as well as the degree of the conviction about having a serious illness. Health anxiety has a close and obvious relationship to distress and function where those with high levels of health anxiety have significantly greater levels of distress and disrupted function (Lucock and Morley, 1996; Barsky et al., 1998). In one study of health anxiety, as an example, primary care patients seeking physical therapy for pain had significantly higher levels of health anxiety than did normal controls (Hadjistavropoulos et al., 2001). Further, personality profiles that measure health anxiety also consistently show pain patients to have elevated levels as compared to normal controls (Hadjistavropoulos et al., 2001).

Health anxiety is a specific form of anxiety and appears to affect pain in similar ways. The anxiety has a special focus on somatic sensations and thus it propels an increase in attention and vigilance to such signs.

For example, individuals with high levels of health anxiety begin to focus on the negative and emotional features of the physical sensations when exposed to a cold pressor pain test (Gramling et al., 1996). This focus also results in accompanying increases in distress and suffering. Bear in mind that in a review of the evidence, it was found that anxiety and fear were clearly associated with higher pain intensity as well as dysfunction (Asmundson and Larsen, 2000). In addition, health anxiety is related to several physiological changes that may enhance pain stimulation and perception (Hadjistavropoulos et al., 2001).

Importantly, health anxiety also affects behavior, that is, the way the patient responds to the pain. Those with high levels of health anxiety typically respond by seeking reassurance and avoidance. For example, those with high health anxiety are more likely to seek medical care which may be regarded as a form of reassurance seeking (Kettell et al., 1992; Leventhal et al., 1996). Those with high levels of pain-related fear, for instance, are more likely to avoid certain movements and are more highly disabled by their pain (Vlaeyen et al., 1995b).

FEAR AND WORRY

Fear may be considered an important extreme example of anxiety. A natural result of a focus on somatic threats to one's health may be fear. Fear is characterized by an extreme reaction that prepares us for a "fight or flight" response. It is also associated with dramatic physiological changes such as blood flow being oriented to internal organs (the person turns "white"), sweating, trembling and facial expressions. In connection with fear are a set of cognitions including negative appraisal. Fear seems, in fact, to trigger certain cognitions. As with health anxiety, fear results in increased vigilance, as well as physiological and behavioral changes. All of these may be expected to affect pain perception. As will be seen later in the book, fear has been highlighted in the so-called fear-avoidance model of pain perception where fear and avoidance are at center stage.

Worry is closely associated with anxiety and fear. Worry is characterized by frequent cognitive intrusions where the person considers "what if" possibilities (Barlow, 2002). Typically it involves ruminations that are quite negative and aversive (Eccleston et al., 2001). As seen in the previous chapter on attention, for chronic pain patients this means a repetitive preoccupation with threatening thoughts about pain and its effects (Eccleston and Crombez, 1999). Worry may be considered the result of a basic anxiety and the spiraling arousal it creates. However, worry may actually be a more persistent form of anxiety in that it has self-perpetuating qualities (Barlow, 2002). In fact, worry may be viewed as a way of coping with and avoiding anxiety (Craske, 1999). Indeed, worry is associated with higher levels of anxiety, cognitive interruptions and difficulties in attentional control (Rachman, 1998). Pain patients may worry about the consequences of their problem (if I don't get better, I may never be able to work) or the "what if" in terms of action (what if I fall; what if I lift too much and hurt my back) or causes of the problem (what if it is cancer).

Worry appears to be a natural reaction to a threat that "gets out of hand". Just as with anxiety and fear, worry is seen as a natural reaction to a threat. The important role worry normally plays is to maintain attention to a possible threat. If you are walking in a neighborhood known for robberies, worry may help keep you alert to such dangers and thereby serve a useful purpose. However, for the patient with long-term pain, there is no such concrete threat. The problem, then, is that the pain may signal an impending threat to health and well-being, but there is no distinct stimulus to react to. In other words, pain may trigger worry even though there is no value in maintaining vigilance. This worry then becomes problematic in itself because it is aversive and increases awareness of bodily sensations including the pain.

A recent study illustrates how worry is related to persistent pain. This investigation used daily ratings of pain-related worry as compared to worry about other things to understand the process better (Eccleston et al., 2001). Thus, 34 patients with persistent pain completed a diary over a 7-day period concerning pain worry and worry about other things. A comparison showed that pain-related worry was more difficult to dismiss, more distracting, more intrusive, more aversive, and demanded more attention than nonpain worry. Moreover, the usual pain-related worry lasted about 20 minutes and was triggered by an increase in pain. Thus these results support the idea that worry for pain patients is an emotion directly related to attentional processes described above as well as to cognitions that will be described in more detail in the next chapter.

STRESS AND TRAUMA

No discussion of the emotional aspects of pain perception would be complete without considering the concept of stress. As a matter of fact, many theories of musculoskeletal pain include stress as a major factor. Stress is a reaction to a perceived threat (a stressor) just like anxiety. However, while anxiety is thought to be related to the individual's psychological set, and may be excessive, stress is usually seen as an immediate reaction to stressors in the environment. Stress is a normal emotional reaction to life events which is characterized by feelings of being pressured or overwhelmed. For many pain complaints such as neck and back pain, there may be no physical trauma that triggers the pain and the individual may even have relatively light physical work. However, stress levels may link the work situation to the pain. Thus, because stress can bridge the gap between physiological injury and pain, it is an important theoretical factor in accounting for neck, back and shoulder pain.

Many accounts of the role of stress in pain perception focus on the neurological changes that occur in our bodies when we are stressed. Indeed, our biological reaction to stress involves a sophisticated system of stress regulation (Seyle, 1950; Chrousos and Gold, 1992). Stress may well act upon the stress-regulatory system which in turn produces lesions of muscle, bone, nerve or other tissue giving rise to pain (Melzack, 1999). For our purposes, we may remember that stress affects us physiologically through a system that directly affects a variety of symptoms such as pain. This model of stress and pain underscores once again the integration of physiological and psychological processes.

There is a large body of evidence that shows a link between stress and neck and back pain (Linton, 2000c; Lundberg and Melin, 2002). One form of stress concerns "life events" where incidents such as a death in the family or an economic crisis are assessed. Several studies have reported a relationship between these events and a variety of health problems including pain (Ogden, 2000; Walker, 2001). Perhaps the clearest evidence, however, has regarded stress at work where work-related stress has also been consistently shown to be related to pain, especially neck and back pain (Bongers et al., 1993; Hoogendoorn et al., 2000; Linton, 2001). Indeed, a study of physiological markers of stress showed that white-collar workers increase their level by 50% during work as compared to non-workers, while blue-collar workers have an increase of 100% (Lundberg and Johansson, 2000). Moreover, increases in perceived stress have also been shown to increase muscle tension, demonstrating an interaction between psychological stress and physiological reactions that may lead to pain (Melin and Lundberg, 1997). Stress or strain is thought to be caused by a combination of high demands at work and a low level of control (Karasek and Theorell, 1990). For example, a job with high demands such as to produce a high quantity in a short period of time that also provides little control over the work, such as an assembly line, would be predicted to produce high levels of stress. The stress would in turn affect us physiologically such as via the muscles and pain would be the result. This might be particularly true when psychological stress is mixed with physical load (Lundberg and Melin, 2002), such as is evidenced in people doing repetitive work.

Even though stress might explain why some people experience musculoskeletal pain, we might wonder why some people with similar work do not. One factor that influences the experience of stress is the balance between the effort we put into the task and the reward received. This has been formalized in the "effort–reward" model of stress (Siegrist, 1996) where the combination of high effort and low reward is clearly associated with a variety of symptoms.

Remarkable associations between psychosocial factors at work including stress and back pain have also been demonstrated (Bongers et al., 1993; Hoogendoorn et al., 2000; Linton, 2001). As an illustration, we reviewed 21 studies that first measured the psychological work variable and then followed participants to observe the future result (Linton, 2001). The follow-up was normally done one year after the first assessment. One way of examining the role of stress is to look at the relationship between self-reports of "feeling stressed" at the baseline and the subsequent effect on back pain at the one-year follow-up. In fact, I found that overall ratings of stress at work at baseline were consistently related to future back pain problems in these studies. A second way of examining this relationship is to look at the key elements of a stress model. Thus, the demand–control model was used to see whether high demands and low control were related to future back pain problems. Indeed, there was evidence that stress factors such as work demands, control and pace were related to future back pain.

An intriguing mechanism for linking stress to pain is muscular activity. The question is by what mechanism mental stress might cause back or neck pain. The answer is through muscular activity. As seen above, mental stress has been shown to influence muscle activity by increasing muscle tension (Melin and Lundberg, 1997; Westgaard and Winkel, 2002). We also saw that mixing physical load and stress might enhance this process. Why, then, might relatively light work such as sitting at a computer result in neck pain? One answer is that it produces constant firing of low-threshold motor units in the muscles (Lundberg and Melin, 2002). We normally think of muscle contractions as being large, obvious changes in the muscles. However, with low-intensity physical load such as is common in sedentary work, some muscle units may be firing constantly. This means that such motor units in the muscle will be firing constantly until they are completely relaxed. In other words, even though the work is not strenuous, some motor units will be constantly firing; these motor units may cause pain in the muscle. Thus, rather than the injury being a result of one huge load that injures the muscle, e.g. lifting something very heavy, it is the result of long periods of low-intensity work.

Regardless of the model considered, increased muscle activity appears to be a notable part of the link between emotional factors such as stress and pain.

Trauma and abuse

An increasing body of evidence has linked personal trauma to pain. The trauma often includes a distinct psychological component and is exemplified by sexual or physical abuse. However, even traumatic accidents may have a relationship to pain perception. Take, for example, whiplash-related pain where the neck pain is associated with an automobile accident. This entails a slow-moving or stationary vehicle being hit from behind. In this scenario, an accident may give rise to neck pain as well as to a post-traumatic stress disorder (PTSD). Although all car accidents may have some psychological sequel, PTSD involves the persistent re-experiencing of the event accompanied by symptoms of physiological and psychological arousal. Patients attempt to avoid thoughts, activities and situations associated with the trauma in order to control the negative stress it arouses. As a matter of fact, PTSD is relevant to patients injured in a traumatic way such as car accident victims and it is related to a host of variables such as pain and function (Geisser et al., 1997). Thus, there seems to be a relationship where pain problems are enhanced by the PTSD. Post-traumatic reactions are also common in other types of trauma such as abuse.

Extensive research also indicates a connection between physical and sexual abuse and pain perception. The report of sexual or physical abuse is clearly tied to an increase in a variety of pain problems. For example, those experiencing abuse more frequently have problems with pelvic and stomach pain (Drossman et al., 1990; Fry, 1993; Scarinci et al., 1994). Interestingly, a relationship has also been discovered for musculoskeletal pain such as back pain (Wurtele et al., 1990; Drossman, 1994; Leserman et al., 1998). For example, we compared pain patients who reported abuse with those who did not report any abuse (Linton et al., 1996b). Although both groups were seeking care for their pain problem, the group reporting a history of any sexual or physical abuse had much worse scores on almost all of the over 20 assessment measures. In other words, patients reporting abuse clearly had more severe symptoms and consequences of their pain than did patients not reporting abuse. The results, while impressive in size, might be related to biases in a patient population. The question was whether abuse affects pain perception in "healthy" people.

Research on the effects of abuse on pain perception took a new turn when individuals in the general public were included. This allows a direct comparison between those with and those without a pain problem. Consequently, I studied the link between abuse and back pain in a large sample of people from the general population (Linton, 1997c). We compared those reporting no back pain during the past year to those reporting symptoms. First, let it be perfectly clear that abuse was *not* found to be a strong risk factor for men. This may be due to a different reaction for men, or to a hesitancy in reporting sexual abuse since it typically involves homosexual relationships. However, *for women,* a history of self-reported abuse was a substantial risk factor for pain. As an example, a report of sexual abuse increased the risk of back pain by more than four times and the report of physical abuse increased this risk by over fivefold. Interestingly, physical abuse such as being hit by someone was as potent as sexual abuse. It is also worth noting that the abuse was normally not ongoing, but had occurred earlier in life. Moreover, there was no observable difference between the report of abuse during childhood or as an adult in terms of pain perception.

Does abuse cause pain?

Although a connection has been shown between abuse and pain, it is not certain that abuse actually *causes* pain. Most of the research has involved designs where those reporting abuse are compared to those not reporting abuse or where patients with pain are compared to those without pain problems. This opens the door for other differences that may prejudice results. Those reporting abuse, for example, may have different lifestyles than those not reporting abuse. Of particular relevance are such variables as social status, income, education level and substance abuse. Any one of these variables might muddy the direction of the relationship between abuse and pain. Further, pain might even increase the reporting of abuse, for example, because the patient is more intensely seeking an explanation for the problem.

In order to determine the direction of the relationship, it is necessary to observe people over time in order to determine better how abuse might affect the development of a pain problem. To tackle this problem, we identified 422 females who reported either no or low levels of back pain (Linton, 2002b). A standardized questionnaire was used to determine self-reported sexual and physical abuse during childhood and as an adult. One year later, these women were contacted and it was determined whether they had developed back pain or pain-related functional problems. For those already suffering pain, self-reported abuse had little effect on the development of the problem over the course of one year. However, for the

group with no pain, sexual and physical abuse were associated with future pain and functional problems. Self-reports of abuse increased the risk for developing pain or functional problems one year later by as much as fourfold. Therefore, this investigation suggests that abuse might be a factor in the etiology of such pain problems.

How does abuse affect pain perception?

There are several ideas about how abuse might affect pain perception. A straightforward interpretation is that those suffering abuse are not able to negotiate effective coping strategies. Thus, abuse would not necessarily lead to more frequent pain, but it would affect how well the person deals with the problem. Think about a person suffering abuse and the related problems this person may have such as low social status, low education levels, etc. Consider further that the majority of people at some time or another suffer from back or neck pain. How well equipped would the person with a history of abuse be at coping with this pain in comparison to those not having such a history? It may be that those with a history of abuse are not as well prepared to cope with a pain problem.

Another explanation put forward is that the person having suffered abuse is more vulnerable for a pain problem. This might entail a physiological susceptibility, but also a psychological vulnerability to the development of a pain problem. In this scenario, pain might be detected "earlier" and the consequences of the pain might be greatly enhanced.

Still another possible explanation is that the combination of physical and psychological trauma disrupts the normal discrimination of body signals (Scarinci et al., 1994). In this model, the psychological (and perhaps physical) trauma of abuse affects how stimuli are interpreted. In a nutshell, the person is said to begin to interpret neutral or other "nonpain" stimuli as painful. Some experimental evidence supports this view. For example, those reporting abuse have been compared to controls (no reported abuse) in a laboratory investigation of pain perception and discrimination. Pressure is applied at various levels ranging from barely discriminable to quite painful. These levels are established on an individual basis and then a series of "new" stimuli are given. The results show that those reporting abuse have more difficulty in discriminating between a painful stimulus level and a neutral one as compared to the controls. In short, those reporting abuse often report pain even though the stimulus level is below their own established threshold for pain. This suggests that the pain perception system is disrupted.

A final interesting explanation associates pain perception for those having suffered abuse with inhibiting emotions (Pennebaker, 1990). The reasoning is that because of the very negative affect involved, people suffering abuse or other trauma attempt to hold back the associated emotion. In a sense the memory and associated emotions are held in check as a way of coping with its unpleasantness. In this model, this avoidance is said to increase stress and awareness of other symptoms. Thus inhibiting the emotions associated with abuse takes energy, creates stress, and heightens awareness of somatic symptoms. Whatever explanation is pondered, it is clear that abuse or trauma may constitute an extreme stressor that may affect pain perception.

MOOD AND DEPRESSION

Depressed mood and pain are imminently linked. However, to understand this relationship we need to ask how an emotion like mood influences pain perception. Although we may suspect that depression causes pain to be perceived more intensely, it is also apparent that suffering chronic pain should affect our mood negatively. Further, feelings of depression are by no means universal for pain patients (Clyde and Williams, 2002). Nor is there a proportional relationship between the pain and mood. The complexity is further delineated by the fact that depression sometimes precedes the pain, but sometimes the onset is after the pain (Dohrenwend et al., 1999). How, then, does the relationship between depression and pain work?

The nature of the relationship between mood and pain

There is considerable evidence to show an intricate tie between mood and pain. Indeed, patients with persistent pain often report symptoms congruent with a depressed mood such as feeling tired, having difficulty initiating activities and feeling "blue". Because of this link, some people have assumed that depression may "explain" the development of chronic pain. In addition to promoting the unjustified view that these pain patients are to "blame" for their pain, there are empirical reasons for re-examining the relationship (Clyde and Williams, 2002). Today we realize that the relationship between depression and pain is neither simple nor straightforward.

Certainly, many studies indicate that chronic pain patients do in fact have higher rates of depressed mood than do people in the general population (Romano and Turner, 1985; Williams and Richardson, 1993; Banks and Kerns, 1996). Although it is difficult to provide exact numbers, somewhere between one and two thirds of chronic pain patients are said to suffer from a depressed mood.

However, it is important to realize that depression and mood have different connotations that are important to distinguish when considering pain. "Depression" is reserved for a psychiatric state and there are strict criteria for diagnosing someone as being depressed. These standardized criteria for a major depressive episode are shown in Table 5.1. Note that it

Table 5.1 The criteria for diagnosing depression according to DSM-IV.

A. Five or more of the following symptoms have been present for two or more weeks and represent a change from previous functioning:

    (a) depressed mood, most of the day, nearly every day and/or

    (b) markedly diminished interest or pleasure in all, or almost all, activities most of the day, nearly every day

    (c) significant weight loss or decrease/increase in appetite nearly every day

    (d) insomnia or hypersomnia nearly every day

    (e) psychomotor agitation or retardation nearly every day

    (f) fatigue or loss of energy nearly every day

    (g) feelings of worthlessness or excessive guilt

    (h) diminished ability to think or concentrate

    (i) recurrent thoughts of death, recurrent suicidal ideation

B. The symptoms cause clinically significant distress or impairment in social, occupational or other functioning.

C. The symptoms are not due to the direct physiological effects of a substance or general medical condition.

D. The symptoms are not better accounted for by bereavement.

involves a depressed mood most of the day, nearly every day for at least two weeks, as well as several other symptoms. Note also that there is overlap in the symptoms associated with depression as well as with pain.

Consequently, although a depressed state may change, it does so relatively slowly and not on a day-to-day basis. On the other hand, "mood" refers to how we are feeling from day to day and may range from ecstatic to irritable or blue. Though we may be in a bad mood for a while, these feelings tend to change rather rapidly. Further, mood is usually thought of as being influenced by current ongoing events: getting a raise boosts mood, while failing a test deflates it. The difference between mood and depression is often missed in discussions concerning pain. While pain and mood are related, we may wonder whether pain is actually related to clinical depression.

Mood affects pain perception

There may be several mechanisms operating that link mood to pain perception. First, a depressed mood is believed to lower our threshold and tolerance for pain. Several experimental studies have manipulated mood and then studied its affect on pain perception. When mood is depressed, these studies generally show an increase in the reporting of pain symptoms and a decrease in pain tolerance for experimentally induced pain. For example, Zelman et al. (1991) found that when participants' mood was made worse by reading depressive statements, pain tolerance was reduced. On the other hand, when mood was improved by reading elative statements, pain tolerance was also increased.

A second mechanism by which a depressed mood may influence pain perception is cognitive evaluation. This will be examined more thoroughly in the following chapter on cognitions, but suffice it to say here that depression is related to a cognitive processing set where there is a tendency to interpret events negatively. In fact, depressed patients have a propensity to interpret events negatively so that certain, diffuse sensations are more likely to be reported as pain (Pennebaker, 1982). Therefore, those with a depressed mood may interpret a given sensation as painful, while they would experience it as something else given an elated mood.

Pain affects mood

Persistent pain is associated with mood changes. Although acute pain seems to naturally elicit anxiety and fear, long-term pain is associated with depressed mood. Just as we have seen that anxiety seems to have survival value, a depressive mood may also increase our endurance. Depression might have helped us to survive in that it reserves resources and elicits help and sympathy. Further, isolation and withdrawal might reduce the chances for further damage or harm.

Pain is a salient stressor and may lead to depression. Indeed, a basic tenet in the psychology of pain is that suffering pain over long periods of time may be related to the development of depression (Romano and Turner, 1985; Von Korff and Simon, 1996; Clyde and Williams, 2002). The fact that persistent pain does not always cause depression might be explained by differences in vulnerability (Banks and Kerns, 1996). Take into account the fact that persistent pain often is experienced as unrelenting, and results in disability and considerable secondary loss, and it is easy to see how pain may influence mood and depression. All this causes a disruption in the person's life and may trigger a depression.

The connection between mood and pain also involves function. It is well known in the depression literature that depression is associated with a decrease in activity levels. This is also true for patients in pain. As an example, one study experimentally influenced mood states to study the effect on function (Fisher and Johnston, 1996). When a depressed mood was induced, this was associated with greater functional problems and disability. However, when mood enhancement techniques were employed, this was related to improvements in function and reduced disability. Therefore, mood appears to have a direct link to function and activity.

Pain and depression are interrelated

Several factors become apparent when examining the relationship between pain and depression. First, the relationship is not a straightforward causal one. Second, suffering persistent pain does not always result in the development of depression. Third, depression and pain may be better understood if pain is viewed as a potentially potent stressor. Fourth, vulnerability to depression may explain why some people do not develop depression even though they experience long-term pain. Finally, there may be several pathways by which pain and depression co-occur as well as influence one another.

One way of understanding the link between emotions and pain, and especially between depression and pain, is to consider cognitive processes where emotions play an integral part. In fact, emotions shape how we interpret our pain. Interpretation is an essential part of the experience of pain and is colored by anxiety as well as mood. Let us consider how cognitions work in the process of appraising what our pain means as we move to the next chapter.

EMOTIONAL ASPECTS IN THE CASE OF HANK

Hank is very aware that his pain problem has interacted with his emotional state. It's no fun having persistent pain. Looking back to when the pain first began to be a problem, Hank was optimistic that he could handle the problem well. He was quite confident that it would heal and he could get back to normal life again. However, as the problem recurred and persisted, he began to lose that confidence. He could not understand why he couldn't manage the problem. He also became irritable. He sometimes shouted at people and made sarcastic remarks that were definitely not typical of him.

Because the pain problem affected his function, Hank also felt guilty about the duties he was not able to do. His routine at home changed rather dramatically and he no longer did his normal chores. This meant that his wife had to pitch in to get things done. It also meant that his children had only half of a father. Hank felt quite guilty about this.

Since Hank was not getting better and yet very little progress was being made in terms of his treatment, Hank became frustrated. He could not get a handle on the problem and others, who might, did not seem to want to. Things were definitely not going Hank's way.

With time, Hank and even his family began cutting down on family, social and leisure activities. It seemed to be too much. And the mental energy needed to organize and actually do an activity began to be a barrier for Hank. Thus, he visited friends and relatives a lot less. He also virtually gave up his most active hobbies and his interest in sports. As the positive side of life began to diminish, the problem really started to affect Hank's mood. In fact, he felt downright depressed. Some days it was hard to get out of bed and face the new day.

Hank noticed that the changes in his mood seemed to also affect his pain. Some days he felt rather blue and then the pain could get especially bad. However, on some days he was more cheerful and had fun and he noticed the pain a lot less. His family frequently invited him to participate in activities such as going to a movie, taking a walk or having a picnic. Although Hank was concerned about getting more pain afterwards, he did agree that he felt better while doing these things with his family.

Other emotions

People suffering pain are known to experience a wide range of emotions. Most research deals with depression and anxiety, but many other emotions appear to be prevalent. These can include irritation, frustration and anger. Modern theories of pain such as the gate control theory and the neuromatrix theory suggest that intense negative emotions can increase pain by altering descending and central pain modulation systems. Furthermore, negative emotions can complicate treatment interventions by disrupting relationships with healthcare professionals. And it can disrupt the patient's support system by creating turmoil in interpersonal relationships such as with family, friends and workmates.

Anger is an example of an additional emotion that appears to be important, but where much less attention has been paid than to anxiety or depression (Greenwood et al., 2003). Anger is sometimes difficult to define because it is confused with hostility or aggression. However, anger refers to an aversive emotional state that can range in intensity from mild irritation to rage (Smith, 1994). Furthermore, anger is distinguished by physiological arousal, certain facial expressions, and impulsiveness toward aggression. It is a reaction to perceived unfair treatment or harm. Indeed, anger has been found to be related to a variety of pain problems ranging from persistent back pain and chest pain to cancer pain (Greenwood et al., 2003). Those with high levels of anger have higher levels of pain intensity.

SUMMARY

We have seen that pain signals, through ties in the brain, are directly associated with a variety of emotional responses. Indeed, the experience of pain in its very essence involves emotional reactions. Some particularly relevant emotional responses include various aspects of negative affect such as fear, worry and a depressed mood. Pain in fact often results in considerable distress. These emotional responses are interactive and play an important "motivational" role. Emotions are integrated into the pain experience system and are closely linked to how we interpret our pain cognitively as well as how we respond behaviorally.

CHAPTER 6

Interpreting pain signals: cognitions

When I feel the sharp, shooting pain, I know I can't go on. I know that it will get worse and worse.

—Patient with whiplash

LEARNING OBJECTIVES

To understand:

- pain signals are interpreted via the central nervous system and meaning is given to the stimulus;

- how we interpret the stimulus influences our reaction;

- interpretation is influenced by emotions such as anxiety and mood;

- interpretation is a cognitive process where various patterns of thinking influence the experience of pain;

- the cognitive process reflects previous learning and cognitive sets like catastrophizing;

- the interactive nature of cognitions with emotions and behavior.

Once a "pain signal" has been attended to, we need to evaluate and attach meaning to it so that appropriate action might be taken. Sometimes this system may falter and we may experience an insignificant stimulus, such as light pressure to the arm, as severe pain. Or we may fail to determine that a serious injury has occurred because we feel little or no pain. Every year some people die of untreated heart disease that almost certainly has produced pain, because appropriate treatment was not sought. Likewise, the diagnosis of cancer may occur relatively late because some people may not interpret the pain symptoms as serious enough to consult a doctor. Undeniably, reacting to every nociceptive stimulus in the same way would not be very efficient; just imagine reacting the same way to a bad cut and a pinprick. Nor would such reaction provide the greatest survival value. In some way, we need to make sense of the numerous signals that may come to our attention so that a suitable response can be made.

Interpreting the meaning of the pain signals is a critical part of the psychological reaction to pain. The meaning we attach to the stimulus is highly influenced by our emotional state and our cognitive set. As seen in Chapter 5, emotions are intertwined in the process of discovering and interpreting pain signals. Thus, a depressed person will tend to have a more negative appraisal of the stimulus than a happy-go-lucky person. Moreover, the way we process the information cognitively will also influence the interpretation. The beliefs we hold and our cognitive style have bearing on our interpretation. In this chapter we will examine a variety of variables that influence how we interpret pain stimuli. As with other aspects in our model of pain perception, we will see that emotional and cognitive processes are dynamic, interactive and bidirectional.

THINKING AND INTERPRETATION

How we think about our pain affects our perception of it. Once "pain" signals are recognized, they need to be interpreted to give them proper meaning. This cognitive processing is highly related to the emotional aspects described in Chapter 5 and it is instrumental in regulating our behavior. In fact, how we view nociceptive signals may dramatically affect our experience. This is probably why certain strategies like "think of something else" have long been employed as methods for controlling pain. Cognitive processing occurs rapidly and often without conscious thought. Simply put, they form thinking patterns or habits in the way we interpret the signals. Because this cognitive processing tends to form "thinking habits", we often call this attitudes or beliefs about pain. These are basic assumptions that we all hold. Examples may be the idea that "pain is dangerous" or "if I hurt, something must be injured". These are important because they may significantly influence how we truly experience the pain.

DOES "THINKING ABOUT SOMETHING ELSE" HELP REDUCE PAIN?

The effects of cognitions on pain experience were dramatically underscored in a clever experiment (Sullivan et al., 1997). Participants in the study were subjected to a cold-pressor pain induction procedure where they immersed a hand in ice water for 60 seconds. However, one group was asked to suppress all thoughts about the procedure before the pain test. The comparison group was given no such instruction. Thoughts and pain were recorded. Amazingly, those attempting to suppress their thoughts actually thought more about the procedure and experienced more pain than the controls! Thus, while being engaged in something interesting may focus attention on something besides pain and thereby possibly reduce the pain, active suppression of thinking about pain may actually be counterproductive.

Cognitions help us to connect our emotions with behaviors. We have seen above that how we are feeling emotionally affects our experience of pain. For example, higher levels of depressed mood or anxiety result in less pain tolerance. The emotions in turn are related to patterns of thinking. Depressed mood may result in negative interpretations of neutral events; we may turn normal events into catastrophes. Likewise, anxiety may increase vigilance for pain sensations in our body and result in endless worry. However, cognitions are also linked to behavior. The meaning we bestow to a stimulus affects what we do about it. Thus our thinking patterns *set the stage for a behavioral response*. If we believe that our pain is caused by a dangerous disease, we probably would seek professional healthcare. On the other hand, if we believe that the pain is the natural result of a little too much exercise, we may simply expect it to get better and not seek professional help. In this section we will examine some of the main ways that cognitive processes work and how they affect our experience of pain.

Cognitive processes involve a number of mechanisms. These are not mutually exclusive, but rather are highly integrated. Therefore, the conceptions below often overlap. Here are some basic cognitive mechanisms that are quite relevant for understanding pain.

BELIEFS AND ATTITUDES

We all hold a number of beliefs that are related to our health and specifically to pain. Ordinarily, we think of beliefs in religious, social or perhaps political contexts. However, we also hold certain assumptions about how pain works and what it probably means to feel a given painful stimulus (DeGood and Shutty, 1999). Beliefs serve the useful purpose of aiding in rapid interpretation of stimuli and they seem to provide a shortcut that helps our brain process the enormous amount of incoming stimuli in a more efficient manner. They provide a sort of automatic interpretation of the stimuli and thus these stimuli do not need lengthy processing in the brain. As a result, beliefs can be quite beneficial. One reason is that they are based on earlier learning such as earlier experiences. However, we may sometimes develop an attitude that is not entirely helpful or perhaps even downright detrimental. This is because of certain learning processes. For example, we may develop a questionable belief based on a single, very unusual experience (I ate a bad donut, therefore all bakery goods are bad). Moreover, we also learn through other media than direct experience such as what we read, see on TV and hear from friends and relatives. Finally, we may cognitively apply a "correct" belief to the "wrong" situation. The belief that one should rest when ill is advantageous when we are suffering the aches of a fever, but may be detrimental if we are suffering muscle aches from the back. Consequently, while beliefs are ordinarily helpful, we may sometimes develop attitudes and beliefs that are not particularly successful.

Beliefs focus on three vital aspects of the pain. The first concerns *the cause of the pain*. It is imperative from a survival perspective to know what the cause of the pain is so that appropriate measures can be taken. Thus, it is natural that we focus on the cause. The second aspect is the *expected consequence or meaning* associated with the pain. This provides a gauge as to the urgency of the problem as well as important information on how to best deal with the pain.

Consider this essential example. You wake up one morning and have a sore throat. If this feels similar to other times you have had a cold, you may interpret the pain as caused by a cold and the consequence to be minor (in a few days it will go away). However, if you have severe jabbing pain even when you are not swallowing, this might be interpreted very differently. Not only will this pain activate emotional responses such as worry and anxiety, but our thinking pattern may result in another interpretation. You may interpret this pain as the result of a potentially dangerous "killer" virus and the expected result might be a serious illness and a threat to your health or survival. This example illustrates that the way we interpret the painful sensation is closely linked to emotions, but also sets the stage for what we do about it.

The third aspect is *expectations about how best to cope with the pain*. As seen in the sore throat example, whether we seek professional care or engage in other ways of coping with the pain is associated with our beliefs. Beliefs, then, are employed in the processing of painful stimuli and help us to quickly interpret the meaning of the pain. While usually helpful, they may sometimes also be detrimental.

A number of beliefs that may hinder recovery have been identified for patients suffering neck, shoulder or back pain (DeGood and Shutty, 1992, 1999; Burton et al., 1999b; Vowles and Gross, 2003). DeGood and Shutty (1999) describe four dimensions of beliefs that are typically associated with chronic pain. These beliefs may enhance or hinder treatment results. They include beliefs about the cause of the pain such as whether it is strictly somatic or rather due to multiple factors. In addition, the beliefs concern diagnostic and treatment expectations such as whether these will actively involve the patient (versus being done to the patient) and whether they will "fix or cure" the problem (versus rehabilitate).

Negative beliefs are tied to coping behaviors and ultimately treatment outcome. For example, a group of researchers in Britain found that the longer a person had been off work for back pain and the greater the number of previous episodes, the more negative the beliefs (Symonds et al., 1996). In turn, those with more negative beliefs were also more negative about rehabilitation and return to work. Thus, there is mounting evidence indicating that negative beliefs are associated with more healthcare, more medication use, more time off work and a generally unfavorable outcome (Szpalski et al., 1995; Symonds et al., 1996; Vlaeyen and Linton, 2000). Indeed, beliefs seem to be powerfully related to actual behavior and outcome. This is why the patient's own beliefs about the future are potent. For example, a very good predictor of future disability is the patient's own belief about their ability to return to work (Carosella et al., 1994; Linton and Boersma, 2003).

Let us look more closely at some beliefs that may hinder the recovery of patients suffering pain (Main and Spanswick, 2000; Burton and Waddell, 2002; Jensen et al., 2004).

"Hurt is harm"

Many patients believe that if they feel pain it automatically means that there has been a serious injury. The person then tends to interpret pain as meaning that something has been badly damaged in the body. While there is an obvious reason to believe that pain is caused by tissue damage, this belief focuses on the injury as being permanent and/or resulting in permanent vulnerability. This interpretation may greatly influence behavior. For example, patients holding this view tend to seek more diagnostic assessments and avoid anything that they believe will increase the pain (since it damages the body).

"Being active will increase the pain", "Rest is the best medicine"

A surprising number of patients with various musculoskeletal pain problems strongly believe that being active will increase the pain. A corollary of this belief is that rest will be an effective coping method. Although pain may sometimes be exacerbated by strenuous activities, in the long run resting is detrimental to recovery. Indeed, maintaining everyday activities and participating in exercise is an effective treatment while bed rest is harmful (Waddell et al., 1997). This belief, then, may lead to the patient using ineffective or perhaps even detrimental ways of coping with the pain, e.g. resting and avoiding activities.

"Need to find the cause of the pain"

Here the patient believes that the pain problem can never be properly dealt with unless the "true" cause of the pain is found. Although numerous examinations may be conducted, the patient may still believe that the actual cause has not been found. This is often because the pain simply does not disappear. Moreover, the patient may receive explanations of the pain but believe that they are not correct. Again, this is often related to the expectation that finding the cause will automatically result in a cure.

"A good doctor can cure"

We all hope for a treatment that will cure our pain. However, sometimes a belief develops where this is seen as the only option. The patient believes that an expert can provide a treatment that will cure the problem. This leaves no room for chronic diseases or normal recurrent health problems. The result may be that the patient repeatedly seeks treatment in hope of a cure. This is detrimental if the best treatment involves self-care methods where the patient needs to be engaged in the treatment. It also creates problems for pain conditions that are recurrent because the patient is seeking pain relief whereas the help that may be given focuses on other aspects such as function.

"Must be 100% recovered in order to resume activities/work"

The patient may improve slowly over time. In some situations complete recovery such as being pain-free is not common. In many pain conditions there is a "gray zone" between being completely sick and being completely well. The belief that one must be 100% recovered before resuming normal activities draws the conclusion that an attempt should not be made, even during very extended recovery periods, to resume normal activities including work because it will result in failure. In a number of painful conditions including back pain and fractures, the recovery period can be quite long. For adults, full recovery can take months. In addition, recovery from such problems unfortunately may never be totally complete. It is relatively common to have some lasting effects. Consequently, patients holding this belief typically avoid and resist resumption of normal activities. This seems to be tied to the idea that they are permanently fragile (susceptible to injury) and that going back too soon will result in a (re)injury. Thus, holding this belief may actually hinder recovery and the attainment of a good quality of life.

EXPECTATIONS

The beliefs we hold mirror our expectations. These may exert a powerful bearing on our experience of pain (DeGood and Shutty, 1999). Certainly, we often have an idea about the cause of the pain, its treatment, as well as how long it should take for recovery. As we have seen above, our beliefs may influence our interpretation of the pain as well as our choice of how to deal with the problem. Thus, some beliefs are truly related to what we expect to happen with our pain.

Expectations may drive coping behavior even in the absence of actual feedback. The expectation that participating in an activity (such as running) will increase pain intensity may in fact be related to avoiding the activity. While the activity (running) may never be attempted, the expectation of the results maintains the avoidance. In a similar way, a whole host of expectations may generate behaviors.

However, a determinant of our experience of pain is *whether our expectations are fulfilled*. We may expect, for instance, that we will fully recover from a bout of neck pain in 3 or 4 days. Epidemiology tells us that this is a very optimistic expectation. When the expectation is not fulfilled, this may generate further negative cognitions and motivate behaviors that may not be particularly helpful. For example, we might begin to believe that it must be a very serious injury because it does not get better as fast as expected. This might in turn generate behavior. For example, based on the expectation that neck pain needs to be treated by rest to avoid further injury, we might employ a treatment like a neck collar. While this treatment fulfills the expectation, it may have little or no actual benefit. Thus, whether an expectation is fulfilled can have clear effects on cognitive processing, emotions and behavior.

EXAMPLES OF PAIN BELIEFS

These reflect the beliefs described in the text.

- The pain I feel is a sign that damage is being done.

- No one has been able to tell me exactly why I'm in pain.

- I count more on my doctors to decrease my pain than I do on myself.

- Back pain means long periods of time off work.

- Medication is the best treatment for my pain.

- I consider myself disabled.

- I trust that doctors can cure my pain.

- I expect my pain will get worse and worse.

- Rest is an effective treatment for back pain.

COGNITIVE TRAPS: NEGATIVE AUTOMATIC THOUGHTS

In the processing of incoming signals we cognitively try to make sense of the experience. We employ various "thinking sets" to help provide a framework from which to interpret events. This is a normal and helpful process. However, for a variety of reasons some patients may employ cognitive patterns that misrepresent actual events or probable future events. The patient may fall into a cognitive trap where the interpretation is tantalizing and well connected with the emotional state, but where a consistent "error" in interpreting reality is made. Thus, the term "cognitive errors" is sometimes employed to describe these ways of thinking. Another way of viewing these is *negative automatic thoughts*. This thought pattern resembles a filter which systematically distorts one's view of the world. The negative automatic thoughts result in only allowing negative, distorted interpretations of events.

Negative automatic thoughts seem to exist as a part of our response system to stress (Barlow, 2002). Negative automatic thoughts provide for a sort of tunnel vision and the negative interpretations may have some survival value. Responding quickly (as in "automatic") and as though even a minor signal is very serious (as in "negative") might have allowed our Stone Age ancestors to escape or avoid predators and other dangers. However, this fast and automatic processing also increases the probability of false alarms or, if you will, errors. As a consequence, a patient may develop a pattern of negative automatic thoughts that misrepresent the true picture and hinder recovery. In their worst form, the negative thought may hold a small grain of truth but otherwise be grossly distorted. The two following examples are particularly relevant for pain perception.

Catastrophizing

This is an exaggerated negative orientation toward pain where a relatively neutral event is irrationally made into a catastrophe (Sullivan et al., 1995). In essence the person imagines the worst possible result that could happen, but accepts it as the given result. Catastrophic thoughts are usually stated as assumptions:

- "If the pain does not get better, I will end up in a wheelchair."
- "The pain will get worse and worse."
- "If I move my back I will wear it out."
- "This pain shooting down my leg is a sure sign that I will become paralyzed."

Catastrophizing seems to affect mood negatively and also to be associated with a variety of problems that hinder recovery and make treatment more difficult. For example, it has been shown that catastrophizing mediates distress reactions to painful stimulation (Sullivan et al., 1995; Vlaeyen and Linton, 2002). In addition, several researchers have found that catastrophizing is closely related to pain severity and function (Vlaeyen and Linton, 2002). As an illustration, Burton and associates (1995) assessed patients seeking primary care for their back pain. They then followed these patients for one year to determine the development of functional pain problems. They found that a tendency to catastrophize at the initial assessment was the best predictor of problems one year later! In fact, it was more than six times better at predicting future disability than the best of the clinical measures employed. Similarly, in a study of patients seeking care for dental hygiene treatment, it was found that catastrophizers, as compared to those who do not tend to catastrophize, experienced more pain and distress during the procedure (Sullivan and Neish, 1999).

Consider how catastrophizing thoughts might affect our interpretation of exercise. To test the idea that catastrophizing is related to future behavior, Sullivan and associates (2002) asked healthy volunteers to do exercises known to result in muscle stiffness and soreness. First, catastrophizing was measured and then exercises were performed. Two days later participants were asked to exercise again. Catastrophizers were found to do fewer exercises on the second occasion. Furthermore, catastrophizing was also related to negative mood and increases in pain intensity ratings. The experience of pain associated with normal exercises, then, was substantially influenced by catastrophic thought patterns.

Taken together, the evidence from a considerable body of research shows that catastrophizing is related to emotional distress, increased pain and disability (Sullivan et al., 2001).

Overgeneralization

Another form of cognitive distortion is overgeneralization. Rather than make a neutral evaluation of the situation, the person makes an exaggerated, negative conclusion that is applied to a whole host of situations. Although the basic assumption may have a small grain of truth to it, the assumption is rigidly generalized to many or all situations. In fact, there is no truth to this overgeneralization. Some examples will help clarify what these cognitions might entail:

- "When I get irritated no one can stand me!"
- "Because I have pain, I will never be able to work."
- "If the pain doesn't get better, all of my friends will desert me."

- "I will never be able to manage this pain without painkillers."
- "I shouldn't do any activities that cause my pain to increase."

In each of these examples, there is some truth to the basic statement but the application is dogmatic and far outstrips reason. It is true that when someone gets irritated they are less pleasant to be around. However, this does not mean that *everyone* will react that way, nor does it mean that *every person will avoid me*. Take the last statement as another example ("*I shouldn't do any activities that cause my pain to increase*"). Certainly some activities may increase pain. Likewise, large increases in activities typical of the "weekend warrior" may unnecessarily increase pain intensity. However, drawing the conclusion that one shouldn't do any activity that might cause any increase in pain is clearly exaggerating a point. In fact, some increases in pain are normal and may actually be a sign that the exercise is resulting in positive changes in the muscles.

HOW DOES HANK THINK ABOUT HIS PAIN?

Hank does not really understand why he has pain or exactly how he should deal with it. The fact that the pain has recurred and persists has made him anxious, frustrated and depressed. Moreover, he feels guilt and stress because he is having difficulty working as well as doing his share of the household chores. Hank really wonders what is going on in his back. He cannot accept that he could have this much pain without something being seriously wrong. The way the pain shoots down his leg and the way his back locks makes Hank believe that the disks must be worn out. This provides a picture in his mind's eye of the vertebrae rubbing against one another, sometimes pinching a nerve (and thus the shooting pain) and sometimes locking together. Indeed, the doctor did tell Hank that his back was aging and suffering from wear and tear. Hank expects that a good assessment could get to the bottom of the problem. For example, taking images of the back should show the doctors exactly where and what is wrong. Further, because of the worn-out disks, Hank expects bending and twisting movements to hurt. He also believes that it is best to conserve his movements as each movement brings him one step closer to the day his back will be entirely worn out and he won't be able to use it anymore.

CONTROL AND SELF-EFFICACY

People who believe that they can take command of their pain problem themselves tend to fare better with their pain than those who feel helpless (Walker, 2001).

Nearly every theory of psychology includes the concept of mastery over the environment. It is sometimes referred to in terms of "locus of control", that is, a set of beliefs about the causal relationships between one's own actions, as opposed to those of others, and the likely outcomes. Some people believe they can control their pain problem to a large extent, while others believe that only others, such as doctors, can treat or cure the pain. This may have considerable effects on how the patient actually copes with the problem. Indeed, perceived lack of control is highly associated with the psychological distress that patients with chronic pain suffer (Walker and Sofaer, 1998). Interestingly, it is the feeling of having control, rather than the objective actual control, that appears to be important (Walker, 2001). For example, a cancer patient may believe that he or she has considerable control and this is associated with longer survival. However, it is not certain that the patient in fact has very much control over the disease process at all. Thus, the belief in itself may have an effect on pain and pain-related variables. Obviously, the belief may also be related to how well the patient actually deals with the problem.

The feeling of being able to control the pain is closely linked to the concept of self-efficacy. Here the effects of previous learning are cognitively combined with expectations to form a belief in one's capabilities to organize and execute a course of action to obtain a given result (Walker, 2001). In other words, perceived self-efficacy is the belief that one can successfully perform a specified behavior such as to deal with the pain (Abraham and Sheeran, 1997). Health locus of control involves both the cause of the pain, and also how it might be coped with. Patients are sometimes classified as having an "internal" orientation where the event (pain) or its successful remediation is perceived to be in the control of the person themselves and an "external" orientation where the pain or its remediation is believed to be outside the person's control (Abraham and Sheeran, 1997). Self-efficacy beliefs are indeed related to successful performance: those believing that they can successfully perform a specified behavior actually perform better than those who do not hold such beliefs (Bandura, 1991; Schwartzer and Fuchs, 1996).

Not surprisingly, the belief that one can control one's own pain is critically linked to pain perception (Jensen et al., 1994). For example, in a study of pregnant women, self-efficacy was found to be related to the use of pain medication during childbirth (Manning and Wright, 1983). Similarly, higher self-efficacy scores have been found to be related to increased physical activity for patients with chronic pain (Kores et al., 1990). Certain physical tests for chronic pain patients have been seen as "objective" measures, but Estlander et al. (1994) found that the patient's self-efficacy, i.e. their beliefs in their ability to do physical activities, was the best predictor of actual test performance. Moreover, there is also a relationship between self-efficacy and actual disability for musculoskeletal pain (Mannion et al., 1996; Johansson and Lindberg, 2000). In short, many studies with a variety of patient populations have demonstrated that self-efficacy beliefs at an early stage of the problem are closely related to functional disability and suffering (Shifren et al., 1999; Brekke et al., 2001).

Our beliefs in whether we can influence our pain, then, are related to the coping strategies we select, how emphatically we pursue these strategies, our beliefs and expectations about their effects, and ultimately how we experience the pain.

INFORMATION BIASES

Cognitive processes may also bias the very information that we process in our brains. The processing of incoming information from the world around us is an active process that is not always particularly accurate. Our senses may be deceived by our minds such as when our beliefs, memories and expectations color the interpretation of incoming information. Emotions, as shown above, play a major role in this selective processing of information. Let us look at how this works.

Information about our pain is cognitively assessed and the perception and evaluation of a perceived threat is a primary cognitive function (Pincus and Morely, 2002). As a result, how we handle the incoming information is central to our interpretation of our pain. Cognitive evaluation is a complex process that is said to be guided by automatic cognitive processes (Pincus and Morely, 2002). Basically, if every nerve signal was to be selected and evaluated consciously, we would have little time for anything else. As a result, "schemata" are used as a shortcut for evaluating information. A schema contains a bank of stored information and serves as a template for interpreting incoming information. When incoming information matches a template it receives priority processing and it plays a role in how we interpret and remember it. This is illustrated in depression where people clearly remember more negative events (as compared to healthy controls) and this enhances ruminating and guilt (Pincus and Morely, 2002).

Three forms of cognitive bias influence pain perception. First is *attention bias*. Information about pain that matches a schema is given priority and thus attention is focused on pain-related signals. This has been demonstrated in research employing the emotional

Stroop task. Participants are presented with words printed in various colors like blue, yellow or red. They are then asked to name the color of the print while ignoring the actual word (example: word "needle" printed in blue color, correct response is blue). Words that have special significance are known to create a block and take longer to name. For example, a needle phobic will take longer to name colors when the words are "injection" or "vaccination". Likewise, studies of chronic pain patients show that pain biases attention toward pain-related stimuli (Snider et al., 2000; Keogh et al., 2001).

A second cognitive feature is *interpretation bias*. The cognitive schemata are hypothesized to hold a range of information including previous experiences and beliefs. Consequently, when new information is handled, these play a role in interpretation where a bias concerning pain may exist. Indeed, patients often interpret their situation negatively as seen above in catastrophizing. Here we are concerned with how the processing of signals may be biased. The reasoning suggests that one example of this bias is in how ambiguous information may be interpreted negatively. To examine this, researchers employ the following clever test. Hononyms (words that are pronounced the same but mean different things) are presented and the pain patient is asked to write down the words they hear. Several words are relevant for pain such as flu/flew; groan/grown; pane/pain. Indeed, experiments with chronic pain patients show a clear bias toward writing down the pain-related words (Pincus and Morely, 2001). Thus, based on cognitive processes, even the simply incoming signals may be biased in the meaning we give them.

A third cognitive feature is *memory bias*. What we remember is truly selective and in the pain context there is a propensity for chronic pain patients to remember pain-related information. Memory tests show that chronic pain patients, as compared to healthy controls, remember more pain-related words than neutral ones (Pincus and Morely, 2002). This is shown in recall bias where participants are presented with a list of words where some are neutral (grass, happy) while some are pain-related (hurt, ache). Chronic pain patients tend to remember more pain words than do healthy controls.

OVERDOERS AND UNDERDOERS: THE FEAR-AVOIDANCE MODEL

An enticing model has been developed that underscores the importance of emotional and cognitive factors while integrating them with biological and behavioral aspects. It is usually referred to as the "fear-avoidance model", but has more recently also been named the "pain-related fear and avoidance" model. The impetus for the model was the observation that patients with pain problems have very different approaches to movement and activities than healthy people. Clinicians typically report that some patients with pain overdo activities, while others have difficulty even getting started. As a result they may be called overdoers or underdoers. Until recently it was difficult to explain these behaviors, but this model may be one important step in understanding better how we approach rest and activities when in pain. The model also integrates biological, emotional, cognitive and behavioral aspects.

The central idea in the model is that fear of pain results in avoidance and creates a vicious circle (Asmundson et al., 1999; Vlaeyen and Linton, 2002). The fear is closely associated with cognitive factors like catastrophizing. Once initiated, the circle is self-maintained and thus it may catalyze the problem into a persistent, long-term disability. Figure 6.1 illustrates the model. A biological signal such as a trauma initiates the experience of pain. A "normal" reaction is illustrated on the right-hand side. Here, the pain is perceived as a warning signal and appropriate levels of fear are evoked. Soon the person begins moving the painful body part to see how much movement can be attained without severe pain. The person confronts the pain, if you will, to establish boundaries for movement. By doing this repeatedly, mobility and strength are regained and the person recovers from the injury. This is the usual course.

Sometimes, however, a different path is followed as illustrated on the left side of Fig. 6.1. In this instance the pain is perceived as a threat and this results in catastrophizing thoughts, for example that the pain must depend on a severed nerve or that one will end up handicapped. The catastrophizing is closely associated with pain-related fear. This fear influences cognitions and behavior. For example, attention is turned toward the body and any signs that the feared outcome may actually be happening. This vigilance in itself may increase the pain. Moreover, it activates the body's defense system including muscle tension which may also increase pain levels.

The fear sets the stage for the avoidance of certain specific movements. The avoided movements or activities are those included in the feared catastrophic outcome. So, if the person is afraid that a nerve is being pinched and might be cut off, then twisting and bending movements believed to pinch the nerve would be avoided. Because the avoidance occurs in anticipation of pain rather than as a response to pain, these behaviors have a tremendous capacity to persist as there is no opportunity to correct the (wrong) expectations and beliefs from learning experiences. In other words, if one never attempts to do a given movement, such as lifting or bending, it is impossible to learn that it is not dangerous.

The avoidance in turn results in a reduction in activity level. In the long run the person may reduce their activity level considerably, including work, leisure and social activities. This is also connected to emotional states and a depressed mood may develop. Of course, this emotional distress also affects pain perception and results in less tolerance and greater intensity. Consequently, as the vicious circle develops it becomes more and more self-maintained and difficult to stop.

The model illustrates nicely how biological pain signals, emotions, cognitions and behaviors interact. Indeed, this model highlights the role of attention in the form of vigilance, emotions like fear, and cognitions like beliefs and catastrophizing in pain perception. It links these to how we behave and the consequences this behavior may have on pain perceptions as well as future cognitions and emotions.

Fear avoidance and disability

Considerable research has examined the model to test its applicability (Vlaeyen and Linton, 2002; Asmundson et al., in press). An essential basic finding is that fear-avoidance beliefs are definitely related to disability (Crombez et al., 1999; Vlaeyen and Linton, 2000). Typically, chronic pain patients holding high levels of fear-avoidance beliefs are significantly more disabled by their pain than those who have relatively low levels of these beliefs. For example, we investigated the consequences of back pain for nursing personnel by comparing those who continued to work and those who took some time off work because of the pain (Linton and Buer, 1995). These participants were matched for pain intensity, pain duration and workload. The results showed that those who were off work had higher levels of fear-avoidance beliefs and behaviors.

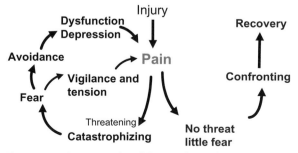

Figure 6.1 The pain-related fear and avoidance model. This model highlights the role of cognitions, emotions and behavior in the development of pain and dysfunction. (Based on Vlaeyen and Linton, 2000.)

For example, they believed that the pain was directly related to activity levels, that they had little control over the pain, and they tended to focus more on their pain.

Early on it was established that fear-avoidance beliefs about physical activities and work are strongly related to disability one year later (Waddell et al., 1993). A surprise in this study, however, was that fear-avoidance beliefs were actually the best predictor of disability outcome and were a more powerful predictor of outcome than either biomedical or other pain variables. This led the authors to conclude that "the fear of pain and what we do about it is more disabling than the pain itself" (Waddell et al., 1993). Another salient illustration of this is presented in a study by Mannion and colleagues (2001). In a multivariate analysis, they demonstrated that while pain accounted for about 20% of the variance in disability, psychological factors (distress, fear avoidance, coping) accounted for 36%. Thus in this case, the fear of pain might be said to be more disabling than the pain itself. In turn, this would suggest that fear avoidance would be a unique risk factor. In fact, several researchers have found similar relationships and therefore suggest that pain-related fear is more strongly related to functional problems than the pain itself (Vlaeyen et al., 1995b; Waddell, 1998; Crombez et al., 1999), refuting the earlier notion that disability is simply caused by the pain (Vlaeyen and Linton, 2002).

Some research indicates that anxious patients or patients holding fear-avoidance beliefs tend to overpredict pain levels associated with doing an activity. For example, in one study patients were asked to predict how painful it would be to perform four specified exercises and they subsequently performed the exercises (Crombez et al., 1996). Patients with high levels of fear-avoidance beliefs overpredicted the actual pain experienced when doing the exercises. This coincides with other studies that show that anxious participants more often overpredict pain than nonanxious ones (Arntz et al., 1990, 1994).

Vigilance

Fear and catastrophizing are also related to attention. As described earlier, pain demands attention. In this case, the emotional and cognitive factors also prime attention so that one is vigilant to any threat in the feared, catastrophic scenarios. Indeed, a few studies indicate that patients with high levels of fear-avoidance beliefs or who avoid back-straining activities are also highly attentive to back sensations (Crombez et al., 1998b; Vlaeyen and Linton, 2002). This attentional vigilance is done at the expense of other tasks such as employing coping strategies. Thus, this vigilance increases the probability of "discovering" a painful stimulus and it also decreases the probability of employing other coping strategies.

Performance

One of the main features of the model is that pain-related fear generates avoidance behavior that will result in reduced activity levels. In fact, several investigations have found such a relationship. For example, a significant correlation was found in a study where fear of pain was measured and participants then performed a range of motion test (McCracken et al., 1992). Take careful note of this next study as well (Vlaeyen et al., 1995a). Chronic back pain patients were asked to lift a 5.5 kg weight and hold it until pain or discomfort became too great. Levels of fear-avoidance beliefs were closely associated with how long patients actually held the weight! In fact, fear-avoidance beliefs and anticipation of pain were found to be the strongest predictors of performance on standardized strength tests (Al-Obaidi et al., 2000). Fear-avoidance beliefs, then, are associated with actual performance. Thus, it is not surprising that these in turn influence everyday activities and may lead to substantial disability.

Fear avoidance in the development of persistent pain

Some authors have suggested that fear avoidance may be one mechanism by which a bout of back pain may develop into a persistent problem. Certainly, evidence from cross-sectional studies shows that one of the most powerful predictors of self-reported disability levels is in fact pain-related fear (Vlaeyen and Linton, 2002). Although there is good evidence that fear avoidance is associated with disability in patients with chronic pain (Linton, 2000b; Vlaeyen and Linton, 2002), certain criteria must be met if fear avoidance is to be employed as a predictor (Linton and Boersma, in press). First, the fear avoidance must precede the chronicity, i.e. we must be able to measure the fear avoidance in the acute/subacute stage of the pain problem. Second, the fear avoidance must be related to the development of the pain and disability problem, that is, it should predict who will actually develop a problem.

Some information does suggest that fear-avoidance beliefs may be present early on and long before a chronic disability problem has been noted. In a study of 917 people in the general population, our research group found evidence to support the idea that some people do harbor fear-avoidance beliefs and catastrophizing (Buer and Linton, 2002). Participants completed questions taken from the Fear-Avoidance Beliefs Questionnaire and the Pain Catastrophizing

Scale that were slightly reworded so that people in the general population could answer them. Although the levels on average were much lower than in a clinical population, a normal distribution was found. The results showed that fear-avoidance beliefs as well as catastrophizing occurred in this general population of nonpatients. While the levels were deemed to be "moderate", some participants nevertheless had the maximum points possible! Significantly, a relationship was reported between fear-avoidance beliefs and current activity levels as well as between catastrophizing and current pain. Similarly, in a cross-sectional study comparing samples of patients with acute and chronic pain, it was found that fear avoidance was present in both samples (Ciccone and Just, 2001). Moreover, fear avoidance was strongly related to disability, explaining about 40% of it.

Several other studies have also shown that fear-avoidance beliefs precede the disability and therefore might be a prominent mechanism in the development of a pain disability (Linton and Bradley, 1992; Klenerman et al., 1995; Linton et al., 2000; Sieben et al., 2002). In summary, there are many studies that demonstrate a relationship between various fear-avoidance beliefs and the development of disability.

Do fear-avoidance beliefs predict disability?

The next question is whether fear-avoidance beliefs or behaviors actually predict future pain and disability problems. To investigate this, we selected 415 people from the general population who reported no spinal pain during the previous year and we asked them to complete a questionnaire assessing fear-avoidance beliefs and pain catastrophizing (Linton et al., 2000). Subsequently, we followed these people for one year to determine who suffered an episode of back pain during this follow-up. We discovered that people with high scores on the fear-avoidance scale had twice the risk of suffering an episode of back pain and a 1.7 times higher risk of lowered physical function at the one-year follow-up. What is more, catastrophizing was also related, increasing the risk for pain or function by 1.5 times. Thus, we were able to show that fear avoidance was related to the future inception of back pain and associated functional problems and we concluded that fear-avoidance beliefs might thereby also be useful in the assessment of patients with musculoskeletal pain.

Fear avoidance has been found to predict future disability in a number of clinical studies as well. A particularly relevant study examined 300 primary care patients who were seeking help for acute low back pain (Klenerman et al., 1995). Patients were examined and psychological and physiological data were collected.

The participants were then followed for one year to determine functional problems. The fear-avoidance variables were found to be the best predictor of outcome, clearly underscoring that the fear avoidance was a precursor rather than a consequence of the disability.

A study from the United States provides additional evidence indicating that fear avoidance early on is a significant predictor of the development of pain and disability (Fritz et al., 2001). To examine the predictive value of fear-avoidance beliefs, 78 subjects with work-related low back pain were followed over the course of 4 weeks. The participants were evaluated an average of 5.5 days after injury and they completed a battery of tests including fear-avoidance beliefs. Disability was measured with a questionnaire as well as by the ability to unrestricted return to work. The results showed that fear-avoidance beliefs were significant predictors of future disability problems even when initial levels of pain intensity, impairment and disability were controlled.

An intriguing study has examined how pain-related fear develops during a new episode of acute back pain (Sieben et al., 2002). In this study, 44 patients seeking care for acute back pain completed diaries on a daily basis during a two-week period. These patients were followed over the course of one year to determine outcome. The results are fascinating. First, pain-related fear was found to develop in three distinct patterns. During the two-week period, 39% of the patients had a descending level, 35% a stable level and 30% had an increasing level of pain-related fear. Importantly, the group with an increasing level during the first two-week period demonstrated significantly more disability and pain at the follow-up. Consequently, the authors conclude that those with an increasing pain-related fear pattern were at risk for developing disability problems.

We investigated the role of fear in the development of pain problems in a group of patients seeking acute care for fractures (Buer et al., submitted). Within 24 hours of the wrist or ankle fracture, participants completed a battery of questionnaires that included fear-avoidance beliefs and catastrophizing. Patients were then followed at 3 and 9 months post fracture to ascertain how well they had recovered in terms of sick absences, strength, range of motion, pain intensity and self-rated degree of recovery. As with the Sieben et al. study above, the results demonstrated different patterns in the development of fear avoidance. We compared scores at intake with those at the 3-month follow up. Those with high scores on fear avoidance (low to high or high to high) were then compared to those with "low" scores (high to low or low to low) to see if this had an effect on the 9-month outcome.

We found that those high on fear avoidance were 3.5 times more likely to suffer pain problems at the follow-up.

It is logical that high or increasing levels of "fear avoidance" beliefs and behaviour are related to future problems. In our study of fractures some patients expected that the pain would go away shortly after the cast was in place. Moreover, they believed that once the cast was removed, they would enjoy full function again. However, for typical adult patients with such fractures, full function may not be achieved until several weeks or months of practice to regain mobility and strength. Thus, increases in fear avoidance seemed to be related to unmet and in particular to unrealistic expectations that triggered more catastrophizing and fear. Certainly, many of these patients wondered what was wrong with their wrist/ankle because movements (still) caused pain and mobility was not 100% restored!

Taken together, these studies show that fear avoidance seems to be related to the actual development of persistent pain and disability. Thus, it represents an important contribution to our understanding of pain and the process of chronification. It also may provide an important key for the early detection of problems and ultimately the prevention of persistent pain.

Overdoers

Although chronic pain is often associated with disability where the sufferer has low levels of activity, some patients with pain conditions may overdo it. A central concept is that overdoers have a long history of being overactive and striving for a perfectionistic optimal productivity (Arntz and Peters, 1995; van Houdenhove et al., 2001). While research on "underdoers" has increased during the past decade, there is still relatively little information on "overdoers", probably because they do not tax the healthcare system in the same way. The salient conception for these patients is the expectation of being immediately able to return to work or maintain high levels of activity even though a recent injury has occurred. For example, the patient may continue to practice sports at a professional level, because of unrealistic expectations, even though he or she is 50 years old and has suffered an injury that normally takes weeks to heal. Rather than starting at a low level of activity and working to regain strength and mobility, overdoers attempt to maintain or even increase previous achievements. This problem may in turn be related to stress where the person may well be a high achiever. In fact, patients who do little at the present may have been overdoers earlier on. Thus, the patient may exacerbate the problem by overdoing activities that disrupt healing.

Although there is little research concerning overdoers, there is ample evidence suggesting that the decisions we make about participation in activities are interesting. These decisions are highly influenced by psychological processes and not just the pain. Whether we participate in an activity as well as how long we participate is associated with expectations and cognitive processes such as the so-called stop rules described below. We seldom stop an activity because we physically have to. Think about the following experimental example. Chronic pain patients were asked to perform exercises such as riding a bike to tolerance and the duration of time was recorded. If patients biked until their pain became intolerable, we would expect them to stop at random times. However, the results showed that patients biked until they reached even time units such as five or ten minutes! (Fordyce, 1976).

An interesting question is how overdoers control their pain while active. It appears that these people lose contact with the feedback loop and ignore or disassociate the pain from the activity. Indeed, athletes are well aware of this and train mentally to withstand the body signals of tiredness and pain to maximize performance. By focusing attention on performance rather than pain, the sensation may be reduced. Further, by cognitively interpreting the pain signals as a sign of performance improvement, the pain may also be ignored.

Stop rules

Why do we decide to continue an activity or discontinue it? The reason for discontinuing an activity is related to cognitive "stop rules" (Vlaeyen and Morley, 2004). In other words, we all have certain rules we set for ourselves concerning how much we can do with no ill effects. Some, for example, may attempt to do "as many as can" while others may adopt a more "feel like quitting" approach. Think about these approaches when doing a particular task such as stuffing envelopes or running. When do we decide to take a break? After a particular amount of time or when we feel pain? Or perhaps after an achievement, e.g. finishing the race or the job. These are incorporated in a process highly influenced by our emotional and cognitive state. In fact, one model that may be quite relevant is the Mood-as-Input paradigm (Martin et al., 1993). It maintains that task persistence as opposed to avoidance or escape is related to the interaction between mood and the stop rule employed.

In addition to mood, one particular factor that may influence stop rules is exposure to high levels of stress. Indeed, some scientists believe that high stress levels and the related frantic pattern of activities might lead to overdoing it and exhaustion which in turn may develop into a chronic pain problem (Teasell and Bombardier, 2000). The typical patient would have a long history of working under stressful conditions as well as managing a home and family. When injured, this patient would have difficulty in adjusting activity levels and simply continuing regular (high) levels of

---

HANK AND "FEAR AVOIDANCE"

Hank has always been an active person and he has thought of himself as tolerating more pain than most. However, Hank discovered that certain movements were just about impossible to perform when his back was acting up. Hank believed that the disks were worn out and that this pinched nerves and caused the vertebrae to "lock" together. Further, he understood that the more he used his back the faster he would wear it out completely. Consequently, Hank avoided extreme bending and twisting movements such as picking something heavy up from the floor. This seemed to ease the pain as well and it also seemed to reduce the number of times he got the terrible "shooting" pains. With time, however, Hank noticed that it took less to trigger a problem and therefore he began avoiding any bending or twisting and furthermore he avoided lifting and carrying things as well. This soon developed so that he needed to avoid any sudden movements or activities that involved heavier work or energy. By avoiding these activities, Hank believed he was coping with his pain. In actual fact, Hank saw a direct link between his activities and the pain. Since the pain, especially the bad bouts he sometimes had as well as the shooting pain, was so negative, he was really keen to avoid it. His strategy was to reduce the pain as much as possible. Nevertheless, his pain had not gotten better. Despite the extended avoidance, he was not better. If the truth be known, he was actually suffering more pain now than previously. In addition, he was finding it difficult to participate in activities that he could easily perform before he had a pain problem. This depressed Hank. Although he believed his strategy would be helpful, he was beginning to realize that something had gone wrong.

---

work and activity. This might then hinder healing and lead to fatigue and more difficulties. This description, however, comes surprisingly close to that of burnout.

SUMMARY

This chapter has highlighted the role of cognitions in pain perception. Cognitions are integrated into an astounding system where biological, emotional, cognitive and behavioral aspects work together so that we can effectively cope with nociception. Pain signals are processed in the nervous system, and this process is highly influenced by the emotional and cognitive state of the individual. In addition, pain also affects us emotionally and cognitively, so the relationship is bidirectional. Anxiety and mood are two emotions strongly related to pain perception. Increases in anxiety or negative mood generally result in less pain tolerance. Our pattern of thinking also influences how we interpret the pain signal. For example, beliefs that pain automatically means harm may negatively influence our interpretation and enhance anxiety. Further, cognitive thought patterns like catastrophizing also influence interpretation. In this case, catastrophizing enhances a negative interpretation where the consequences of the pain are seen as being dire although the true danger is minimal. Here again emotions and cognitions interact. A model that incorporates the interaction between various factors is the fear-avoidance model. The model describes "normal" processing of nociceptive stimuli, but also the development of fear. Fear is associated with catastrophizing and vigilance that in themselves may enhance the pain. Moreover, the fear leads to avoidance of movements that may also result in activity reductions that in turn negatively influence mood which lowers pain tolerance. An integrative model stresses the role of biological, emotional, cognitive and behavioral factors working together and influencing each other interactively.

Learning to cope: behavior in pain and health

I have a lot of pain sometimes, but I have learned how to manage it. I can cope with it.

—Cancer patient

LEARNING OBJECTIVES

To understand:

- pain may be viewed as behaviors such as taking medicine, resting or seeking care;

- pain behaviors are influenced by emotions and cognitions, but above all by their environmental consequences;

- most pain behaviors are learned;

- learning involves the immediate results of a behavior such as a positive reinforcement (increases behavior) or punishment (decreases behavior);

- learning paradigms illustrate how various problems may develop;

- learning is important because learned pain behaviors may be altered and treatment may key on this to help the patient cope better with the pain.

Most of the things we do when we are in pain are learned behaviors. Taking a pain pill, resting or seeking medical care are all examples of learned behaviors. It is true that some behaviors are reflexive like pulling your hand away from a hot stove. Yet in modern society most of the behaviors we engage in when we are in pain are influenced directly by learning. In this chapter we will examine the concept of pain behavior and how learning affects these pain behaviors. As part of the highly integrated pain system, emotional and cognitive states as well as the biological state work together to help us quickly learn how to deal with pain. While emotional and cognitive processes set the stage for certain behaviors, the environment, through the consequences the behavior produces, steers whether the behavior will continue. Accordingly, coping is learned behavior. This has enormous implications for understanding pain patients. And it has enormous implications for treatment. If pain behaviors are learned, then they might also be altered. Indeed, learning techniques are an indispensable tool in the treatment and prevention of pain problems.

PAIN BEHAVIOR

The things we do when we experience pain may be viewed as a set of pain behaviors (Fordyce, 1976; Keefe and Williams, 1992). Earlier we dealt with the fact that pain is more than biology, but one may rightly wonder how it can be considered to be a learned behavior. The answer is that it is not any single behavior. Consider, though, that pain is expressed as behavior: we complain that it hurts, limp, and hold the "hurt" body part. This pain behavior has a clear link to emotions (we might be afraid or irritated) and cognitions (we may expect it to go away, or believe it is caused by a virus). As we will see below, it is also influenced by the results it produces.

Pain is observable when it is expressed behaviorally. Pain behavior, then, is any act or behavior we engage in to control our pain, or that communicates our pain to others. Think about how we normally know if someone is not feeling well. Usually we do not see the disease, but instead we recognize that the person is sick by the way that she or he is acting. We may also get information from what the person tells us. So, we know if someone is ill by what they do, how they do it, and what they say. Indeed, if you came upon a person suffering acute illness, the first thing you might notice is that they are slumped over, breathing heavily, acting "strange" and the like. In other words, the discriminating factors that would tell you that they are ill is their behavior rather than the disease itself. All of these behaviors may be considered to be *pain* or *illness behaviors*.

A pioneer in the field, Wilbur Fordyce, was instrumental in defining pain as behavior (Fordyce, 1976). He worked in a rehabilitation clinic with pain patients who had suffered for many years and were highly disabled by the pain. For these patients, no additional medical treatments were available; medical treatments had been exhausted and everything had been tried. He reasoned that further medical investigations and treatments were bound to fail because the problem was how these patients were dealing with their pain. He argued that a central problem for these patients was their behavior, that is, the way they dealt with the pain problem. In fact, the overt expression of pain through behavior appears to be the most salient and relevant aspect of a patient's presentation (Sanders, 2002).

Fordyce (1976) delineated some typical behaviors that characterize patients with persistent pain problems. Today, these have been observed in clinics around the world. As an example, consider these four common categories of pain behaviors:

- A general reduction of normal activities.
- An increased consumption of medications and devices to control pain.
- Nonverbal motor behaviors that communicate pain such as limping, grimacing or rubbing the painful site.
- Verbal complaints including moaning, sighing and reports of pain intensity.

Accordingly, pain is not any *one* behavior, but a set of behaviors that communicates our pain to others.

However, pain behavior is a central link in our pain perception and attempts at coping. Normally, pain behaviors allow us to learn how to deal with the situation in the best possible way. Remember that most people, most of the time, deal very effectively with their pain. Nevertheless, occasionally learning processes may lead to behaviors that are successful in the short term, but that lead to long-term problems.

CAN PAIN BEHAVIORS BE LEARNED?

Most of us consider pain behaviors to be the result of an internal painful cue. A jab in back pain, for example, might result in a grimace, an "ouch!" and a change of position. Clearly, the perception of pain including the emotional and cognitive processes in Chapters 5 and 6 may initiate a behavior. Whether the behavior continues, is altered or stopped, however, depends on how well it works, i.e. its consequences. Consider the following experiment that we conducted to test the idea that pain behaviors can be influenced externally (Linton and Götestam, 1985a).

Participants were healthy volunteers who knew they were going to be in a "pain experiment" (Linton and Götestam, 1985a). They sat in a chair with a blood pressure cuff around their upper arm. The experimenter stood behind the participant and could manipulate the pressure in the cuff. Participants were told there would be a series of trials and they were asked to rate their pain intensity after each trial. On the first trial the relationship between pain intensity and pressure was determined by increasing the pressure until the pain reached a standardized level of (medium) pain. Thereafter, the participants were told that the pressure level might be the same as, more than or less than the first trial. During the next few trials, however, the pressure level was exactly the same in order to obtain a baseline and control for habituation effects. Then the experiment began, as may be seen in Fig. 7.1 where it is marked by a line in the graph. As Fig. 7.1 shows, the pressure level was then in actuality systematically decreased. Participants rated their pain

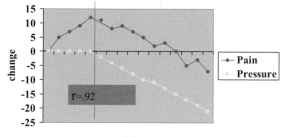

Figure 7.1 The results from a pain experiment where neutral feedback was provided after each trial. Note that as the stimulus intensity (pressure) decreases, so do the pain intensity ratings. (Based on data from Linton and Götestam, 1985a.)

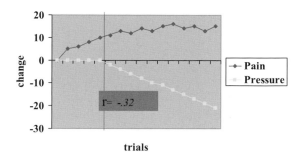

Figure 7.2 The effects of contingent feedback on pain reports. After each pain rating, feedback was provided (positive for increases in pain ratings). Note that the pain ratings increase despite the fact that the stimulus intensity is systematically decreased! (Based on data from Linton and Götestam, 1985a.)

on each trial and the experimenter merely thanked them for each rating. The results were as expected: when the pressure decreased, so did the pain intensity ratings (Fig. 7.1) and the correlation was quite high ($r = 0.92$). Interestingly, the baseline indicated an increase in ratings that is probably due to habituation and the expectations surrounding a "pain experiment".

In the next part of the experiment we attempted to increase pain ratings despite decreases in pressure by manipulating feedback, i.e. the consequences (Linton and Götestam, 1985a). Hence we conducted this part of the experiment in a slightly different way to study the effects of learning on pain reports. The experiment began in the same way as above. However, when the trials began with a systematic decrease in pressure, *different feedback was provided*. In the first case described above, intensity reports were greeted with a neutral "thank you". Now, however, an attempt was made to reinforce increases in pain ratings. As a result, when a rating was higher than the baseline the experimenter said "good", but if it decreased or was the same the reply was "hmm, that's strange". The dramatic results are shown in Fig. 7.2. Although the physical stimulus (pressure) decreased in a similar manner as in the first experiment, the pain ratings actually increased. The correlation between the pressure stimulus and the intensity ratings virtually disappeared ($r = -0.32$). Therefore, the feedback provided influenced the pain ratings and we observed increases in pain ratings despite a clear decrease in the painful pressure level. This is one clear example of how environmental consequences influence pain behaviors.

Learning has powerful survival value because it allows us to adjust our behaviors to meet the demands the environment places upon us. It helps us to maximize results. This is a miraculous opportunity to deal effectively with our pain. Accordingly, a set of behaviors may evolve in order to deal with a particular pain problem. Over time this develops into a set of coping strategies (Lazarus and Folkman, 1984). These are ways of dealing with the pain and involve an interaction between cognitive-emotional evaluation of the problem and behavioral methods for dealing with it.

Coping strategies develop where emotions are linked to cognitions that in turn set the stage for certain behaviors. In a sense this provides for a rapid method of dealing with a stressful stimulus. It is not surprising, then, that typical coping strategies for pain involve an integration of emotional, cognitive and behavioral aspects. Consider the strategy of "positive self-statements" (Rosenstiel and Keefe, 1983). The actual behavior being performed is the self-statement, but it entails cognitions (evaluation of what is positive) as well as emotional aspects (positive emotion, e.g. feeling good about an accomplishment). Learning is important, then, for developing and fine-tuning coping strategies.

LEARNING: CONSEQUENCES STEER BEHAVIOR

Let us investigate how learning works. To do this we need to consider the basic elements of how learning occurs (Rachlin, 1976). These paradigms are very useful for analyzing various pain behaviors as well as their links to emotions and cognitions.

The learning paradigm

The basic learning paradigm involves the behavior, the situation in which it occurs as well as the consequences of the behavior. These three aspects are always considered in an analysis of the effects of learning. In fact, the situation, behavior and consequences are central elements in the assessment of pain clinically.

We need to know what the patient does, in which situations, and how this works.

Stimulus

The situation in which a behavior occurs is an important aspect because it serves as a *stimulus*. With repeated learning trials this stimulus situation will signal (set the stage for) a behavior. In other words, it provides a valuable shortcut for the behavior. This makes it possible for us to react quickly, and with relatively little consideration. We learn quickly to discriminate such stimulus signals. For example, children learn very quickly to discriminate between the lunch bell and the fire alarm. When the lunch bell rings, certain behaviors quickly appear (ask what is for lunch, wash hands, line up, etc.) and there is no need to consider what the bell means. Hence, the *stimulus* is a guide for appropriate behavior; it sets the stage for this behavior.

To illustrate this, reflect on the behavior of people with pain in various situations. I have been impressed with the changes in pain behavior one may observe in clinical situations. In the waiting room where the secretary or nurse may engage in small talk or humor, the patient may laugh or talk normally about neutral topics. If we did not know the patient had a pain problem, we might not even notice any pain behavior. However, when the patient comes into the clinical examination or treatment room, more pain behavior may occur. The patient may spontaneously begin to tell me about the pain, and pain behaviors such as a slight limp or grimace may be observed. If a doctor appears and asks how the patient is, this may result in even more pain behavior. However, when the patient leaves, he or she may meet a friend for a snack at the coffee shop and the pain behavior may again decrease considerably. The pain behavior, like any other behavior, is under the "control" of the situation. The situation is a stimulus to tell us what behaviors may be appropriate. This is an advantage as it helps us to steer our behaviors to produce optimal results such as complaining about our pain to the doctor and not as much to a friend.

In fact, studies indicate that people do display more pain behaviors in certain situations than others. In one interesting study, for example (Cinciripini, 1984), pain patients were first interviewed by a "student" dressed in plain clothes. Subsequently a doctor, in white, took over the interview. Unbeknown to the patient, the number of overt pain behaviors such as verbal complaints and nonverbal movements (grimaces, holding body part, etc.) were recorded during both interviews. Dramatic differences were observed where the patient exhibited, as expected, many more pain behaviors in the presence of the doctor.

Behavior

Any behavior may be employed in the paradigm, but in our context pain behaviors and coping behaviors are particularly relevant. It is important to define and isolate the behavioral response because this will clarify the learning paradigm. Moreover, behaviors will be a major focus in most intervention programs. This will also be of assistance in associating the behavior with emotions and cognitions. In fact, discussing behaviors is very useful in starting an assessment because patients are attuned to this. It is much more difficult for some patients to reflect on their emotional states or cognitions, but they are normally aware of most of their behavioral patterns.

In the assessment of pain problems a variety of other behaviors may be important. One example is everyday activities. These make up function. Activities of daily living may be greatly affected by the pain and thus included in the assessment.

Consequences

While the stimulus might be viewed as the antecedent to the behavior, the consequence is what happens afterwards. This consequence is vital for determining whether the behavior will increase in probability. For instance, if we work extra on producing a report and this results in special praise that is experienced very positively, then this will affect the likelihood of working extra hard on a paper in the future.

LEARNING PARADIGMS

The systematic application or removal of a consequence is referred to as *reinforcement*. *Positive reinforcement* is a consequence where things a person enjoys or derives pleasure from are delivered. When positive reinforcement is strictly provided after a defined behavior, that behavior increases in frequency. *Punishment,* on the other hand, involves things a person wants to escape from such as pain, worries or a stressful situation. When delivered strictly after a defined behavior, punishment quickly decreases the frequency of the behavior. Normally, punishment has a rapid effect, but it also results in negative emotions. Being punished for a "wrong" behavior reduces the frequency of the behavior, but may also result in negative affect such as hate or revenge. A special learning paradigm is the avoidance paradigm where we relatively quickly can learn to avoid a punisher.

Figure 7.3 shows how learning affects pain behaviors in various paradigms where reinforcement is contingently applied. Positive reinforcement increases pain behaviors as shown in the figure. Here, a group of friends has gathered for dinner. One person has back pain and complains clearly about it: "Oh, I have been

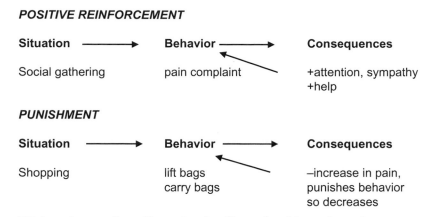

Figure 7.3 Learning paradigms illustrating the effects of positive and negative consequences.

having so much back pain, it's terrible. And it is really hurting right now." This type of pain behavior is typically responded to with attention and sympathy. We may ask about the condition (How did you hurt your back? Have you been to the doctor?) and we often offer to provide assistance (Here let me move the chairs to the table. I can give you a hand with the garden, if you need it. I know a good physical therapist I could put you in contact with). This attention and sympathy is experienced as positive and therefore the behavior is reinforced. This means that it will increase in frequency. Thus, the person is more likely to respond with such pain behavior. The situation or stimulus greatly influences when and where the pain behavior will occur. Thus, *in the same or similar situations, the person will be likely to respond in a similar way.*

Complaining about pain serves an important function and there is nothing innately wrong with this. First, it lets other people know how we are feeling so that they can adjust their behavior to the circumstances. Second, it elicits help that may be necessary if the individual is to survive or get better. Third, it may provide for social support that focuses attention on something other than the pain.

However, in certain situations, complaining about pain develops into a problem in itself. The person may become a bore since every discussion seems to end in pain complaints. Moreover, the pain complaints in themselves may focus attention on the body site and enhance vigilance. Finally, the complaints may trigger automatic negative cognitions and emotions that are a hindrance to initiating more appropriate coping behaviors.

Think about how much positive reinforcement is normally provided in the healthcare system for a variety of pain behaviors. In fact, I suggest that the type and amount of treatment provided for acute pain is directly linked to the amount of pain behaviors the patient displays. A person with few complaints about pain is, for example, unlikely to receive a prescription for a painkiller. Likewise, the person with many verbal and facial pain behaviors is likely to receive more attention, assessment and treatment. Accordingly, positive reinforcement is one mechanism that shapes verbal and nonverbal pain behaviors.

Pain is a particularly effective punisher. Remember from Chapter 2 that the word "pain" is derived from punishment in some languages. Figure 7.3 shows how a negative consequence steers behavior. For instance, a person with back pain may attempt to sit down in the chair at his or her desk. However, the behavior of shifting weight to the chair to sit down results in an excruciating stab of back pain. Because of the negative outcome, we learn that this is not a viable behavior and its frequency usually drops dramatically. We do not sit down in the chair for some time. Again, the stimulus situation steers our behavior so that the behavior does not tend to occur in similar situations in the future.

Avoidance learning

The negative consequences of punishment result in two things. First, we try to escape the situation. Continuing with the example above, we try to get up from the chair as quickly as possible to escape the pain. Second, as shown above, the behavior decreases in frequency. This is because we begin to avoid the situation! Avoidance is a powerful learning paradigm that clearly includes an integration between behavior, emotions, cognitions and biology. Have a look at the example in Fig. 7.4. Based on previous experience with punishment, certain behaviors are perceived as a threat. In this case the threat for the back pain patient is to ride a bike when the person believes he cannot

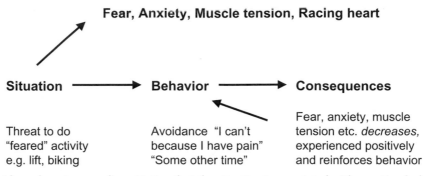

Figure 7.4 An avoidance learning paradigm. Notice that the situation is associated with negative feelings, physiological reactions and thoughts that are reduced when the situation is avoided. This increases the likelihood of the behavior in the future.

do this. This situation is linked to biological, emotional and cognitive responses in the form of fear, anxiety, muscle tension and the like. These are experienced quite negatively. The behavior, then, is to avoid the threatened activity. In this case, the person provides verbal excuses like "I can't because I have too much back pain". The consequence is that when the person successfully avoids the threat, the fear, anxiety, muscle tension and heart rate dissipate. This is experienced as wonderful relief, and thus the behavior is reinforced. This means that in a similar threat situation in the future, the likelihood is increased that this avoidance response will be repeated.

Because pain is a powerful motivator, learning paradigms are particularly important in steering pain behavior. For most people this works exquisitely well. However, in some cases it may result in an undesirable increase in pain behaviors that create more problems than they solve. The intensive, repeated seeking of healthcare, for example, may be related to the reinforcement of this behavior in the early stages of a problem. Further, the attention that complaints about pain produce may sometimes increase the behavior so that it becomes problematic. This may also happen when a person begins to avoid certain activities. The movement may be punished by immediate increases in pain. This in turn may lead to avoidance of the movement, enhanced vigilance, and negative thoughts and emotions. However, if the avoidance is successful, it results in a reduction of these negative aspects which reinforces the avoidance.

SHORT-TERM VERSUS LONG-TERM PERSPECTIVE

To understand the influence of learning on pain behavior, we need to view the learning in a time perspective. Learning is a *normal* process that occurs over

time and has cumulative effects over time. Once we learn a behavior that is successful, we tend to continue it until the results clearly dictate a change. If we view the effects of learning on a short-term basis, the behaviors reinforced are, by definition, helpful. Again, this is the way we adjust our behavior to the demands the environment places on us. Avoiding a movement that causes pain, for instance, is therefore normal and a good coping strategy. We learn to cope and this is a normal learning process.

However, the long-term consequences of a given behavior for the patient can sometimes be quite negative. For example, although complaining about pain may result in direct offers of help and the like, the consequences of complaining frequently and avoiding several movements can lead to the disuse syndrome and a difficult chronic problem. How can this happen? The answer is that *immediate* consequences have much more impact on our behavior than do long-term ones. As a result, small immediate pain reductions are more powerful in steering our behavior than larger long-term consequences. A second explanation is that avoidance behavior, by its nature, is extremely resistant to change and may persist indefinitely (Sanders, 2002).

A third explanation is that if the consequences are gradually reduced in frequency, the behavior tends to become very stable and difficult to change. At first glance this seems to be contradictory. However, in reality a behavior may not be followed by the exact same immediate result every time it occurs. Putting money in a slot machine is one example of this phenomenon. In the beginning it is important to be reinforced by winning. Once this gambling behavior is established, however, it may persist even though the behavior is seldom reinforced and even though the person loses more money than they win! This fact of learning puts certain inertia in our behaviors; they tend to continue until we "learn" another response or the result of the behavior clearly changes.

BOUNDARIES ON LEARNING

Learning exerts great influence on us and yet boundaries to our learning are set by biological, cultural and social factors. We might assume that humans can learn virtually anything. This would be wrong. Through evolutionary processes we have come to be able to learn certain things very easily while other things are much more difficult. Moreover, the social environment has developed to provide limits as well.

Biological limits on our capacity to learn involve genetic programming. Behaviors that are extremely essential for our survival are therefore often "easier" to learn. One example of this is that food aversions are learned in one trial (Rachlin, 1976). If you eat something that makes you very ill, that food will become quite aversive. Most people feel nauseated just seeing or smelling the food. This has obvious survival value in helping us to avoid eating poisonous foods. Likewise, we easily develop an aversion to potentially harmful things like snakes or spiders (Rachman, 1998). There is also some evidence that reducing activities (resting or taking it easy) is easily learned as a reaction to pain. On the other hand, some things are extraordinarily difficult to learn and these often feel unnatural. Although it may be achieved, learning to walk sideways is difficult and most people would revert to usual walking as soon as possible.

The social environment also places restrictions on our learning by setting a framework for what is acceptable. Social pressure is exerted to create mores, customs and traditions for suitable behavior and even ways of thinking. This also affects pain. Consider the pain experienced in childbirth. In the so-called developed countries, childbirth normally results in the experience of pain. For example, in one study 91% of women giving birth reported high levels of pain including 41% who rated the pain as the worst imaginable (Wallenstrom et al., 1996). However, in some cultures, such as the Yap culture in the South Pacific, the women report different or even no specific pain during childbirth (Callister et al., 2003). In this culture women work up until delivery and they go back to work almost immediately after giving birth. Since physiological differences can hardly account for the differences in pain reports, it appears that cultural difference may explain the difference. While women in Western countries are attuned to the fact that childbirth may be painful, the Yap culture does not appear to ponder this point. Moreover, while it is acceptable to complain of pain and even to plan for pain-relieving procedures during delivery in developed countries, the Yap culture may not encourage or perhaps even tolerate such behavior. So, while childbirth is quite similar biologically, it occurs in very culturally different settings. These cultural factors also affect what is defined to be acceptable as a pain complaint.

Another example concerns men. For men in many natural cultures, complaining of pain for minor cuts, bruises and the like is not satisfactory because it is seen as a symbol of weakness and moral/spiritual degradation. In terms of expressing pain, behaviors such as crying and pulling your hair are appropriate behaviors in some societies while in others they are avoided since they are considered to be signs of weakness.

The decision to seek healthcare is also guided by social factors (Skevington, 1995). Society places demands on what we might deem legitimate to seek care for as well as when and from whom we seek care. Consequently, seeking emergency room care for a scratch would not be approved of in many places, especially if it occurred when other options for care were available. Similarly, seeking care from a psychologist for back pain is not viewed as acceptable in many cultures.

Finally, cultural factors also influence how we react to others who are experiencing pain. In the Western world "sick" behavior is responded to with sympathy and attention; we often want to help the person.

The family is a powerful influence that, like culture, sets limits on our learning (Romano et al., 1997; Kerns et al., 2002). While the society and culture we live in sets general boundaries, the family sets more specific limitations. Reflect on a child complaining of a sore throat at the breakfast table. The family will influence whether the child continues to complain about the symptom as well as what action might be correct. Should the child take medication for the symptoms, or stay home from school? These behaviors are learned, but the family sets the boundaries for when, for example, it might be necessary to stay home sick. Thus, the family as well as society exerts important influences that shape the behaviors, thoughts and emotions that are deemed acceptable when we are in pain.

COPING STRATEGIES

Coping is the term used to describe the strategies a patient uses to deal with their pain. We all employ such strategies even though they may not always be a conscious choice. If faced with a potentially painful situation, such as a medical or dental procedure, we might consider how we would deal with the pain. The strategy we employ might include cognitive ones like attempting to ignore the pain or visualizing that we are Superman and consequently will not be bothered much by such small amounts of pain. The strategies might also include behavioral ones such as relaxation or verbal comments (I will tell the dentist when it starts to hurt). While this example provides the time for contemplation, this is not always the case in real-life situations. Nevertheless, we react with coping behaviors. Coping strategies then may be evoked through conscious or even unconscious processes.

Coping strategies are learned and involve an integration of the emotional, cognitive and behavioral systems. As we have seen in earlier chapters, painful stimuli set off emotional and cognitive processes. In order to provide immediate responses to the painful stimuli, there is a sort of direct connection to beliefs and emotions that steer our coping. Emotions help to steer our cognitions and negative emotions tend to stimulate more negative expectations and thoughts. Thus, if we believe that pain is always very harmful, this would be connected to coping strategies such as escaping or avoiding. Normally, this also involves thought patterns where we may deal with the pain cognitively such as either by catastrophizing or using self-statements that are positive ("I've tolerated a lot more pain than this before"; "I will certainly be able to handle the pain, it's only for a couple of minutes").

Learning experiences help to fine-tune our coping strategies. When a particular strategy works, then it reinforces the behavior and the coping strategy involved. An interesting aspect is determining if the strategy "works". Because we often are trying to minimize or avoid pain, it is often difficult to know how effective the coping strategy was as compared to some other strategy. In other words, we do not know what the resultant pain would have been had we not employed the strategy, or had we employed another strategy. An example illustrates this. Suppose the dentist warns that a procedure may cause some intense pain. You decide to try to remain calm and use a relaxation technique. In fact, the procedure is not very painful and you might naturally draw the conclusion that the strategy you employed was helpful. However, perhaps the dental procedure simply did not produce nociception. Moreover, another strategy might have been much more helpful. This type of paradigm lacks important feedback links.

Because we often attempt to avoid or escape pain as in the example, the coping strategies we learn are not necessarily the most effective. In fact, some strategies may actually cause more pain.

Another aspect of coping is that short-term positive effects may actually have long-term negative effects. This is because some strategies may be quite effective in reducing acute pain, but lead to a change in behavior patterns that enhances disability. For example, taking a painkiller is usually quite effective in reducing pain, but taking them regularly for a long period of time may produce side-effects, addiction or habituation. Similarly, resting often reduces acute back pain. However, in the long term resting may contribute to a weakening of the muscles, more pain and the development of the "disuse syndrome".

Coping entails any method a patient employs to deal with or adjust to their pain (Rosenstiel and Keefe, 1983; Boothby et al., 1999). As a result, specific coping strategies will not be dwelt upon here; the more common ones are listed in Table 7.1. However, the concept is important when we communicate with patients and

Table 7.1 An overview of some common coping strategies.

Coping strategy	Description
Catastrophizing	Excessive and exaggerated self-statements or thoughts ("I expect the worst")
Praying/hoping	Placing the solution to the pain problem in others or future events ("I have faith in doctors that someday there will be a cure for my pain")
Reinterpretation	The actual pain experience is changed to give it another meaning ("I don't think of it as pain, but rather as a dull warm feeling")
Ignoring	Attempting to think of something else, that is, not to think about the pain ("I try not to think about the pain")
Distraction/diverting attention	Attempting to focus attention on something other than the pain ("I try to think of something pleasant")
Positive self-statements	Rephrasing to put the pain in a positive light. Often contains positive self-efficacy ("I know I can deal with the pain")
Distracting activities	Attempting to use activities to distract from the pain, but not exercise treatment ("When in pain, I try to do chores or hobby projects")

attempt to engage them in self-help treatments. Patients usually understand the idea of coping, and may well take a very positive view of the idea of learning to cope better.

SUMMARY

Learning exerts a powerful influence on our behavior, but also on our emotions and cognitions. It is a vital process that allows us to adjust to our environment and the demands it places on us. Indeed, most pain behaviors are learned and the connection between biological, emotional and cognitive processes is highly integrated. As a result, learning influences the entire organism and not just an isolated behavior. However, the immediate consequences of a given behavior is the mechanism that governs it. In addition, the antecedent conditions such as the setting are important cues that tell us when a particular behavior is appropriate.

Learning paradigms are amazingly useful in understanding how a pain problem develops. These paradigms provide clues as to how habits develop that may enhance recovery or augment disability. Thus, we may understand better how patients react and cope with their pain by studying learning paradigms.

Because most pain behaviors are learned, this creates a tremendous treatment potential as learning can also alter these behaviors. Consequently, treatment programs may utilize learning paradigms in developing effective methods for dealing with pain problems. Moreover, psychological treatments based on learning highlight the fact that the target of treatment is not just the experience of pain intensity, but the entire realm of the problem including emotions, cognitions and behaviors.

CHAPTER 8

An integrated model

The psychologist asked me to describe my pain; how I felt deep down inside, what I did to deal with it. I sure didn't know about that, all I knew is that the pain affected every millimeter of me and I was doing what I could to manage.

—Carpenter seeking help for pain

LEARNING OBJECTIVES

To understand:

- that pain entails a highly integrated system;
- this system consists of biological, emotional, cognitive and behavioral aspects;
- painful stimuli from the environment place demands on an individual;
- learning helps us to adjust to these demands and steers the system to become effective;
- the model presented represents an integrated, pliable and resilient system that is highly effective in dealing with pain;
- the psychological processes are normal and help us to provide better care;
- the psychological processes empower the patient because they provide ample opportunity for change, i.e. to deal with the pain more effectively.

In this chapter we will penetrate an integrated model of pain that serves as a heuristic aid for understanding pain perception. This model incorporates a biopsychosocial conceptualization, but focuses on how the psychological aspects work and interrelate. Thus, it highlights a psychological perspective on pain perception. By examining this model closely you may integrate the various psychological factors described in the previous chapters. Thus, this model will help you to understand better how psychological factors affect pain perception, and it will provide you with a relatively simple framework to remember and utilize this information.

THE PSYCHOLOGICAL MODEL

Figure 8.1 shows a modern view of pain perception from a psychological perspective. It provides a cross-sectional view of what happens when we react to a painful stimulus. The starting point in the model is some sort of injury that produces nociceptive stimuli in the nervous system. These nerve impulses ascend to the brain and are processed there. Here psychological factors are intertwined with biological processes. These processes are controlled in part by emotional and cognitive aspects. In order to be fully relevant, these nerve signals need to be brought to awareness. Chapter 4 highlighted how this is done. This is an interesting part of pain perception because the brain receives thousands of impulses and it is selective in bringing things to consciousness. Since pain has survival value and is a warning signal, awareness may be steered to the painful stimulus. Attending to the stimulus may also increase awareness and suffering. Vigilance may also increase the probability of becoming aware of pain stimuli. Indeed, coping strategies like distraction are common methods people use to cope with pain.

Once a stimulus has been attended to, it must be interpreted; that is, we must try to make sense out of what the signal actually means. The interpretation process involves complex cognitive and emotional aspects that color our perception. Thus, a stimulus that may appear to be quite harmless (an increase in heart rate) may nevertheless be interpreted as extremely noxious (severe chest pain) if it is interpreted as the first sign of a heart attack. This is a vital part of the pain perception process as the interpretation of the stimulus is a key to what action we should take.

Once some meaning has been given to the pain, we may "plan" how to deal with the situation. Coping strategies are ways of dealing with painful stimuli and may include cognitive or behavioral action. When a strategy is put into action, we have behavior. According to the laws of learning, this behavior will have an effect demonstrated in the results or consequences. The consequences thus provide feedback which in turn determines whether the behavior will be repeated in the future: successful behaviors increase in probability while unsuccessful ones decrease in probability. Finally, as indicated by the arrows, the feedback not only affects the behavior, but also the cognitive and emotional processes. Thus, we learn how to deal with pain. This feedback also provides information for forming future emotional and cognitive reactions. For example, feedback will "tell us" whether the anxiety we felt and the catastrophizing thoughts ("I might die of a heart attack") when we felt an increase in heart rate were actually helpful. And, in turn, feedback will be provided for the attentional processes.

There are factors that set limitations. These boundaries highlight the role of social factors like the culture and family we belong to. These set a framework for what is construed as acceptable beliefs, interpretations and behaviors when we are experiencing pain.

As may be seen in the model, then, the psychological aspects are truly integrated to form a pliable and resilient response to pain. This represents the normal psychology of pain. In fact, biological and psychological factors work hand in hand to help us deal effectively with the demands the environment places on us. Thus, the human species is highly developed for dealing with the aches and pains of everyday life as well as with the pain caused by diseases. This does not mean that we can avoid or control all pain. It does mean that we have an amazing capability of perceiving and interpreting bodily signals so that the most appropriate action may be taken most of the time. The end result is a marvelous system that is highly effective in dealing with pain.

A normal process

The model that I have outlined clearly represents what might be termed the normal psychology of pain. This is central as many patients as well as professionals consider the psychological aspects of a patient's problem

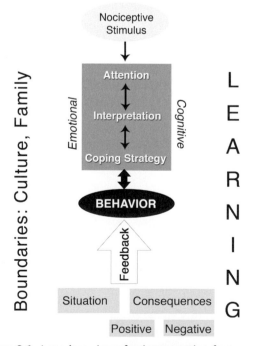

Figure 8.1 A modern view of pain perception from a psychological perspective. The text provides a detailed description of the process.

to be the result of "abnormal" psychological factors. This view is not only wrong, it is also destructive since it reinforces the separation of psychological and biological factors. It also tends to point the finger of fault at the patient. Clearly, however, psychological processes are involved in all pain perception. This has untold value in helping us to respond to the situation in an effective manner. Without the normal psychological processes described in this model, our ability to survive would be greatly impaired. It is imperative, then, that we consider the usual, normal way that psychological factors influence pain perception if we are to capitalize on this knowledge in the clinic.

Advantages of the psychological model

The model I have developed here has several distinct advantages. First, it appears to provide the best available description of the experience of pain. This after all is a key goal of cultivating a psychological model. Second, it provides a framework from which to understand how biological and psychological processes are integrated.

This takes a giant step from a simple medical model. Further, it helps to eradicate us from a dualistic approach where pain is either "physical" or "mental". Third, this model provides incredible insight into the process of pain perception. For this reason, we may exploit it when developing interventions for pain. To be sure, this model is utilized extensively in the second part of the book where we examine the implications of the model for clinical practice. By better understanding how pain works, we are in a better position to develop new methods for assessing, treating and preventing disabling pain. Finally, this model provides impetus for empowering the patient. I have underscored the idea that the pliability of the system allows for change. Patients may therefore learn new ways of thinking about their pain and in behaving, i.e. coping with their pain. This opens the door for new treatments, but also for preventive strategies and self-help programs. Indeed, it may truly give patients the power to take command over their situation and cope with their pain in the best possible fashion.

PART

2 | Implications for clinical practice

I could have hurried a lot less and still been in time for my deathbed.

—Vilhelm Moberg, *A Time on Earth* (1984)

While Part I focused on grasping the psychology of pain, Part II is concerned with applying this knowledge in the clinic. The need for using psychological aspects is evident in Part I, but how do we address these? The definite aim of Part II is to help you become a better clinician by assimilating psychological principles into your practice. An in-depth understanding of the psychology of pain has great implications for clinical practice. Using the models and information in Part I provides enormous potential for improving the care we provide for patients. While making us better clinicians, it also allows us to empower our patients so that they may develop health self-care routines. Employing psychological principles runs the range from the first time you meet the patient to rehabilitation or the care of the chronically ill.

In this section, we begin with the first visit. This is unusual. The majority of textbooks begin with the really difficult cases of persistent pain and disability and present programs for rehabilitation. However, the best way forward seems to be with early, preventive interventions. Some reason that most acute pain, e.g. acute back pain, resolves quickly and does not constitute a problem. However, the basis for the development of chronic problems may be sowed during the very first visit. To be sure, we may turn the table around and assert that excellent care, which naturally includes a psychological perspective, is a key to preventing the development of long-term problems. Addressing psychological aspects early also appears to work better than waiting until the problem has progressed into a persistent one. To underscore the importance of this, we start with the first visit and proceed from there.

However, to recapitulate Part I and provide a more detailed background from which to understand the implications of a psychological approach to pain, we begin Part II with a chapter on why chronic pain and disability develop. Think about two people who injure themselves in a similar way. Let us presume that the nature of the injury is basically the same. However, one may recover rather quickly and experience few problems, while the other may develop extensive difficulties and is clearly distressed by it. What might explain the difference? In understanding why a pain problem sometimes develops into a persistent one with associated disability, we also gain insights into how we might best deal with patients.

By starting at the beginning of a problem, Part II also places the emphasis on early, preventive interventions. This is strategic. The medical model is infamous for concentrating on the treatment of known disease. However, for pain such as spinal pain, a real problem is the development of long-term pain and disability. Another model is therefore needed. We will explore how early, preventive interventions may be employed in healthcare situations with a wide variety of patients. A program for using certain techniques from the start will be emphasized and subsequently we will explore how this might be combined with early identification and the initiation of cognitive-behavioral interventions to better serve patients.

Above all, Part II aims to help you develop your proficiency to enhance the patient's own self-help skills. You will not become a psychologist or therapist by reading this book. However, Part II will help you to learn how to integrate relatively simple psychological techniques into your usual practice. Doing this can have great impact. In fact, we will also briefly examine exactly what the effects of using such methods are. We will weigh the costs and benefits of doing so.

CHAPTER

9

Why does persistent pain develop?

I never thought I would ever be this disabled. It just seemed to creep up on me; one day I woke up and realized I had a big problem I couldn't handle.

—Patient with fibromyalgia

LEARNING OBJECTIVES

To understand:

- persistent pain problems develop over long periods of time and involve not only pain, but also dramatic changes in lifestyle and function;

- musculoskeletal pain (and many other types) are recurrent in nature, and this provides many opportunities for learning;

- the biopsychosocial system for pain perception is extraordinary in helping us efficiently to deal with pain normally;

- the process of development where a small number of people develop reactions (coping strategies) that are successful in the short term but devastating in the long run;

- the process is influenced by different factors, and the individual course from acute to chronic;

- because changes occur gradually, the patient may not be aware of the process until it is too late;

- the process of development offers many opportunities for intervention. In fact, many alternatives are available that are not utilized (take step back, see many ways of dealing with a given situation).

With the models from Part I, a new answer may be given to a central question: why does a seemingly normal acute pain problem develop into chronic disability? Despite the dire need for prevention, surprisingly few analyses of this process have been available. Yet identifying the mechanisms involved might well provide new insights that culminate in more effective interventions. Innovative studies have now identified a number of risk factors and a picture of the development of chronic pain is emerging. However, it is still a riddle where each piece of evidence must be meticulously fitted together into the image on the puzzle. Fitting the new evidence into a theoretical model should help us to see the "whole picture" more clearly even though a relatively large number of the pieces of the puzzle are not yet available.

The purpose of this chapter is to develop a model of the development of chronic pain based on the data available and to cast it into a psychological perspective with the models developed in Part I so that we might promote preventive interventions. Once again, this chapter spotlights back and neck pain because they are so common and relevant. However, the processes described are meant to be applicable to the development of persistent pain and disability in general.

A DEVELOPMENTAL PROCESS

To understand persistent pain and disability, it is helpful to view it as a developmental process since psychological factors interact with biological factors and work over time to produce the cognitive, emotional and behavioral changes defining the syndrome. Curiously, the psychological reactions associated with acute pain are normally effective in adjusting to the pain until healing occurs and the pain subsides. A surprising number of people, moreover, cope with persistent pain so well that they require little sick leave or healthcare (Linton, 1999b). For a minority of people, however, the cognitive, emotional and behavioral reactions are not sufficient and may, in themselves, actually contribute to the development of persistent pain problems. These work over time and while short-term gains may be achieved, the long-term results may be overwhelming.

WHO GETS BACK PAIN?

Back pain seems to be a very prevalent problem, but who exactly gets back pain and how does it start? To answer this question, we conducted a study in the general population (Linton et al., 1998) and repeated it to be absolutely sure that the results were correct (Linton and Ryberg, 2000). Questionnaires were sent to 3000 people randomly selected from the census in central Sweden between the ages of 35 and 45. The response rate was good (78.5%) and an analysis of nonresponders showed that the data obtained were representative.

We found that 66% reported an episode of back pain during the past year. Women reported back pain slightly more often (69%) than men (63%). However, the pain varied considerably. Pain intensity, for instance, varied from very mild to nearly unbearable and the average reported pain was 4.2 on a 0–10 scale (Table 9.1). With consideration of the effects shown in the table, we reckoned that 25% of the population had a significant problem.

Our study also demonstrated that a relatively small number of sufferers consume huge amounts of the

Table 9.1 The effects of back pain in the general population.

Variable	Mean response
Usual pain intensity	4.2*
Worst pain intensity	7.0*
Degree of functional problems	4.5*
% taking sick absence because of pain	19%
% taking more than 15 days in past year	8%
No. of healthcare visits for pain (all)	3.7

*0–10 scale.

available resources. For example, 6% of those reporting back pain accounted for 41% of the healthcare visits reported. These patients had an average of over 20 visits during the past year! Moreover, of these 6%, many had been off work because of their pain during the past year. In fact, 45% of them reported more than 90 days of sick leave during the previous year for back pain.

What is the typical onset of back pain? We might think that a traumatic accident such as a heavy lift is the reason. However, the data do not support this idea. Instead, the onset is often not related to any specific activity, accident or movement. For example, in one study 51% reported the onset of their back pain to be spontaneous, while 17% reported it starting during normal activities, and only 32% reported onset due to an accident (Lloyd et al., 1986; Crombie et al., 1999).

This is in contrast with what people attribute the cause of their pain to. In a recent report based on national statistics it was shown that most people believe their pain onset is related to an accident or other factors at work (Waddell, 1998). While 21% of men reported an accident at work as the cause, an additional 35% attributed it to working conditions and a further 27% to an injury elsewhere such as while working at home.

We investigated the factors to which workers attributed their back pain (Linton and Warg, 1993). We surveyed 145 workers at the same workplace concerning their beliefs about back pain and its prevention. The results showed that employees were convinced that back pain is work-related. Moreover, specific aspects of work were regarded as particularly important in the etiology of back trouble. Blue-collar workers reported the following hierarchy of work factors:

1. Work pace.
2. Poor posture.
3. Lack of interest from management.

4. Monotonous work.
5. Heavy lifts.
6. Physical/ergonomics of the workplace.
7. Risk-taking.
8. Lack of proper work organization.
9. Improper work techniques.
10. Lack of safety devices.

The factors that blue-collar workers reported were different than those of management. For example, management did not believe that heavy lifts were particularly important, and moreover they believed that individual factors such as personal problems, poor physical condition and the like were more important than workplace factors.

We also examined the effects of job satisfaction on the report of back pain. As can be seen in Fig. 9.1, there was a strong relationship. Those who were satisfied with their job had half the one-year incidence of reported back pain compared to those who were not satisfied. The figure shows a reasonable "dose-response" effect: the more satisfied the worker, the less frequent the report of back pain. It is important to remember, however, that job satisfaction does not directly cause pain. However, it may reflect a conglomerate of work variables and may even include some that overlap with physical work. Still, it is important to know that workers see their problem as being related to work, and that job satisfaction is linked to the reporting of back pain.

THE TIME FACTOR: ACUTE, CHRONIC OR RECURRENT

Time is a crucial factor as it provides a framework and plays a role in the chronification process itself. The development of chronic pain may be described in a series of stages (Skevington, 1995; Gatchel, 1996) that were detailed in Part I. These are generally referred to as *acute pain*, which is generally defined as pain up to about 3 weeks, *subacute pain*, considered to be between 3 and 12 weeks, and *persistent or chronic pain*, defined as more than 3 months' duration.

Although the above stages of pain development serve as a heuristic aid, it is vital to understand that musculoskeletal pain is almost always *recurrent*. Even if typical bouts of back pain get significantly better rather quickly and most people return to work within 6 weeks (Reid et al., 1997), the rate of recurrence is high and most sufferers will experience several episodes of pain during the course of a year (Von Korff, 1994). In addition, it is rare indeed for someone with no history of such pain to be off work for 6 weeks or more on the first episode. Rather, persistent problems tend to develop over extended periods of time in which recurrent bouts become more frequent and the duration longer (Philips and Grant, 1991; Rossignol et al., 1992; Von Korff, 1994). More than 50% of patients with acute back pain will experience another occasion within a year (Nachemson, 1992), and prospective studies indicate that almost half will still have significant problems 6 to 12 months later (Philips and Grant, 1991; Von Korff, 1994; Linton and Halldén, 1997). Finally, although patients may expect an episode of back pain to be resolved in a matter of a few days, research indicates that it takes an average of 8 weeks for patients in primary care with an acute episode of back pain (van den Hoogen et al., 1997, 1998) (Fig. 9.2).

Recurrent bouts mean learning opportunities

Persistent pain problems do not occur suddenly as the result of a single event, but rather they develop in an interaction with the environment. During the recurrent bouts people will attempt a variety of ways of coping with the pain and the resultant disability. The intensity of the pain itself may alter emotions, thoughts, beliefs and behaviors. These changes are shaped by the interplay among biological factors, the environment, and

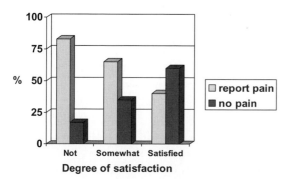

Figure 9.1 The relationship between job satisfaction and self-reported back pain. (Based on Linton and Warg, 1993.)

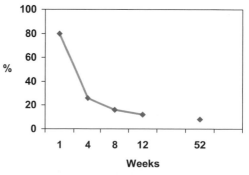

Figure 9.2 Percentage of those off work for back pain after an acute bout. Note that most people return to work within a few days or weeks, but after about 12 weeks a small proportion remain off work and become disabled.

our behavior, emotions and cognitions. Without a doubt, learning is the foremost mechanism by which the environment impinges upon the development of persistent pain.

Because pain usually is not constant, but instead varies considerably over time, each "bout" of the pain offers an opportunity for learning. This is a powerful way in which we adjust our behavior and the associated cognitions and emotions to the stress to which the pain subjects us. As we saw in Chapter 7, short-term consequences are more powerful in shaping behavior than are long-term consequences.

One implication of this is that coping strategies that are successful in immediately reducing our pain will be reinforced. Resting is one thing that often reduces acute back pain. While this is often a useful strategy, in a few cases it may become a dominant strategy because the short-term reinforcement of reduced pain overrides the long-term problem of the disuse syndrome. The fear-avoidance model described in detail in Part I nicely accounts for how this may happen and includes biological, emotional, behavioral and cognitive aspects.

The typical course of a bout of back pain

About 85% of the adult population will have a bout of back pain that leads to work absence or a healthcare visit, but how long does it take for the problem to subside? We have seen in this chapter that people generally return to work within at most a few weeks. It has also been suggested that although one may return to work, this does not mean that the problem has vanished. A study from England sheds light on recovery rates because they followed patients who received care from their family practitioner for back pain to see recovery rates (Papageorgiou et al., 1996). Three months after the consultation only 27% reported complete recovery. While an additional 28% were improved, 44% remained the same or were worse!

Recurrent bouts of pain are common. In one investigation, those seeking care for acute, subacute or chronic back pain were studied to see how many suffered recurrent problems (Waddell, 1998). This was measured one to four years after the initial problem. The results are sobering. 70% of those with acute problems at presentation reported recurrent pain, while 80% of those with subacute problems reported this. As expected, 95% of the chronic patients reported continued bouts of back pain. Indeed, another study calculated the probability of further bouts of back pain based on the time since the last attack (Biering-Sörensen, 1983). They found that the shorter the time since the last episode, the higher the probability of a recurrent attack. For example, when the time since the last attack was less than a week, the probability of an attack during the next year was 76%. However, if the last attack was between 1 and 12 months ago, the probability fell to 52%. Once back pain has been experienced, the likelihood of a recurrent episode is quite high.

Thus, while back pain may improve, the typical course of the problem highlights recurrent bouts and relatively long time periods for recovery.

Psychological risk factors in the transition from acute to persistent pain

One way of approaching the development of persistent pain is to examine the risk factors associated with it. In this way we might isolate variables that seem to be instrumental. Psychological factors are known to play a significant role in chronic pain (Skevington, 1995; Main and Spanswick, 2000), but they also appear to play a fundamental role in the *transition* from acute to

---

THE DEVELOPMENT OF PERSISTENT PROBLEMS FOR HANK THROUGH LEARNING

Sitting is often difficult for back pain patients and Hank was no exception. Because of acute pain, Hank was reluctant to sit. When he first attempted to sit down normally, he got an intense jolt of pain that seemed to shoot down his thigh (Hank was punished for sitting properly). He tried to adjust his sitting and found that if he sat on only one buttock, leaned a bit forward, and put some of his weight on the armrest, then he experienced much less pain (reinforced this way of sitting with pain behaviors, e.g. guarding, bracing). Because this resulted in a great difference from his first attempt, Hank realized that with his back condition this was a much better way of sitting. The next couple of times Hank sat down he used this new method and found that it worked well (reinforcement by avoiding pain). Indeed, a couple of times while working, he inadvertently moved to sit more normally and felt more pain. Although this behavior was very successful in the short term, let us consider the results over time. As Hank successfully avoids pain by sitting in an "awkward position", his attempts at sitting normally become less frequent. However, healing—even if it is a relatively slow process—is occurring, but Hank does not experience this (for sitting) because he no longer attempts to sit normally. Moreover, think about the effects of sitting in the position Hank has taken. After just a few days of sitting like that the muscles and other tissue will adapt to that position. Consequently, when Hank attempts to sit normally again (after several days), the change will feel "funny" and may in itself cause discomfort because different muscles, etc., are being used. Thus, what seemed to be an ideal coping strategy for sitting turns out to be a problem for Hank's function in the long term.

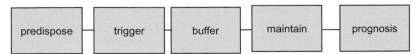

Figure 9.3 Various ways in which psychological factors may affect back pain.

chronic problems. In fact, psychological events appear to be quite instrumental in the transition from an acute injury to a chronic disability (Turk, 1997; Burton et al., 1999a; Linton, 2000c).

Figure 9.3 illustrates how psychological variables may intervene at several stages in pain perception and behavior. Some factors may *predispose* a person to be in pain while others may *trigger* or initiate the problem. Psychological factors are often involved in *maintaining* or catalyzing the problem. Learning, for example, may result in lifestyle changes that appear adaptive but which may maintain the problem in the long run. Resting may be reinforced by reductions in pain as well as sympathy in the short run. However, although this learned behavior may become well established over time, resting may in the long term result in reduced mobility, poorer physical condition and contribute to negative mood. Moreover, factors like depression may be related to *treatment prognosis*. Finally, *buffer* factors such as social support and active coping strategies may help people to withstand their pain problems. Certain factors, e.g. anxiety or depression, might well be involved in several of these stages but some factors will apply only to one. Let us determine which psychological factors form the base from which development might be understood.

Several authors have reviewed the vast literature concerning psychological risk factors for back pain. For example, Weiser and Cedraschi (1992) looked at articles relating psychological variables to chronic pain. They appraised 16 investigations involving a variety of populations. They found that distress and cognitive beliefs were related to the outcome as were stress and job satisfaction. A similar evaluation of the literature (Turk, 1997) found that pain severity, distress, maladaptive coping, passive cognitive beliefs and job satisfaction were related to outcome. A more comprehensive appraisal included 44 cross-sectional studies and 15 longitudinal ones (Bongers et al., 1993). First, this review found that the results for back pain were nearly identical to the results for neck, shoulder or musculoskeletal pain. Second, this review confirmed that individual psychological factors as well as workplace factors are related to pain.

To isolate which psychological factors might be involved in the development of persistent pain, we conducted a systematic review of the literature that focused on prospective studies (Linton, 2000b, 2000c). Prospective designs are characterized by the fact that they first measure the psychological variable and then follow participants to determine outcome. In this way, the effects of a particular psychological variable in the *development* of the problem may be better ascertained. The literature search isolated 37 such studies that were deemed to be of relatively good quality (Linton, 2000c). In fact, 26 of the studies first measured psychological factors either in healthy individuals or acute back pain patients and subsequently followed participants over several months to determine how the pain problem developed. These 26 studies are therefore particularly interesting for models concerning the development of persistent pain. A summary of the studies is shown in Table 9.2. It shows that various psychological factors were consistently related to the onset and development

Table 9.2 A summary of the psychological risk factors isolated in a review of the literature.

Risk factor	No. of studies	% finding factor to be a significant risk
Stress, distress, anxiety	11	100
Mood, depression	16	87
Fear avoidance, coping style	9	89
Fear-avoidance beliefs	4	100
Perceived future problems	2	100
Cognitive coping	4	100
Pain behavior, function	7	86

Based on Linton (2000b, 2000c).

of back pain problems. These specifically include stress or anxiety, mood, fear-avoidance beliefs, coping strategies, and pain behaviors and function.

One might suspect that psychological factors are confused with other variables such as workplace factors or medical factors. For example, it might be that people who feel stressed do so because they have a lot to do at work and this, rather than the experience of stress, is the real cause of the pain. However, in my review I found that 18 studies actually controlled for medical or workplace (ergonomic) factors. This entails measuring such other variables and then adjusting the results in light of them. Fifteen of the 18 studies still demonstrated a clear, significant relationship even when potential confounding variables were included in the analysis.

The significant psychological risk factors isolated represented cognitive, emotional and behavioral variables (Table 9.3). For example, cognitive variables such as fear-avoidance beliefs and catastrophizing were stable features having a particularly significant relationship with the development of dysfunction. Further, anxiety, distress or stress were related to back pain in every study that investigated them. Similarly, mood and depression were unfailingly reported to be significant risk factors. Behavioral aspects included coping strategies and high levels of pain behavior and dysfunction were related to poor outcome. Similar findings have been reported in other reviews of the literature

(Turk, 1997; Pincus et al., 2002). Thus, psychological variables affecting the individual seem to be pivotal in the transition from acute to chronic pain.

THE ROLE OF THE WORKPLACE

Work plays a central role in the advance of persistent pain because patients typically have difficulties maintaining or returning to work. In long-term back pain problems, work disability is a common feature. Indeed, the workplace is often viewed as an important element that *causes* back pain. For example, when asked, the vast majority of patients will report that their back problem is related to their work. This may involve an identifiable injury or a more gradual process. Further, some scientists maintain that other workplace factors like job satisfaction are strongly related to return to work after a back pain problem. They point to the fact that some patients return while others do not, even though they do the same basic work. Thus, it is intriguing to examine the literature on the role of psychological workplace factors in disability due to pain.

To shed light on the scientific evidence, some reviews have scrutinized the available literature. I inspected several hundred articles in order to locate prospective studies where a psychological workplace factor was first measured and outcome was assessed at a later time point, usually one year later (Linton, 2001). This produced 21 such studies that investigated the role of a wide variety of factors prospectively. Table 9.4 provides an overview of the relationships. Overall the evidence was compelling that psychological factors at work do indeed influence future pain and disability. For example, strong evidence implicated job satisfaction, monotonous work, social relations at work, work demands, stress, and perceived ability to work. However, it should be noted that job satisfaction was often assessed with a single question and usually was a composite of many of the other more specific factors including demands, control and social relations at work. In addition, moderate evidence that control, work pace, the belief that work is dangerous to future back pain and disability were also related to the development of future problems. It seems clear then that the psychosocial work environment is related to future back pain and resultant disability.

Other reviews in the literature draw similar conclusions. For example, Bongers et al. (1993) found that a lack of social support and low levels of control over one's work were related to back pain, while Hoogendoorn et al. (2000) found strong evidence that social support at work and job satisfaction are risk factors whereas there was less evidence for work pace and content. Indeed, the American National Research Council

---

CONCLUSIONS ABOUT PSYCHOLOGICAL RISK FACTORS BASED ON THE SCIENTIFIC EVIDENCE

1. There is strong evidence that psychological variables are strongly linked to the transition from acute to chronic pain.

2. There is strong evidence that psychological variables generally have more impact than biomedical or biomechanical (workplace) factors on back pain disability.

3. There is strong evidence that attitudes, cognitions and fear-avoidance beliefs are related to the development of pain and disability.

4. There is strong evidence that depression, anxiety, distress and related emotions are related to pain and disability.

5. There is evidence that poor self-perceived health is related to chronic pain and disability.

Table 9.3 Overview of some psychological variables believed to be important in the development of chronic pain.

Psychological factor	Description
Pain behaviors	
Overt	Various ways in which one communicates to others that we are experiencing pain. Examples are grimacing, bracing and rubbing.
Activity/function	Low levels of daily activities and high levels of "down time" signify a problem, but not necessarily related to pain level.
Avoidance	A learning paradigm where certain activities, places, etc., are avoided. Behavior is maintained by reduction in fear or anxiety. Patients may avoid activity to reduce fear.
Cognitions	
Beliefs about pain	Strongly held views about pain and illness containing both cognitive and affective components. Socially and culturally generated and modifiable. May include beliefs about pain control (locus of control), pain modification (self-efficacy), health professionals and efficacy of treatments.
Catastrophizing	One of a number of maladaptive strategies for coping with pain, commonly related to the etiology of depression. Believed to be related to fear-avoidance vicious circle.
Cognitive distortion	Systematic errors in the thinking of people, particularly in the depressed. This may take the form of making arbitrary inferences or drawing mistaken conclusions in the absence of evidence. They may magnify the significance of an unpleasant event and minimize or discount a pleasant one. Commonly found in relation to pain and disability.
Locus of control	Beliefs concerning the place where the control of pain is based, e.g. personal responsibility for pain control, pain control by others (e.g. doctors) and pain control through chance happenings or misfortune. These beliefs may be the foundation for action to seek pain relief.
Coping strategies	A number of ways of managing or deflecting unwanted stress or pain. These may include cognitive (distraction) and behavioral (take pill) aspects and they may be passive (hoping) or active strategies (relaxation).
Control	Belief that it is possible to respond to influence an aversive event. Desire to predict such an event. Control and predictability influence pain perception.
Attention	A type of vigilance or monitoring activity that can be harnessed in coping strategies either to divert or distract from the source of stress or to focus directly on the pain, stress or anxiety. Choice of strategy depends on the circumstances.
Helplessness	A style of beliefs predominantly used by those who are prone to depression whereby negative events such as the onset of pain tend to be seen as likely to persist and generalize.
Emotions	
Mood	Depression, anxiety, but also fear, sadness, anger and frustration are associated with pain and disability. More likely to be a consequence of pain than a precursor to it.
Anxiety/somatic anxiety	Increased physiological arousal together with cognitive components like worry that enhance the detection of painful sensation and maintain perceived pain. Thus, a target for treatment. Somatic anxiety refers to the distress and concurrent symptoms.

Continued

Table 9.3 Overview of some psychological variables believed to be important in the development of chronic pain.—cont'd

Social	
Gender	Similarities and differences in the way women and men respond to pain sensations, interpret them and report them and styles of obtaining treatment. Formed in part by social and cultural frame.
Social comparison	Comparisons made with other people with different diseases or health states or with self (ideal self) at different times defined by health events, within the lifespan.
Social support	Any input directly provided by another person or group which moves recipients toward the goals they desire. For pain may be positive or negative.
Spouse relations	The interpersonal relationship between pain patient and spouse and the effect that this has on pain behaviors. A solicitous spouse may increase pain behaviors.
Workplace	Relationships at work with management as well as coworkers may influence perceptions of injury as well as pain and disability.
Work management	The way in which a workplace organizes and deals with pain problems and rehabilitation may influence pain perception and behavior.

Based on Linton and Skevington (1999).

recognized in their report that several work-related psychosocial factors were associated with musculoskeletal disorders (National Research Council, 2001). Consequently, psychological and social factors at work appear to play a significant role in the development of persistent pain and disability.

Table 9.4 A summary of psychosocial workplace risk factors for back pain.

Factor	No. of studies	% finding it a risk
Job satisfaction	14	93
Monotonous work	6	66
Work relations	6	83
Perceived demands	3	100
Work content	1	100*
Control	2	100*
Pace	3	66
Perceived stress	3	100
Perceived ability to work	3	100
Belief work is dangerous	2	100*
Emotional effort	2	100*

Based on Linton (2001).
*Insufficient number of studies to draw a firm conclusion.

Workplace factors as a barrier to return

Often when the workplace is viewed as a source of the pain, even if it does not cause the pain, there may be barriers that make a return to work difficult. These obstacles point to several problems that may arise which make it difficult for the individual to actually begin working again. These may include factors like a fear that returning to work will result in reinjury, or worries that not being able to work properly will create more work for workmates.

Moreover, people engage in new lifestyles during their time off work and this may also create barriers. Although we know relatively little about what people actually do while off work, clinical experience and the literature demonstrate that people quickly adjust to the situation and develop new daily routines. For example, the individual may get up later, have a more leisurely breakfast, and ease into activity during the morning. This routine could be in sharp contrast to a typical work day which requires an early start and relatively hard work from the beginning. Thus, simply breaking lifestyle habits to get to work may become a barrier. The idea of barriers to return to work has been exemplified by Chris Main and his associates and seems to be a central aspect in the role of work (Main and Spanswick, 2000).

To understand barriers better, we developed a questionnaire to measure such obstacles and then tested it on a clinical back pain population. Participants were off work for musculoskeletal pain and first completed the questionnaire. We then followed the participants for 9 months to analyze how their responses related to their actual return to work. To construct the questionnaire we isolated 87 items that represented nine scales of possible barriers. We found that the items were truly related to outcome. Factors such as expected perceived ability to return to work, social support at work, expected physical workload and harmfulness were isolated. All in all, with the most relevant items from the questionnaire we could correctly classify 79% of the participants in terms of their actual return to work! In other words, the barriers we identified were highly related to return to work and support the idea that they may form obstacles or barriers to return.

Working despite pain: integrating physical and psychological aspects

Another way of looking at the relationship between the individual and workplace risk factors was underscored in a study we conducted with practical nurses at a large hospital (Linton and Buer, 1995). By means of a survey we located women with back pain. When examining the data we discovered an interesting fact: some had been off work frequently with their pain, while others had not. We wondered what this might be related to and set about the task of investigating. Because the nurses might have very different physical work environments, we first checked this aspect, and subsequently we looked at how much pain they were experiencing. We even checked to be sure that those not reporting being off work for back pain might have been off work due to other illnesses, but found no support for this idea. Thus, we obtained women who were matched in terms of their work situation (such as type of ward, amount of lifting) and their experienced pain, but some of them had been off work more than 90 days during the past year, while others had not missed a single day.

We proceeded to study the differences between these groups to see how the one group worked despite having considerable pain. Interviews were conducted that indicated that these women were also more active in their everyday and leisure life. They were not resting at home to make up. How did these women cope? We found that those working had different ways of dealing with the pain problem emotionally, cognitively and behaviorally. Differences between the groups were seen for function, pain beliefs and coping strategies. Those off work had stronger beliefs that pain was directly related to activities (fear avoidance), they participated in fewer activities, they believed that they had little control over their pain, that their health was poor, and they tended to focus on the pain rather than function.

The interface between the worker, her or his individual make-up and the workplace has been delineated by Feuerstein and associates (Shaw et al., 2002). They point out that workplace ergonomic factors may set the stage for certain behaviors and reactions from the individual worker. Depending on the individual's situation and coping strategies, the ergonomic exposure may lead to a problem. It is an interesting model that unites information about ergonomics, body mechanics, psychosocial workplace factors and individual psychological factors.

CASE STUDY: HANK

Hank never dreamed that he would have trouble returning to work. However, with the severe pain he experienced in the beginning, it seemed impossible to remain at work. Indeed, his doctor suggested being off work and provided a sick leave certificate. At first Hank found it awkward to be at home during a work day. His family was away at work and school and he was alone and could do what he wanted. In the beginning that wasn't much. Hank took it easy. He read the paper, watched TV and caught up on reading. After a few days he was determined to do more so he sometimes went for a walk or did some small jobs around the house. He also visited his shop to work on hobbies. Hank also frequented a local coffee shop where he could meet a couple of friends, and he began to take responsibility for errands such as going to the bank. He picked up the children from school and spent some time with them. And he tried to get supper going so that it would be ready when his wife came home. While this routine worked, Hank found it necessary to rest often and to do the activities in his own way and at his own pace. It was comforting to be able to take pain medications or rest whenever he needed to.

Hank learned that his employer had found a substitute to work for him. This fellow was a nice guy and a good worker. This was good for the workplace, but Hank felt annoyed that they had replaced him so quickly. Hank talked to his supervisor when he needed to tell him that he would be off a little longer. Hank also discussed going back to work with him. The authorities were suggesting that it was time for Hank to get back to work. His supervisor seemed to understand, but wondered whether Hank was actually fit to do the job. Hank was doubtful himself. He worried that working would cause more pain. Further, he was concerned that if he came back but couldn't manage, things would be even worse. His supervisor would not like it, they would get behind at work, and the substitute would be gone. Hank found it difficult to find the energy to make the necessary effort to begin working again.

THE ROLE OF THE HEALTHCARE PROFESSIONAL

The role of patient factors is often under the microscope in discussions of the development of persistent pain, but the role we play as healthcare professionals appears to be imperative. Indeed, there are at least two major ways in which our role influences outcome. The first is in our interaction with the patient where our own reactions may influence the course of the patient's problem, and the second is in how we implement new techniques such as psychosocial aspects into modern healthcare.

The way we deal with patients is crucial for good care and treatment outcome (Piasecki, 2003). Here, our reactions may influence how successfully we communicate with the patient and what messages are given. We have found that healthcare professionals basically have similar reactions, beliefs, emotions, etc., as do patients. In one study, for example, we looked at the fear-avoidance beliefs that healthcare professionals may hold. We used questionnaires that are employed to assess a patient's beliefs, but rewrote items so that they would be relevant for professionals. The results were startling. Although a majority of the professionals did not hold extensive "fear avoidance" beliefs, roughly 30% did hold such beliefs. For example, over two-thirds of general practitioners and physical therapists believed that one should advise patients to "avoid painful movements", and more than half believed that patients should not do monotonous work. More results are shown in Table 9.5.

The results of our study were also shown to be related to reported practice procedures. Importantly, the risk of using inappropriate techniques increased with the level of fear-avoidance beliefs that the professionals held. Although sick absenteeism may be a result of pain, it is not a treatment in itself and experts have underscored the risks of placing patients on the sick list (Waddell et al., 1997; Waddell, 1998). Nevertheless, those with high levels of fear-avoidance beliefs in our study were 2.5 times more likely to report that sick leave is "a good treatment" for back pain. In addition, being high on fear-avoidance beliefs also decreased the likelihood that clear information about activities was provided by over threefold. Thus, the attitudes and behaviors that we healthcare professionals have might well influence outcome. We will return to these factors in the following chapter.

The second way we professionals play a role is in how well we implement the newest findings such as incorporating a psychological perspective into practice. Naturally, there is a time lag between the first reports of a new, effective method and its clinical application. However, research suggests that when it comes to psychological techniques there may be particular cognitive, emotional and behavioral problems that hinder implementation. We found that although professionals may generally be aware of psychosocial factors, there was a lack of specific knowledge about which factors are relevant and how they might be utilized (Overmeer et al., 2004, in press). Implementation also seems to be steered by beliefs and in our clinic we have identified several such beliefs as examples. Professionals may believe, for instance, that dealing with psychological factors is not their job, or that one should not bring up topics unless you have a treatment to provide for it. Such beliefs will certainly set boundaries for what issues are brought up and dealt with.

FACTORS SHAPING THE PROCESS OF CHRONIFICATION

Earlier we dealt with how learning forms our emotions, beliefs and behaviors; in this section we shall investigate important factors that shape the process of chronification. Indeed, the integrated system we have already examined is the major force in the development of chronic pain. To understand how learning impinges on us over time, several factors need to be accentuated because they are instrumental in this learning.

Process

First, though it is understandable that we tend to view the development of chronic pain as a linear happening that occurs relatively rapidly (e.g. 3 months), and that is directly related to a specific injury, it actually involves a process of change over relatively long periods. As we saw above, the recurrent nature of musculoskeletal pain sets the stage for learning and the gradual development of persistent pain and disability. In turn this gradual change seems to be related to cognitive and learning factors. Bear in mind that we are discussing a process rather than a single event!

Table 9.5 Examples of fear-avoidance beliefs and the percentage of general practitioners (Drs) and physical therapists (PTs) who endorsed them.

Assertion	% agreeing	
	Drs	PTs
Stop activity if it hurts	17	32
Should not do monotonous work	58	51
Avoid painful movements	67	69

Based on data from Linton et al. (2002b).

Unique to the individual

Although I highlight the general principles involved in the development of a persistent problem, it is important to emphasize that the process is in point of fact unique to each individual. What is more, the differences between people may be quite large. While anxiety and fear avoidance may be important for one person, monotonous work and a poor relationship with a supervisor may be decisive for another. Likewise, the pertinent risk factors may change over time. For example, anxiety and fear may be crucial in the acute stage, while depression and catastrophizing may become more important as the problem becomes nonrelenting. The time line may be different as well. While one person may fall into a persistent problem relatively quickly, another may struggle for years before the problem becomes chronic. The path to a persistent problem, then, is distinctive for each person.

Gradual lifestyle changes

The recurrent nature of back pain allows ample opportunities for learning, but a key appears to be that changes occur so slowly that the individual does not realize the devastating effects and therefore allows the development to continue. The process is gradual. Rather than the "straight line" often depicted in the literature, the road to persistent pain is crooked. It is not unusual to have some periods with little or no pain. With small alterations taking place during bouts of pain, a change in lifestyle may occur. However, because of the gradual nature of the change, the person may not be aware of the process until a major development is already a fact. Bear in mind that gradual changes in lifestyle are particularly difficult to perceive, as was presented in Chapter 7. Therefore, on a cognitive-perceptual level, individuals may not become aware of the type and size of the change until it is quite advanced.

Contributing to this is the expectation that the pain will reside quickly and "normality" will soon be restored. Patients may thereby incorporate coping strategies such as rest, taking medications and the reduction of social activities because they believe they will only be temporary. As an illustration, a father who normally plays with his small children each day upon returning home from work may stop doing so when faced with back pain. He may believe that the pain will soon subside and then the play may be resumed exactly in its usual form. While this is but one small lifestyle change involving a few minutes, it is quite likely that other small changes will be made in other sectors of this man's life. When these small changes are pieced together they involve a major change. The gradual character of the change may then

shortcut feedback so that the problem continues to develop.

The role of injury and its resultant pain

Psychological models might be criticized because they always seem to assume that an injury has occurred, but often ignore this injury once the nociception has been initiated. Indeed, many psychological models seem devoid of the role of nociception. Nevertheless, we know that the intensity, duration and quality of the pain seem to influence our psychological reaction. Thus, an intense "jolt" of pain is experienced very differently than a mild "ache".

These nuances have direct relevance for our understanding of the development of long-term pain problems. First, as we saw in Part I, pain sensations generate reactions including central emotional processes. Intense pain that is quite unlike earlier pain experiences is, for example, linked to fear and worry. This may in turn elicit beliefs (it must be dangerous or it wouldn't hurt so much). In addition, worry enhances vigilance which influences whether pain signals will be detected. Vigilance and worry, if sufficiently strong, are said to result in misinterpretations, i.e. where nonpainful signals such as pressure of movement are interpreted as painful. So the intensity of the pain is likely to influence development since it is related to so many aspects of the pain experience.

Second, the pain signals from an injury are related to how the problem might best be dealt with. Coping is postulated to be directly related to the idiosyncrasies of the pain sensations. Distraction may work wonderfully to cope with low-intensity pain, but might be relatively useless for very intense pain. This may be the direct result of the fact that intense pain physiologically is programmed to elicit our attention or to the fact that it is difficult to initiate or maintain many types of coping such as distraction as intensity increases.

Critical events

Certain critical events seem to account for the apparent "jumps" in the development of long-term pain problems. Learning does not ordinarily occur at a smooth even tempo. Performance tends to stagnate and then is followed by an abrupt improvement. This is typical of most skills such as learning to read or play the guitar. Sometimes these jumps are triggered by certain events. In our discussion, critical events are decisive experiences that result in a new belief and/or behavior, or a "jump" in the enhancement of it. In this section we will concentrate on negative thoughts and behaviors, but "positive" critical events also apply to the recovery process. A negative critical event might occur when a patient attempts to return to work and the supervisor states, "Your back is too weak for this work". This event might be critical in changing the patient's beliefs about his or her back and ability to work ("If my supervisor doesn't believe I can do the job, I must be in really bad shape").

Another example might involve a visit to a healthcare practitioner. Let us assume that the person with back pain expects to get something to relieve the pain and that the pain will go away within a few days. The provider, however, states that there is probably degeneration in the spine and that the person needs to rest to protect the back. This might trigger a dramatic change in beliefs and behavior where the patient now begins to entertain the thought that the pain may not subside, that permanent functional problems will develop and that it is necessary to restrict movement in order to "save" on wear and tear.

Critical events emphasize that development occurs in hops, leaps and bounds rather than in an even, linear fashion. The increments may be of various sizes. Here again, we see the individual nature of the development, as the exact events that trigger the critical events appear to be peculiar to the individual.

Dynamic process

The development of a persistent pain problem is by its very nature vibrant. However, to date, most models of chronic pain have been rather static, probably because such models are easier to understand and test. Consequently, if we are to understand how and why chronic pain develops, we need to consider longitudinal aspects. Static models are quite good at isolating important variables and demonstrating links between them. This is vital for understanding which factors are involved in the development. However, static models are poor at elucidating the *process* involved. Indeed, if we consider the number of variables that may be important in the development of chronic pain and then multiply them by a time unit such as hours or days, a tremendous number of events can occur. To understand development, then, we need to know more about how these processes start and progress. A good model will incorporate dynamic aspects, although we certainly could not expect a detailed description of every possible road to a chronic problem.

Learning is an important concept as it incorporates a dynamic view. Thus, the person's interaction with pain as well as the interaction with the environment is included in a learning approach. Modern theories of learning include cognitive and emotional aspects. Their advantage is that they serve as an aid in understanding the dynamics of the process since different stimuli, thoughts, emotions, behaviors and consequences may be placed into the scheme. In this way an individual's situation may be entered into the scheme and analyzed to determine a reasonable explanation for the development. At the present, however, it is more difficult to generate scenarios of common paths for the development of persistent pain disability. Such information is vital in order to be able to identify people at risk of developing persistent pain as well as to develop effective preventive interventions. As a result, more work needs to be done so that we may understand better how a persistent problem develops.

Overview of why chronic pain may develop

The development of long-term pain problems is a complex, multidimensional process where psychological factors in an interaction with the environment play an important role in enhancing or catalyzing the development of the problem. The evidence suggests that once a painful injury occurs, the environment impacts and shapes our behavior, emotions and cognitions through psychological factors. These in turn influence the course of development. Usually this is advantageous and quite often the person copes adequately and recovers. However, sometimes the process results in further development of the problem. Thus, psychological factors interplay with other types of variables. Rather than being static, the development involves a dynamic process where critical events trigger changes in beliefs and behavior. Small resultant changes in lifestyle may then gradually proceed without alarming the individual since they do not perceive the change. The recurrent nature of musculoskeletal pain is an important element as it presents numerous opportunities for learning.

Thus, psychological factors are important in the development of a persistent pain problem. They are comparatively powerful in predicting disability and they may offer important insights as to how such problems might be prevented.

IMPLICATIONS

Even though the model in this chapter is far from complete, it nevertheless synthesizes our current knowledge on how and why chronic pain and disability occurs. This model paves the way for new and better methods for managing pain and disability.

Targets

My model of the process of development indicates one decisive truth: *if psychological factors are truly a key part of the problem, then addressing these factors might be an effective intervention.* Rather than exclusively choosing medical targets such as pain relief or increased mobility, psychological aspects are important goals for intervention.

We may first wish to think about the implications for the goals we set in caring for our patients. My model, supported by the literature reviewed above, emphasizes the tremendous importance of dealing with the psychological aspects of the problem. This means tending to the behavioral, emotional and cognitive aspects as well as the biological ones. Consequently, it may be as important to set targets for resuming activities as it is to have goals for decreasing pain intensity. Likewise, it may be crucial to deal with a patient's fears and worries in order to maintain good quality of life. Moreover, since these factors are all part of an integrated system (as shown in Part I), dealing with the correct targets may gain benefits in a variety of areas. Therefore, if psychological factors are driving the process forward, this may well necessitate interventions that address these.

Early identification and intervention

One advantage that this model has, is that the process of development presents many opportunities for early intervention. Moreover, it suggests that the path to chronic pain is by no means a set one. It is pliable; it may be stopped. As a consequence we would do our patients a great service by helping them to alter development in the direction of a chronic problem. In other words, we might apply the knowledge we have to provide early, preventive interventions. There is no obvious reason to wait until the problem becomes established and persistent. There is every reason to begin early on when opportunities for change are greater, and the pattern is not yet well established.

How might we best achieve early interventions? It is a troublesome question because so many people suffer some sort of pain problem. In fact, nearly everyone at some time in their life has a problem with their back. How could we possibly provide early interventions for all? The answer is in a systematic approach to care.

The subsequent chapters in this book deal with providing the right intervention, to the right person, at the right time point. In a nutshell, we will see that psychological factors may help us identify patients who are likely to develop persistent pain and disability. Thus, we may then concentrate our limited resources on the "right patient". Moreover, we will explore how the application of psychological aspects can be incorporated into "normal" patient care so that we indeed may identify problems and targets early on. We will look at simple methods to employ at the very first visit, as well as more advanced methods that may be needed once the process has advanced. By putting this system together, we might well dramatically improve our care and empower patients to best manage their pain.

CHAPTER 10

Communicating with patients

LEARNING OBJECTIVES

To understand:

- that good communication enhances understanding, compliance and patient satisfaction;
- that patient models of their pain steer their expectations of assessment, prognosis and treatment;
- that patients usually seek care to obtain an explanation, reassurance about the seriousness of the problem, information about reactivation (function) and pain relief (cure);
- common reasons why professionals do not implement psychological factors into their practice.

To obtain skills:

- in developing a "shared understanding" of the problem with your patient;
- in empathizing with your patient;
- in educating your patient;
- in engaging your patient to active participation;
- in specific types of interviewing skills to obtain pertinent psychological information.

Of all the techniques that may be available for enhancing treatment effects, communication is probably the most valuable. It is a prerequisite for nearly all pain treatments, particularly those with a focus on self-help or psychosocial issues. If the patient does not understand, believe or feel engaged, it is unlikely that she or he will follow the treatment advice or be satisfied. In fact, a surprising number of outcomes improve for a wide variety of ailments when healthcare professionals communicate effectively (Stewart, 1995; Di Blasi et al., 2001). Moreover, communication is the principal determinant in patient satisfaction with care. When communication is effective, patients perceive the care they are receiving as being a high-quality intervention and they are generally quite satisfied (Piasecki, 2003). Conversely, the main reason patients give for low satisfaction is poor communication (Worthlin, 1995). Finally, adherence to follow advice is enhanced by good communication (Piasecki, 2003).

Communication skills encompass psychological aspects of pain and certainly can be learned. These skills lend us a hand so that we may understand better the patient's situation and needs. They facilitate empowering the patient. By achieving clear communication we may establish a "shared understanding" with the patient of the problem, its likely cause, and avenues for intervention. What is more, these skills assist us in establishing relevant goals and targets. Fortunately, we can all improve our communication skills by honing some relatively simple behaviors.

In this chapter we will explore how we might better communicate with our patients. We will examine some models that will help us to grasp what patients want from a clinical visit as well as what might disrupt communication. Then basic skills will be brought forward that are known to enhance communication in a healthcare situation.

DISTORTED COMMUNICATION—A TWO WAY STREET!

Communication is truly a two-way street. It involves the healthcare professional as well as the patient. Both come into the situation with certain expectations, beliefs, worries and so on that may have an impact on how effective the communication is. To exemplify this, consider how Hank communicates with his doctor in the example below. It is also illustrated in Fig. 10.1.

As illustrated in the figure, when Hank is going to the doctor he is really worried about his back and wondering what is wrong. He holds several "fear avoidance" beliefs, some catastrophizing, and he is quite vigilant to the pain and suspects that the vertebrae are chipped or ragged-edged causing damage to the muscles and nerves that are tearing against them. The doctor ordered images of Hank's back and the purpose of the visit is to see the results. However, the cognitive and emotional aspects of Hank's problem are going to affect his communication. Although Hank is normally a good listener, the state he is in will significantly affect what he hears and how he interprets this. In turn, this will affect what Hank gets out of the consultation, the message he takes home.

First, patients remember only a small proportion of what is said during a consultation. Studies suggest that some information is never taken in, while other parts are quickly forgotten. As a rule of thumb, roughly 25% of what we say to a patient will not be registered. An additional 25% will be forgotten before the patient leaves the clinic. Thus, only about half of the information we provide may actually be remembered. And what is remembered will be subject to interpretation.

The message taken home after a consultation is influenced by two major factors that are steered by our cognitive and emotional state. The first is *selective listening*. This means paying more attention to parts of the conversation that are of particular interest. In Hank's case, he will be likely to pay more attention when the doctor talks about things that address his fears and worries, such as something being wrong with the vertebrae. Further, he may take in more readily aspects that relate to or support his cognitive beliefs, for instance, that a wrong move might be harmful. In a sense, Hank's ears grow to elephant size when the doctor speaks about the spinal cord and what might

Communication depends on the patient and HCP!

Anxiety
Fear
Vigilance
Fear avoidance

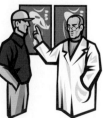

Anxiety, Fear—mistakes
Fear—Hank's reaction
Desire to treat
Desire to be professional

Selective listening
Misinterpretation

Unclear
Double messages

Figure 10.1 An illustration of factors affecting the communication between Hank and his doctor. Note that emotional reactions influence how clear the message is as well as how it is interpreted.

be wrong with it. On the other hand, his ears seem to diminish to "mouse ears" when the doctor addresses other aspects like the fact that the changes observed are normal or that exercise would be helpful. As may be deduced, the emotional fear and worry in connection with the beliefs steer what is heard as well as how it might be interpreted. Simply put, we naturally fit new information into our own model of what we believe.

The second factor influencing the message taken home is *misinterpretation of ambiguous information*. As with selective listening, this is a normal process that we all use to filter and process information efficiently. When a message is not clear, our psychological state colors our interpretation. Consequently, when a neutral or vague statement is made, it will be interpreted negatively. Imagine a doctor telling you that "we do not know for sure what the long-term prognosis is, but people manage". How might you interpret this message? A catastrophizer would certainly judge this to mean that there is a big risk he will not get better and in fact that he probably will get much worse.

Vague information may simply be unclear, but in healthcare settings it frequently contains *double messages*. Because we may not be certain ourselves or do not want to take responsibility, we may provide information that actually has two opposite messages. Let us imagine that a patient asks whether he may go skiing given his current back condition. The physical therapist replies: "Being active is good for your back, but you wouldn't want to overdo it." How might this statement be construed? Again, if the patient is anxious or fearful about movements leading to injury, it would be understood in a negative way: don't go skiing! Medical situations present great challenges in providing clear messages since the answer to patients' questions often depend on the circumstances. For example, the physical therapist might provide such a statement (above) because she feels that shorter cross-country skiing would be fine, while it might be too early to do the hard training professionals undergo. Yet, for the patient, the nuances disappear and the message is interpreted negatively.

Like the patient, the healthcare professional is also influenced by emotional and cognitive factors when communicating. We have seen earlier that healthcare professionals may hold some of the same cognitive fear-avoidance beliefs as do patients (Linton et al., 2002b) and these may be reflected in the information provided. Returning to the example, this may also affect the doctor and consequently he may be feeling apprehensive. He wants to convey that the images are normal. However, because he is not sure what is actually causing the pain, he feels uncomfortable. In part, this seems unprofessional: a doctor should know what

is causing the pain. Further, the doctor is sensitive to the patient's feelings and does not want to suggest that "nothing is wrong" with his back. Thus, he feels pressured to provide some sort of explanation. Moreover, the doctor needs to tie this explanation to a treatment; but not really knowing what is wrong makes this very difficult. In the end, these worries, expectations and pressures may greatly influence what the doctor tells the patient as well as how well he listens to the patient's responses. We see that the feelings and beliefs the doctor has here sets the stage for diffuse and quick explanations that a patient may not understand. It is also very easy to provide double messages since the doctor is not clear what the message should be.

PATIENT MODELS OF THEIR PAIN

Patients often have ideas about what is wrong with their back, but these models may be surprisingly naïve. The way patients view their problem—their understanding and misconceptions—guides how receptive they are in communication. Further, these models influence the expectations the patient has in terms of what information is *relevant*. Finally, comprehending the patient's model will help you to better understand the patient's questions and responses. In short, if we understand the patient's model we will be in a better position to communicate.

Yet most healthcare professionals do not understand patient models very well. Schooled in anatomy and physiology we, in comparison to most patients, have extensive knowledge about the way the body works. Our picture of the spine, for instance, is shaped by the pictures, descriptions, films, etc., we have seen and experienced during our training. As a result there is a risk that professionals will underrate or not perceive the concerns of the patient. Because we know that the pain is not a serious threat to health, we may not listen to the patient or understand the patient's concerns. For example, back pain is not fatal and is very rarely attributable to serious disease. But in failing to recognize the patient's model of the problem, we miss important opportunities to communicate and educate. To be sure, failing to grasp the patient's model is to preempt a mutual understanding of the pain problem.

On the other hand, most lay people have a diffuse and inaccurate picture of how their back actually works. To exemplify this I asked students in a psychology class to correctly position a model of two vertebrae with regard to their placement in the body. That is, I asked them to identify which side was inward and which was the outer part we feel when we touch our backs. These students are well educated and grade pointwise among the top students at the university. Although guessing would provide 50% correct, the

CASE STUDY: HANK

Excerpts from the consultation where Hank's doctor explains the results of the imaging tests. Thoughts and interpretations are presented within parentheses.

Hank	Doctor
"So, what exactly did you find?"	*"Well, fortunately no serious damage was found."*
(Hank does not register this as he is focusing on what is wrong with the disk.)	*"There is some degeneration in the L4–L5 area here."* (Points to image.)
(Hank tunes into "degeneration of disk" because it confirms his beliefs!)	*"But this is typical for someone of your age."*
"Oh." (Doesn't quite register as still thinking about ramifications of degeneration. I have worked hard, no wonder this is happening. Hank fears severe functional problems are ahead.)	*"Pain like yours is common and might be caused by the hard work you've been doing, the muscles, or because your back is not quite aligned."*
"I see." (Hank interprets: I should not work, this could be harmful. My back is not only degenerating, but out of line. I at least need an adjustment.)	
"What should I do about it?" (What is the treatment? Adjustment, surgery?)	*"It's good if you can remain active, but you might want to take it a little easy for a few days."*
(Rest until it gets better and the pain goes away.) *"Can I lift things?"*	*"Um, this varies from person to person. You can try to lift some and see what you can manage."*
(Be careful; stop if it hurts.) *"What is the treatment?"*	(Doctor feels pressured and apprehensive.) *"Unfortunately, our options are limited. How much pain are you having?"*
"Quite a lot. I can't hardly do anything and I can't sleep at night either."	
(Hank grimaces and his body language says HELP!)	(Feeling more pressured to do something, but uncertain as to what is best.)
	"I'd like you to try this medication. It is a good pain reliever." (Gets prescription block.)
(This reinforces Hank's pain behavior. The message is: your back is so bad you need more medication.)	*"Here is a prescription that will last you three months with the refills."*
"Thanks a lot doctor." (I must really have a problem if I get medications for three months. I thought it would only take a couple of weeks to get better. How will I ever be able to work?)	

actual number was only 60%! Research shows that the general public has very crude notions of how things inside their bodies work (Linton, 1991, 1992; Asmundson et al., 2001). Yet patients develop ideas and beliefs about what is wrong with their backs. Again, these models are notable because they direct expectations about assessment and communication.

Six basic concepts of back pain

To get a better idea of how patients with back pain view the cause of their problem, we extensively interviewed eight patients (Linton and Boersma, 2004). All of these patients had suffered from back pain a longer period of time and two of them had been "successfully" treated surgically. We asked them a series of open-ended questions to delve into their own conception of their pain problem.

We were then able to reduce what the patients told us to six basic notions:

1. My back pain is mechanical

First, patients had a clear mechanical view of their back and the cause of the pain. No mistake could be made, the back was constructed like a machine. In fact, it was frequently referred to in such terms, and it was also compared to machines such as a car. This is in contrast to the view that the back is a highly evolved biological entity.

2. Something is broken

Second, the pain was seen as being caused by something being broken. Physiological causes were not entertained. As an example, none of the patients made comparisons with other physiological disease processes by likening it to, for instance, a cold or the flu. Instead, the causes involved broken parts.

One model presented, for example, was that the disk was much like a balloon filled with liquid to provide padding between the vertebrae. However, the disk had been punctured—much like the pinprick of a balloon—and the liquid had run out. The consequence was that the vertebrae were now touching each other; grinding and tearing with each movement.

Another patient presented this model. He said that the bones in his back somehow were locked together. He pictured that one bone became hooked around another. This happened when he overexerted himself. Thus, his back periodically became "locked" in place and he lost mobility.

A final example also concerned the bones, the vertebrae. This patient described her back as having gravel in it. More specifically, she reported that there must be pieces of material (bone, sediment or something) in between two of the vertebrae. Each movement meant tearing, grinding and wear. She likened her back problem to putting sand in a mechanical clockwork.

3. A concrete "fix" is needed (or it will be permanent)

To remedy the situation, there was consensus that their back needed to be fixed concretely. Without this "fix", the problem would plainly persist. Given the views above (see 1 and 2), such fixes were seen to be tangible interventions. These were directed toward the believed problem. For instance, the patient viewing his back as being locked pictured manipulation as being a potent method for "unlocking" it. Likewise, the patient reporting gravel in her back imagined that surgery or injections were needed to remove or dissolve these.

4. Emotionally charged

Fourth, the descriptions of the model were quite emotionally charged. This was observed in two ways. In the first instance, these patients used very emotional adjectives to describe their back pain. Typical words were "cutting", "jabbing", "stabbing", "burning" and "shooting". Common phrases were "it feels like someone is pounding a hammer", "chopping with an ax", or "poking a hot needle" into my back. Contemplate what any one of these examples actually implies. Certainly, nerves on fire or having a knife stabbed into your back are terrifying and distressing thoughts.

Emotional aspects were also cogently present as patients described their frustrations. In essence, patients said they experienced their back pain as a horrible/serious problem, but yet they were unable to control it or obtain appropriate help. Obvious signs of distress, heightened vigilance and negative thought patterns were present when patients described how difficult it was to understand their problem and obtain suitable help.

5. Guides expectations about care

The models patients revealed were related to their expectations about proper care. As seen above, patients believed that a tangible fix was needed to cure the problem. However, the models also influenced their perceptions of what might constitute a good assessment and even what types of questions would be appropriate from the doctor or physical therapist. For example, patients had high expectations that the healthcare provider would do a thorough physical exam to locate the cause of the problem.

Interestingly, although patients had mechanical models, they expected a discussion of the psychosocial consequences of the problem. As an example, patients thought that it was quite proper for a healthcare provider to ask about the work and home situation since these were highly affected by the pain problem. Patients viewed these questions as complementary to the physical exam.

6. Incorporate health information to prove model is true

Finally, patients were clever at incorporating the information they received from healthcare providers as "proof" that their model was correct. Patients quoted what doctors and others had said to illustrate and support the model. The examples patients used illustrate the nuances of the communication process.

- "The doctor said my back is pretty much worn out [fill in: "degenerated", "out of alignment", "too mobile", etc.]. It is no wonder, I have worked so long at that job".

- "I suspected there was something really wrong, and the doctor said the disks were shriveled up and didn't provide the cushioning they should".
- "My back is a wreck; my chiropractor said that a nerve is pinched between the bones and that's why I have these terrible pains".
- "I was right about the cause of my back pain, my doctor said it's really a mess. He can't understand how I've been able to work this long".

We see in these examples that information from healthcare professionals has been incorporated into the models as a sort of proof that they are correct.

Effects on communication

The models patients have of their back pain appear to be closely linked with communication. Earlier we looked at how beliefs and emotions affected communication such as in the selection of information that is remembered. The models of a health problem that we may have are linked to how we select information in communication. The six concepts above then may be utilized to help us understand what kinds of information are going to be relevant. That is, by understanding the model, we may better predict what the patient is likely to hear and remember in a discussion. Moreover, we will have important information concerning how the patient might interpret bits of information provided in the conversation. Finally, we might better anticipate what sorts of questions and misconceptions the patient may have.

WHY PATIENTS SEEK CARE

The reason why patients seek care is often related as much to worrying about the condition as it is to the symptoms themselves. Certainly this is true for back pain. Although patients may focus on the pain and other symptoms when asked, deciding whether or not to seek care is often driven by psychosocial factors. Almost everyone has at some time experienced a backache. Yet only a relatively small number will decide to seek care. Why? As you will recall from Part I, pain that is experienced in a very different way catches our attention and in the process also enhances fear and worry. Imagine having suffered some back pain such as the usual muscle ache of overexertion from raking leaves. Now consider pain that feels like a burning wound and that shoots down your leg. Moreover, this pain makes it extremely difficult for you to move about at will; you feel tremendous pain when bending over and when lifting the lightest of materials. Because this pain is so different from previous experiences it draws our attention to it and worry levels increase. Catastrophic thoughts may ensue. Now let us suppose

that a family member encourages you to seek help, you may well do so. Thus, new symptoms that attract our attention and prompt worry are likely to be a reason for seeking consultation.

If a complex array of psychological and physical factors motivate the patient to seek care, what then does the patient want from the consultation? Research has indicated five basic things (Turner et al., 1998; Von Korff, 1999) and they are summarized in Fig. 10.2. Although the reasons in the figure are not in any particular order, a logical first reason to seek care is the reduction of pain. Patients seeking primary care facilities for an acute bout of their pain often report relatively high levels of pain intensity (Cherkin et al., 1996; Turner et al., 1998; van den Hoogen et al., 1998). Thus, patients want pain relief or at least pain reduction. Further, patients are normally anxious and concerned about the cause of their pain. They wonder if something is seriously wrong. If you will, they want a diagnosis or explanation of why it hurts. It is important to understand that patients are not particularly interested in the medical name of the disorder, but rather want to understand why they are feeling this "unusual" and often intense pain. Third, patients may be quite concerned about the progress of their problem and in reinjuring themselves. Patients wonder quite candidly what the best course for recovery is. This involves mundane questions such as whether one should rest and whether doing certain activities will result in injury. Fourth, patients want to know how they can regain function. Again, most patients with acute bouts of back pain have considerable problems with some everyday activities like putting on their shoes or carrying grocery bags. Fifth, patients want to know about the possibility of a "cure", in other words, what the prognosis is as well as what treatment options are available.

Interestingly, Table 10.1 shows that the most frequent reason for seeking care was *not* pain reduction (Turner et al., 1998; Von Korff, 1999). Note that the most common medical treatments are actually less sought out than clear information on the cause of the pain and reassurance that it is not serious. For example,

Purpose of seeking care

1. Reduce pain
2. Anxious about cause
3. Fear of injury
4. Improve function
5. Can it be fixed? (prognosis)

Figure 10.2 The most important reasons patients give for seeking healthcare for back pain.

Table 10.1 A summary of the reasons given for seeking healthcare for patients with back pain.

Aim for the healthcare visit	% of patients
Receive	
Diagnosis	68
Reassurance not a serious disease	52
Medical cure	51
Prescription medication	35
Excused (certified) absence for work	12
To receive information on	
How to manage back pain	85
How to reduce pain without drugs	83
Return to normal activities	81
How to prevent recurrence of back pain	76

Adapted from Von Korff (1999).

getting a prescription was only rated as important by 35%. Similarly, a referral to a physical therapist was important for 30% and a sick leave excuse (certificate) only 12%. Thus, patients find it very important to receive an explanation of the problem and reassurance.

Study the list of desired information provided in Table 10.1. Patients reported that they were interested in receiving various types of information. Among these, how to manage the pain (with or without medications) was highly valued (85%) while information on how to return to activities was a close second (81%). Interestingly, information on how to prevent a recurrence of the back pain was also very important (76%). This study recorded the actual visit to the doctor and then analyzed these audiotapes. Despite the patient's aims for the visit and informational needs, the study finds that these are often not met (Turner et al., 1998; Von Korff, 1999). Moreover, when these needs are met it is often the patient who prompts them as physicians were mainly oriented toward assessing the pain symptoms. In short, the desires and needs of patients are not always met and there is a real need for better communication.

COMMUNICATION, THE CONTEXT OF TREATMENT, AND OUTCOME

The "placebo effect"

Although placebo effects are often seen as a problem that confuses treatment or an unstable effect of a naïve and gullible patient, new research demonstrates that the context in which we deliver treatment is a principal determinant of its effectiveness. Indeed, the so-called placebo provides new insights into the patient–provider relationship and the principles of effective communication.

One of the most legendary effects in medicine is the so-called *placebo effect*. This refers to patients obtaining a treatment effect when they believe they have been given a potent treatment, but when in fact the treatment is inert. A typical example is providing a patient with a sugar pill or an injection of salt water instead of an active pain analgesic. Many times such "placebos" provide pain relief. Early on a variety of healthcare providers as well as healers, witch doctors and the like saw the potential of this effect in clinical practice. A book was published in 1917 that illustrates this interest. It was written for medical practitioners and was entitled *Suggestive Therapeutics* (Munro, 1917). In this book, the author describes a variety of methods to suggest to patients that given health improvements would be observed. This was one attempt to harness psychological forces including the placebo effect.

The "placebo" effect came into disrepute for two reasons. First, many treatments through the years have made wild claims about effectiveness and have asserted a specific mechanism. However, scientific examination has shown many such claims to be false; the treatments in fact did not possess an effect above and beyond the "placebo". Giving certain drugs asserted to be wonder drugs, for example, has been shown to be no more pain relief than an inert pill. Thus, the "placebo" effect became an obstacle to scientifically demonstrating a treatment effect. Moreover, the placebo became a benchmark from which to judge effectiveness. Secondly, placebo effects were "psychologized" so that they became mystical and imaginary. It seemed to suggest that the patient was weak, naïve and not intelligent. Moreover, since the placebo was seen as almost magical, the effect could not be "real pain relief", nor could it last very long. Thus, placebo effects were to be avoided on scientific as well as "ethical" or good practice grounds. However, a reexamination of the facts and modern research have greatly changed our view!

Placebo effects depend on treatment delivery

The concept of placebo suggests that the effect is magically caused by the patient's gullibility, but we now know that it depends on the context of treatment. Thus, the inert pill has no inherent effect, but the way it is administered does. It is not a matter of "tricking" the patient, but rather of providing the treatment in an effective manner. Indeed, it may be said that the effect depends on clear communication that assures and creates a positive expectancy (Benedetti, 2003).

Because the placebo has been viewed as trickery, we may wonder whether it should be utilized in the clinic. It is understandable that clinicians may feel uncomfortable about using such methods and ethical guidelines exist that control the use of placebo techniques. However, in our context, this effect is related to providing clear information and appropriate expectations. By providing good communication, the added effects of expectancy are built in.

In fact, many scientists want to discard the word placebo to underscore the true nature of the phenomenon. For example, Moerman (2002) has strongly argued that the term placebo is misleading since it focuses on an inert treatment, while the true effect is due to the context and the meaning around the treatment. In fact, recent reviews are clear in drawing the conclusion that the context of the treatment, that is, how the treatment is administered and how the healthcare provider–patient interaction occurs, determines the effect on health outcomes (Di Blasi et al., 2001; Benedetti, 2002). When a treatment is given, the healthcare providers' *"words, attitudes, and behavior play an important role in what effect the treatment has"* (Benedetti, 2002, p. 135).

The power of the healthcare provider–patient interaction can have enormous effects. In a classic study conducted in primary care with a variety of patients, Thomas (1987) compared either (1) providing the patient with either an obvious diagnosis and an assurance that the therapy would provide unmistakable relief, or (2) a message that the diagnosis was tentative and the effect of the treatment in doubt. In fact, patients were given the same actual treatments. How did this influence outcome? An evaluation was conducted two weeks later and the group receiving clear reassurance of the effects of the treatment had recovered significantly better than those receiving the uncertain information.

Other studies show that an affirmative suggestion of pain relief has a powerful analgesic effect. In studies of dental patients having a molar extracted, the power of this effect is clearly demonstrated. For example, in one series of studies it was found that the open injection of saline water (salt water with no analgesic effect), provided with the information that the injection would provide relief, in fact gave as much pain reduction as the hidden (computer administered via a tube, patients do not know if, when or how much will be administered) administration of 8 mg of morphine (Levine et al., 1981; Levine and Gordon, 1984). Put another way, openly injecting a patient with a substance that is described as a painkiller (actually saline solution) is as potent as 8 mg of morphine.

The conclusion is drawn that an open injection of morphine, with the information that it is a good pain reliever, is more effective than a hidden injection of the same size *because of the context variables ("placebo" effect)*.

Consider another example that focuses on the effects of communication with the patient and perceived pain intensity. In this study patients with postoperative pain volunteered to participate in a study about postoperative pain treatment. All participants were given an intravenous (IV) administration of a saline solution (inert). In one group, the patients were given no additional information. However, in the second group participants were told that the IV could either be a "potent painkiller or a placebo with no effect". Finally, the third group received a clear message: "You are receiving a painkiller and your pain will soon subside." The results showed a substantial effect of the communication. When patients were provided with an expectation of pain relief, actual pain ratings were lower. In further work it was established that the same level of pain reduction could be attained with considerably smaller doses of medication when patients were provided the expectation that pain relief was imminent (Pollo et al., 2001).

Interestingly enough, the opposite effect of a placebo may be achieved with poor communication. This effect is called nocebo and refers to an increase in pain not directly related to increased tissue damage. In the same way that positive and trust-inducing contexts produce placebo, negative and fearful contexts produce nocebo (Hahn, 1997). Many patients, for instance, have experienced terrible pain during procedures that are relatively painless because of fear and the expectation that it will be painful.

Consequently, the effects of any treatment are in part dependent on the context and atmosphere in which they occur. This greatly influences the expectations and anticipation the patient has. While these effects are often considered to "be in the patient's head" or simply "not real", compelling evidence is accumulating to show that part of the "placebo" effect is related to changes in the brain. In short, the expectation stimulates the brain to release pain-relieving endorphins, the body's natural painkillers. Thus, the placebo is an excellent example of how communication skills may positively impact on pain. Further, it is an outstanding demonstration of how the biological, cognitive, emotional and behavioral systems are integrated.

COMMUNICATION SKILLS

Everyone can improve their communication skills. We have already seen that such skills are appreciated by patients and help to improve patient satisfaction as well as outcome. In this section we will examine the basics of good communication with pain patients. There are several models for presenting this material and we will pursue the main points (Keller and Carroll, 1994; Ottosson, 1999; Piasecki, 2003).

Developing a shared understanding

Effective communication means connecting with the patient and building a partnership. This working relationship builds on a shared understanding of what the problem is, its likely cause, and good methods for tackling the problem. Most patients are very willing to engage positively and they appreciate collaboration with the healthcare provider.

Making contact

The first few minutes of the visit are extremely important as they set the tone for the communication and the patient forms an opinion of the potential value of the visit. "Joining" is the concept of connecting with the patient. This is facilitated by a sincere greeting, e.g. "Nice to see you." Making eye contact and a smile are critical in setting a warm and friendly tone to the atmosphere. To be successful in joining with the patient, it is important to communicate your interest in the patient—to show that it is the person and not the disorder that is important. One way to show this is to converse briefly about another topic (for example, "How is the fishing [or other hobby] going, catch any big ones?"). Showing interest in the patient as a person helps to set them at ease and it builds an environment for open communication.

Setting the agenda

While patients have certain expectations for their visit, the patient typically does not arrive at the appointment with a thought-through agenda. However, patients do come with a story to tell and several concerns. Yet in a normal healthcare situation the patient may only get the opportunity to air one concern. This is because many clinicians use communication styles where the professional "takes over" the discussion and begins to ask a series of "yes/no" questions. Although such questions are sometimes valuable in making a diagnosis, they are inexcusable at the beginning of a visit because they stifle open communication. The result may be a frustrated patient. Moreover, it may result in a frustrated clinician when the patient then brings up a new problem just as the visit was ending.

Ask open-ended questions

The best way to help patients articulate their concerns is to ask open-ended questions. These queries cannot be answered with one or two words, but require some explanation. Several illustrations of the difference

Table 10.2 Open-ended versus directed questioning. Open-ended queries elicit the patient's concerns and help us to schedule our time during a visit. Here are examples of each type of question.

Directed question	Open-ended question
Are you having a lot of pain today?	Could you tell me about how much pain you've been experiencing lately?
Do you take any pills for the pain?	Tell me what kinds of things you do to relieve your pain.
How many pills do you take for the attacks?	Describe for me what is going on when you get these attacks.
So, the pain is your main problem?	How are you feeling otherwise?
Are you able to work?	Tell me more about how the pain is affecting you, like how you are functioning.

between directed questions and open-ended ones are shown in Table 10.2. Notice that the directed questions can all be easily answered with a yes or no or a number, while the open-ended ones require some explanation. This provides an opportunity for the patient to express their concerns and tell you their story.

Listening and confirming

One consultant in communication skills for professionals maintains that there are three steps to good communication: listen, *listen* and listen. In fact, given the time constraints as well as the need to obtain specific information so that a proper diagnosis can be made, it is not surprising that we professionals may find it difficult to listen. However, a relatively short period at the beginning of a visit spent listening and communicating with the patient will save considerable time and effort later on.

Listening means paying attention to what the patient is saying. This is communicated with body language (eye contact, nodding to indicate you have understood, not allowing one to be disturbed, etc.). Looking in the journal or at a computer screen says that these items are more important than what the patient is saying. Also, allowing interruptions such as telephone calls to interfere sends the message that you do not have time for the patient, or that other things are more important. Take the time to listen.

Another central way of letting the patient know you are listening and have understood the problem is *confirmation*. This amounts to summarizing what you have heard to check with the patient that this is correct. It is a way of acknowledging the patient's story. This is typically done periodically during this phase of the visit with short rephrasing:

- "It sounds like your pain is getting worse and this is the reason you have had difficulty working."
- "If I understand your description, this therapy does not seem to be helping you."
- "So, your pain doesn't seem to get worse when you are a bit more active. Is that correct?"

By rephrasing and summarizing you recognize the patient's problem, and confirm that you have really listened to what he or she is saying. Moreover, by gaining the patient's approval of your summary you help to build a shared understanding of the problem. In other words, there is mutual confirmation of the nature of the problem.

Prompting sensitive information

Every pain problem has an emotional, cognitive and behavioral side, but patients are not always skilled at presenting these aspects. In part, this may be because the patient does not expect that you will be interested in these aspects. It may also be due to a lack of training in presenting such aspects in a clear way. And it may be related to the patient's fear that the problem will not be taken seriously if psychological aspects are mentioned. In turn, patients many times signal psychological aspects, but we professionals do not pick up on them. This may be because we do not interpret the message properly or choose to ignore the message because we are not prepared to deal with such issues. Yet this entire book focuses on the value of working with the entire pain problem, including the psychological aspects. How might we use general communication skills to facilitate this?

Prompting is a good technique to help get psychosocial issues on the plan for the visit. In the next section we will discuss other techniques that help to establish rapport with the patient, but here we will focus specifically on bringing up such topics and placing them on the schedule. *Prompting* is a method that lets your patient know that you are interested in sensitive, psychological aspects. It is an active way to help the patient formulate the issue:

- "Sometimes a pain problem can affect other parts of your life, like your mood or your sexual functioning. Do you have any such concerns?"
- "Is there anything else you would like to bring up today?"

- "Pain is often hard to deal with. Tell me about the consequences it is having on the rest of your life".

These phrases open the door for a patient to tell you their concerns. It sends the message that it is proper to talk about such issues and that these may be typical aspects of a pain problem.

Managing time

A big fear that most clinicians have is losing control of the visit and thereby wasting precious time. Indeed, we may have a picture of particular patients going on endlessly about their problems. Yet consider two facts. First, studies have shown that patients have only about 20 seconds(!!!) to tell their story before the doctor interrupts, and starts asking directed (yes/no) questions (Beckman and Frankel, 1984; Marvel et al., 1999). This unfortunately gives the patient the impression that the doctor cares less about them and it also prevents important information from coming up that in turn may be related to poor satisfaction and results. Second, the first two minutes of an interview can be the most decisive and helpful. After two minutes, the clinician typically has a description of the problem and probably a number of questions to clarify what the patient has told us. This is vital for obtaining a good description as about half of a typical patient's concerns are frequently missed. How do we provide the opportunity for patients to take a couple of minutes to describe their problem? And how do we overcome the urge to interrupt?

Luckily, some straight rules can help us to manage time better in patient encounters. Here is a summary:

- Be sure to give the patient the first two minutes by jotting down the time (start, stop) on a paper.
- Before starting the encounter, write down exactly how much time you have to spend with the patient, e.g. 15 minutes.
- Have a clock easily visible to you in the office so you can casually check the progression of the session.
- Do not allow interruptions, e.g. phone calls or questions from other staff.
- Provide a warning a few minutes before the end of the session, e.g. *"We will have to stop in five minutes."*
- Announce the end of the allotted time, e.g. *"We will have to stop now because we have run out of time. Let's schedule your next appointment."*
- Practice. Get feedback from colleagues.

By providing the patient with a couple of minutes to tell the story at the beginning of the visit and following up with open-ended questions, you will have an excellent chance of obtaining valuable information that is needed to set the agenda.

Setting the agenda for the visit

Because visits have time limits, it is good practice to establish a plan for using that time with the patient. This is an essential part of the development of a shared understanding, of connecting with the patient. You will need to understand the patient's expectations about the visit and develop a list of priorities for the session. For example, some statements help to organize the visit:

● "You have mentioned five concerns, which one should we start with?"
● "How should we best use our time today?"
● "What are the most important goals to achieve today?"

These statements send the message that the patient is an active partner in making decisions and that the patient also has responsibility for using the allotted time wisely. Moreover, you may then be able to negotiate how the time will be used at the beginning of sessions.

Taken together, the communication described above helps us to develop a shared understanding with our patients. Naturally, this does not end with the first visit or description of a problem, but continues to develop over time. This shared understanding will serve to help us better deal with the problems with which our patients present.

Empathizing

Empathy is a fundamental way in which to establish a connection with your patient. It refers to sharing an emotional state with another person. And it gives that person a sense of closeness and sharing. Empathy in other words helps us to establish an alliance with our patient. It promotes cooperation and participation.

Empathy may be established in two ways. First, you need to demonstrate for your patient that you in fact see and hear the patient. Second, and more difficult, is showing that you accept the patient and respect her or his views.

We have already dealt with basic methods for letting your patient know that you have understood her or his story, but additional techniques help you to see and hear the patient's *feelings*. Here we need to tune into facial expressions, tones of voice or statements of emotion. By practicing observation for these you will be better able to identify the emotional aspects. Often we get a gut feeling that an issue is emotionally charged, but we fail to pursue it. This may be because we find it uncomfortable or feel that it is not socially acceptable to ask about these topics. However, it is an important part of the assessment and intervention for pain!

Once a cue for an emotional topic has been observed, you may follow this up by inviting the patient to talk about it:

● "You look troubled. Let's talk about what is worrying you."
● "You say that this pain is 'getting you down'; could you tell me more about that."

By observing, asking for and paying attention to the emotional aspects the patient has, you communicate to the patient that you truly understand them.

Acceptance is the essence of empathy. It involves compassion and positive regard. This is sometimes a challenge, particularly if the patient engages in behaviors that you do not approve of. However, acceptance is not the same thing as approval. It is an understanding of the issues and an acceptance that this is the current situation:

Patient: "I know you wanted me to exercise, but I just couldn't find the time".

Professional: "Maybe this was the best decision for you at the time. Let's review your program and progress".

Patient: "I've had such poor care in the past. I should have done more myself, but it just makes me so mad!"

Professional: "It's natural that you feel disappointed since your pain problem has not gotten better. It can be a frustrating experience. Our task now is to see how we can go forward. Let us see how we can begin to deal with this".

These responses all show empathy for the patient because they do not judge the patient. Rather than reprimand the patient or become angry, the professional has accepted the situation and looks to the future to find ways to cope with the problems. This communicates good empathy and helps to connect with the patient.

Educating

The healthcare visit provides an excellent opportunity to educate the patient. But to be clear, patients are not stupid. Instead, they may have misconceptions, beliefs, attitudes that do not match the situation. Sometimes there is a lack of knowledge as well. Most lay people are not well versed in the details of how the body works. The exact content of the education will be particular to the patient. We will deal with specific types of information in the coming chapters. Remember, though, that patients enjoy learning and discovering.

Engagement/adherence

Much of the care we provide for pain patients involves the patient following our advice or recommendations. Often this is blamed on the patient and we imply that they have failed to "comply" with our good advice. A more neutral term is "adherence", since it refers only to whether a regime has been followed and has no implications for fault. More recently, the term "engagement" has been brought forward to underscore that as professionals there are many ways we can actively enlist patients to help in their own treatment.

Yet we know that adherence to even simple regimes is surprisingly low (Ley, 1981; Meichenbaum and Turk, 1987; Turk and Rudy, 1991; Headrick et al., 1992). For example, of those offered an exercise program such as to prevent back pain, around half will decline, and of those who take the offer less than a third will continue for more than a few weeks (Linton et al., 1996a). Improving communication can also help to improve adherence.

A behavioral model for understanding adherence is helpful in dealing with patients. A variation of this model is presented in Fig. 10.3 (Linton, 1992; Ogden, 2000). It shows how the recommendation for a patient to engage in a certain health-related behavior is processed. On the left-hand side are factors that determine whether the behavior will be initiated at all (adherence to try recommendation), while on the right-hand side are factors that influence long-term adherence.

The patient's decision to attempt to follow a recommended course of action is influenced by several factors. As clinicians we need to understand and deal with these. First is the question of whether the patient experiences a threat to their health. For example,

patients with acute back pain often do not see the problem as a threat to their general health. Indeed, while they may experience pain, many expect the problem to resolve with little or no effort on their own part. This can be compared to smokers who realize that smoking sometimes affects health, but at the same time do not believe it to be a threat to their own health. To engage the patient, then, we need to know if he or she believes that the pain problem is a threat to their long-term health and function.

Second, the patient needs to perceive the "health behavior" under discussion as a reasonable intervention. A patient may feel that the pain is a threat to their long-term health, but that the recommended intervention is not appropriate to reduce that risk. This is tied closely to the beliefs with which the patient comes to the clinic, as discussed in Part I of this book. A good example for back pain patients is the recommendation to exercise. Some patients simply do not see how this is relevant. Considering the models that patients have of their back pain (see above), it is not uncommon for patients to expect tangible treatments such as massage, injections or the like. To be successful with a recommendation, the patient needs to believe that the intervention (health behavior in the model) under discussion is a reasonable method to reduce their risk of long-term adverse health effects.

The third aspect on the left side of Fig. 10.3 is the patient's subjective evaluation of the pros and cons of actually doing the recommended health behavior. This may have little to do with the *actual* pros and cons. We all have visions of what may happen should we engage in certain behaviors. For example, a patient may believe that exercise might be marginally helpful for the pain problem, and generally good for his or her health. However, this person may also believe that it will be difficult, cause considerably more pain, and disrupt the daily schedule. To be successful in initiating the health behavior, the patient needs to believe

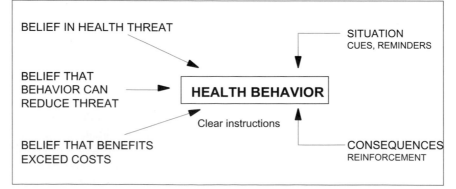

Figure 10.3 A modified version of the health beliefs model.

that the positive effects will outweigh, the negative effects.

The model in Fig. 10.3 illustrates that for patients to initiate a health behavior, they need to believe that there is a risk to their health, that the recommended behavior will reduce this risk, and that the pros are larger than the cons of engaging in the health behavior.

Motivating patients to initiate health behaviors

How do we convince a patient to undertake the recommended health behavior? The answer is that we do not try to simply talk the patient into trying the behavior. Instead, we may help the patient to understand his or her situation and the consequences of different choices. The communication principles in this chapter are the basis of conducting motivational interviewing (Jensen, 2002). To be successful with this in the clinic, we need to assess the patient's beliefs. In addition to showing empathy, educating and developing a shared understanding, there are some important techniques (Jensen, 2002):

1. *Developing discrepancy.* The idea here is to delineate the difference between the patient's current behavior and the important goals he or she has. Encourage the patient to talk about the problem and goals. Reflect on the differences and encourage the patient to do so as well.
2. *Avoid argumentation.* It is essential to avoid argumentation, especially where you are promoting a particular behavioral change and the patient is resisting. This only upsets the patient and provides an opportunity for him or her to develop a host of reasons why they cannot change their behavior.
3. *Roll with resistance.* Rather than argue, you may roll with resistance by changing strategies. A good way is to restate the patient's comments to demonstrate understanding. This may then be followed by a reframing of the situation.
4. *Support self-efficacy.* To change behavior, the patient needs to believe that he or she can take command and achieve the goal. Thus, clinicians need to support the patient's statements and attempts at behavior change. This might be done by examining and reinforcing other behavior changes the patient has previously made. Statements of intent might also be supported.

Eliciting self-motivational statements

A key technique is to educe self-motivational statements from the patient (Jensen, 2002). Table 10.3 shows examples of how this might be done. It involves recognizing the problem and showing concern. Moreover, a good motivational interview will bring forward statements about an intention to change

Table 10.3 Examples of statements that will encourage self-motivational statements.

Strategy	Example of question
Problem recognition	How well are you dealing with your pain problem?
Concern	What concerns do you have about the long-term consequences of your pain?
Intention to change	Of the things you can do, what would you like to see change the most?
Optimism	What things in your life do you feel that you are still in control of? What indications do you have that you could succeed with this?

as well as optimism about its likely success. In short, ideas are developed and the patient is guided along a path of building confidence and excitement about making positive behavioral changes.

Negotiating goals

Although we often have definite recommendations to offer, to ensure adherence we need to negotiate the changes with the patient. This reinforces self-efficacy and enhances successful behavioral change. By employing the techniques above, you will obtain a good picture of what types of changes are realistic. Part of the shared understanding should be a shared idea of what should be done to improve the situation. As a result, the goals for the intervention as well as the details of how it is done are subject to negotiation. If a patient needs to exercise, then, we first need to agree that this is a relevant goal. Realistic expectations of the difficulties and benefits should be discussed as well as previous experiences with exercise. Next, the specific exercise regime should be developed starting at a point the patient believes he or she can manage.

Stages of change

The techniques above are designed to help the patient initiate a behavioral change that will enhance their health. However, we are not always successful. Indeed, motivating behavioral change is a most difficult task. Yet there is reason to believe that our efforts may nevertheless be of help, even when the patient does not initiate the change. Rather than view behavioral change as an all or none proposition, the stages of change model views it as a stair-step process (Ogden, 2000; Jensen, 2002). This model was originally

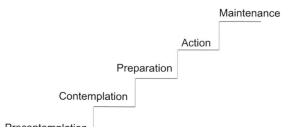

Figure 10.4 The stages of change model. Patients are said to go through these stages in adhering to medical advice.

developed by Prochaska and DiClemente (1982) and postulates that there are five steps to lasting behavioral change (Fig. 10.4). Here are the five stages:

- *Precontemplation*   no change is considered to be necessary
- *Contemplation*   a change is deliberated
- *Preparation*   the change is planned
- *Action*   initiation by engaging in the health behavior
- *Maintenance*   sustaining the change over time

Consequently, even if the behavioral change is not maintained over the long term, the therapy may still result in the patient moving up the adherence ladder. Motivational interviewing may help the patient, for instance, to move from the precontemplation stage to the contemplation stage. This enhances the patient's chances of being successful in the future.

Providing clear instructions

Once an agreement has been reached on the goal of health behavior, clear instructions are needed. In order for patients to follow our advice, they must understand exactly what we want them to do. Fortunately, there are several rules of thumb for providing clear instructions:

1. *Provide as few instructions as possible.* Memory is directly related to the number of instructions received. Thus it is essential to limit the number of instructions provided. Before the session, summarize for yourself the essential instructions. This helps to limit the number of instructions.
2. *Be specific!* Rather than providing general advice, provide specific, detailed information. This means telling the patient *what* they should do (walk, bike, take a pain tablet), *when* they should do it, *where* they should do it and *why* they should do it. Keep in mind that this emphasizes what the patient *should do* rather than what they should avoid.

3. *Group the information into categories.* Use categories to organize the information. Such categories might be "results of the examination", "discussion of intervention", "home work".
4. *Underscore the most important information.* Important messages may be given at the beginning, repeated and explained during the discussion, and highlighted again during a summary. Direct the patient's attention to the most important parts.
5. *Ask the patient to repeat the instructions in his or her own words.* This is an excellent method of checking whether the patient has understood the instructions! Surprisingly, even when the techniques above have been followed to the letter, patients will have missed an important aspect or misconstrued the instruction. By having them repeat the instructions, you can check understanding and correct any misconceptions.
6. *Provide written instructions.* Because patients will remember less than half of what is said in a typical meeting, written instructions should summarize the main points. Thus, the patient has the opportunity to consult and review these written instructions.

Supporting behavioral changes

Unfortunately, most discussions of adherence end when the patient initiates the new health behavior. However, statistics show that commencing a behavior is much easier than maintaining it. The right-hand side of Fig. 10.3 deals with how we can help patients to maintain behavioral changes. The key is to provide sufficient support until the behavior is established and the natural consequences reinforce the behavior.

The situation in which the behavior is to occur needs to be firmly established. This may sound trite, but it is not. In our clinic, we have worked extensively with back pain patients who want to exercise regularly. Some common but surprising barriers have been identified. These include:

- Where should I exercise?
- What clothes should I wear?
- Do I need to take a shower afterwards?
- How hard do I need to practice? Will I sweat?
- What will others think when they see how uncoordinated I am?

To overcome such concerns and firmly establish the new behavior, some techniques may be applied. First, specify where the behavior should occur by providing cues such as instructions or reminders. For example, for one patient who wanted to walk more, we agreed that walking to and from work was a good situation.

To cue this we provided a reminder in the form of a note on his breakfast food box.

A second technique is to ask the patient to perform the recommended behavior during the visit. In this way, you may instruct, correct and encourage the behavior. Moreover, many of the worries patients have will surface and can be dealt with. A rule of thumb is to begin with simple tasks and gradually increase the level. By tailoring the program to the patient's needs and situation you will increase the chances for success.

Most important is to ensure that when the new behavior does occur, it is reinforced! Ideally, this should occur immediately for the best effect. However, many health behaviors have few immediate positive effects. Preventing a new bout of back pain, for example, is a powerful motive, but happens far in the future. Indeed, the positive effects of many health behaviors can take days, weeks or months to observe. Therefore, positive consequences may need to be programmed to support the behavior until these positive effects can be experienced. Also, there is a need to monitor progress so that these gradual changes over longer periods of time can actually be seen.

Programming positive consequences means coming up with a system for providing reinforcement for the new behavior. As clinicians we need to provide a rich schedule of positive verbal encouragement. Family members and friends may also provide such encouragement. In addition, monitoring progress such as with a graph provides feedback that allows the patient to observe changes. Still, these may be relatively weak and they usually involve a time delay between the behavior (e.g. exercising) and the feedback (verbal praise, improvement in pain ratings).

Positive consequences may be programmed by a contract-like agreement. Here a system is developed with the patient to provide rewards for progress. For example, rewards might be provided daily and weekly for following a training program. These rewards are something that the patient treasures: seeing a movie, a chance to relax, a special treat, a new shirt. The key is to tie these rewards to progress. For example, a system might be worked out where a chance to relax, watch a favorite TV show and enjoy a small treat are taken each day that the patient succeeds in doing the exercise program.

Cognitive and emotional aspects are important to deal with. Some behavioral changes will result in negative consequences—at least in the short term. We have found, for instance, that after exercising back pain sufferers actually have slightly more pain (Linton et al., 1996a). The immediate increase in pain is quite small, very natural since it involves exertion, and acceptable to most people. However, if the patient expects the pain to decrease immediately, this will be a disappointing result that may be interpreted as a sign that the exercise is not working. Thus, it is important to deal with these aspects when planning the program.

SUMMARY

By employing the communication skills outlined in this chapter you will be better able to establish a shared understanding with your patient. This is enormously helpful in engaging the patient in the intervention program and provides a framework for adjusting and tailoring the treatment. In the next chapters we will examine more specific approaches for dealing with pain problems.

CHAPTER 11

Managing the first visit

The first visit a patient makes for their pain problem presents a unique opportunity to form a partnership that will enhance treatment results and promote prevention. In fact, the first visit sets the tone for the relationship and the expectations the patient will have concerning future examinations and treatment. It is an excellent situation for conducting an examination, educating the patient and reinforcing self-care. Because pain problems almost always entail a good portion of self-care, it is essential that this be promoted from the first visit. When proper communication techniques are employed, the first visit can lead to a shared understanding of the problem and partnership in resolving it. In this chapter we will examine how the first visit can be conducted to achieve these goals. We will first look at some recommendations and then develop the skills needed to meet these challenges.

WHAT SHOULD BE DONE: SCIENTIFIC GUIDELINES

Because the first visits to healthcare professionals are so important, several authorities have developed guidelines to help us conduct these sessions efficiently. In several countries around the world, top experts have been given the task of examining the scientific evidence and, based on this, elaborating a set of clinical guidelines for dealing with pain problems. Perhaps the most frequent problem addressed is back pain (Koes et al., 2001).

The guidelines recommend several straightforward steps (Nachemson and Jonsson, 2000; Koes et al., 2001). Interestingly enough, these correspond quite well with patient expectations as described in Chapter 10. Based on the recommendations and our model of why patients seek care, consider the following steps for conducting a first visit. The purpose is to identify medical diseases but also to establish a partnership with the patient that will promote self-care.

The first recommendation is crystal-clear: the patient should be given a thorough physical examination. The aim is to rule out any so-called *red flags*. These are biological factors that signal medical problems that need attention. Examples of these are fractures, infection, cancer and the like; recognized important red flags are listed in the box below. If a red flag is identified then further assessment is required, often by a specialist. However, red flags are quite rare, particularly in primary care settings. Estimates vary but are probably less than 1% of such patients. The examination is also important from a psychological perspective. It gives the patient more confidence in the clinician's judgment of what the cause of the problem is. In addition, it provides an opportunity to discuss the problem and obtain a more in-depth understanding of how the patient is experiencing the problem.

A second recommendation is to provide an explanation of why it hurts. Healthcare professionals sometimes feel uncomfortable about doing this because it is difficult to be absolutely sure. The back has many parts and since we cannot directly observe it, any one of a large number of things might cause the pain. On the other hand, patients do not demand a diagnosis in Latin. Rather, they want a reasonable explanation of their pain. Consequently, providing such an explanation can be very helpful. We will deal with how this might be done later in the chapter.

Third, the door should be opened to assess psychosocial factors that may be linked to the problem. Psychological factors that may hinder recovery have been termed *yellow flags* (see Table 11.1). These are signals that recovery may be hampered by any one of the psychological factors described in Part I of this book. Patients normally view these factors as part of the consequences or suffering they experience due to the pain. By employing the communication techniques in the previous chapter, such factors may become a natural part of the interview you have with the patient. Otherwise, simple questions such as *"How is this affecting your work/family?"* or *"Do you think you will have any problems returning to normal activity?"* can be helpful. See Fig. 11.1 for a model of the red and yellow flag concept.

Providing the patient with reassurance that the problem is not serious is the fourth recommendation. As we saw earlier, many patients seek care because the pain is quite different from what they have previously experienced and they wonder if something is seriously wrong. As a result, providing reassurance is seen as a key method for promoting self-care and preventing the development of long-term pain problems. We will deal more specifically on how this might be achieved below.

The fifth recommendation is to help the patient deal with the pain. It is common that patients seeking primary care have quite severe pain such as a rating of 8 on a 0 to 10 scale. This may be accompanied by bouts of very severe pain. Naturally this is not only frightening, but makes normal function difficult. Relieving the pain consequently is central to the

---

RED FLAGS FOR POTENTIALLY SERIOUS MEDICAL CONDITIONS

- Features of cauda equine syndrome (urinary retention, bilateral neurological symptoms, saddle anesthesia)*

- Significant trauma

- Weight loss

- History of cancer

- Fever

- Intravenous drug use

- Steroid use

- Severe, unremitting nighttime pain

- Pain that intensifies when patient is lying down

*Based on ACC and National Health Committee recommendations, New Zealand, 1997.

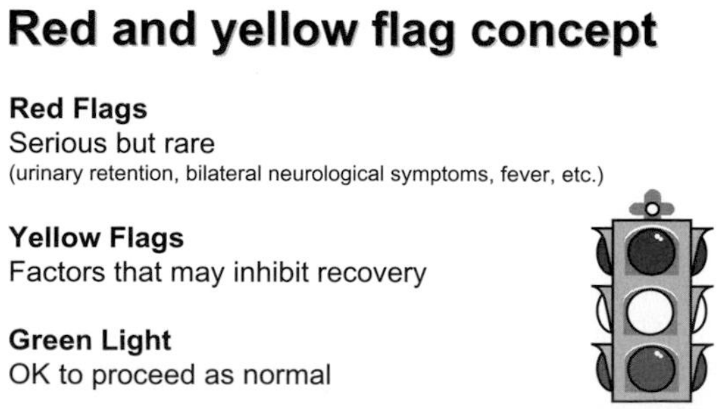

Red and yellow flag concept

Red Flags
Serious but rare
(urinary retention, bilateral neurological symptoms, fever, etc.)

Yellow Flags
Factors that may inhibit recovery

Green Light
OK to proceed as normal

Figure 11.1 A model of red and yellow flags. If no flags are present, this means the patient has a "green" light to go ahead with normal activities and we would expect full recovery.

Table 11.1 An overview of psychosocial "yellow flags" and examples of each category.

Cognitions and beliefs about the pain

Fear avoidance, i.e. belief that activity will cause pain or injury

Belief that pain must be completely abolished before attempting normal activity

Catastrophizing

Belief that pain is uncontrollable

Expectations concerning assessment, treatment and outcome

Belief that one has poor health or is handicapped

Emotions

Fear of pain or disability

Depression and irritability

Anxiety or heightened awareness of body sensations

Stress

Loss of sense of control

Behaviors

Use of extended rest

Reduced activity or withdrawal from activities of daily life

Avoidance

Report of extremely high-intensity pain

Sleep quality reduced since onset of pain

Substance abuse

Family

Overprotective partner

Solicitous behavior from partner

Socially punitive responses

Extent of support in attempts to return to normal activities including work

History of abuse

History of model for chronic pain behavior

Work

Belief that work is harmful

Unsupportive or unhappy current work environment

Negative experience of management or absence of interest from employer

Specific aspects of psychosocial environment, e.g. stress, perceived load, monotony, control, etc.

Compensation

Lack of financial incentive to return to work

Disputes

History of ineffective case management

Continued

Table 11.1 An overview of psychosocial "yellow flags" and examples of each category.—cont'd

Diagnosis and treatment
Health professionals sanctioning disability
Conflicting diagnoses
Diagnoses leading to catastrophizing and fear
Dependency, e.g. on passive treatments
Healthcare utilization
Expectation of a "techno-fix"
Lack of satisfaction with previous treatment
Advice to withdraw from daily activities or work

Based on Kendall et al. (1997).

promotion of a return to normal function and it also pulls the rug from under the fear that may generate a fear-avoidance syndrome. In medical settings, pain relief is associated with pharmacological treatments—pain pills. To be sure, analgesics are quite effective for acute bouts of back pain and are recommended by every guideline to date (Koes et al., 1995). Moreover, the Swedish guidelines go a step further (Jonsson and Nachemson, 2000). In order to maintain function, the Swedish guidelines recommend that patients take analgesics *in order to be active*. Thus, the pain tablets may be taken so that it is possible to participate in everyday activities.

While analgesics are important in relieving pain, nonpharmacological techniques should also be explored with the patient. There are two good reasons for this. First, in order to promote self-care, it is a good idea to have techniques that the patient can do themselves. Rather than developing a reliance on medical treatment, this sends the message that self-care is first-line treatment. Second, patients are interested in other pain-relieving techniques and these may be quite effective. For example, various forms of relaxation (yoga, tai chi and the like), massage (self-conducted or by a family member), heat, cold, rest positions and the like may all be useful methods of relieving the pain. Some of these provide momentary relief while others may provide more long-term benefits. By helping patients find ways of relieving their pain you also send the message that the pain is not harmful and that the patient can manage it.

Finally, providing clear recommendations for reactivation is the sixth recommendation. Back pain frequently necessitates changes in function. It is difficult to bend over, lift, reach and the like. It is normal for patients to wonder whether it is harmful to engage in such movements. Frankly, they do not know whether

they should avoid such movements or persist despite some pain. Providing clear information, then, will help the patient to maintain or regain function. More details on how this can be achieved are provided in the section below.

The six recommended steps above are designed to promote self-care and prevent long-term pain and disability. By incorporating them, the patient will obtain the information they desire and their expectations will be better met. Moreover, important messages will be provided. These are straightforward: *although it hurts, there is no serious or permanent injury; it is not only appropriate but vital to maintain or regain activity. Self-care is the way to achieve this.*

Several information booklets are available that help to underscore the most important points (Burton and Waddell, 2002; Jensen et al., 2004). Although information booklets by themselves are not powerful, they do play an important role. For example, the *Back Book* and *Back Pain: What Everyone Should Know About It* provide very clear messages that may reinforce your message from the first visit. It provides a written version that the patient can refer to again and again. Key messages, reduced to a single page, are also available on the web (www.workingbacksscotland.com).

PROVIDING AN EXPLANATION

It can be very challenging to provide a patient with an explanation of why it hurts. This is particularly true if we demand a 100% accurate diagnosis. As a result, many clinicians opt for telling the patient what *they don't have*. Worse, the patient may be told that *no abnormalities were found*. While both of these options may be medically correct, they do not meet the needs of the patient and they convey inappropriate messages. Consider what the message is when telling the patient that they do not have cancer or an infection. This does not provide a clear message of knowing what is wrong, but instead introduces doubt (the doctor doesn't know). Add to this a statement like *"it could be a disk or it might be soft tissue injury"*. The message is that the professional does not know what is wrong; it might also imply that it shouldn't hurt. This can be alarming! Take the second example: no abnormalities were found. Patients commonly interpret this as meaning that "the professional doesn't think there is anything wrong with me". Rather than reassuring the patient, both of these statements introduce uncertainty and may be interpreted as "the professional does not understand my pain". They set the stage for the patient drawing his or her own diagnosis. Moreover, they set the stage for catastrophizing.

The explanation should be logical and provide a simple explanation of why it hurts. How can this be done without manufacturing the information?

A good way to begin is by summarizing where and what kind of pain the patient is suffering. Still, a logical explanation can be provided. It should, of course, be connected to the physical examination. Thus, the explanation should refer to the particular places it hurts and the way it hurts (*"You had a lot of pain when I put pressure here. This is where the muscle attaches to the bone. Since it hurts when I touch it, it is tender and inflamed"*). By providing a summary of where and how it hurts, you demonstrate to the patient that you have understood the problem. This is a crucial first step.

Next, you may test explanations that are logical and congruent with the patient's symptoms. Normally, the pain is linked to soft tissue processes. There may be inflammation and the patient may consequently have very tight, contracted muscles. The explanation you put forward can be formulated as a hypothesis so that the patient can react to and correct any misconceptions. *"You felt something in your back when you bent down to lift a box. This seems to have caused a muscle spasm. Now, you are sensitive in this region and even relatively light pressure provokes your pain. The tissue is probably inflamed making it tender. A natural reaction is for the muscles around this area to contract to protect your back. However, when they contract this much and as long as you've had this problem, the muscles themselves become painful [presses on muscles to demonstrate] and tender."*

Keep in mind what message you are giving your patient. The explanation above, for example, focuses on soft tissue. An important message to convey is that this naturally heals. Another message concerns the role of activity. As we have seen in Part I, a natural conclusion many people draw is that rest is the most appropriate treatment for pain. While patients should not totally ignore their pain and overdo activities, a central message is to remain active and regain activity levels.

The explanation of the pain might well include logical aspects of why it is important to be active. For example, one explanation is that blood flow is linked to healing. By using the back you increase blood flow, thus speeding the healing time. Other explanations may compare the injury to other sorts of problems where movement is necessary. Recovery after an operation, for instance, shows that getting up and moving about the same day as an operation (even major operations) has led to faster healing and fewer complications. Still another explanation is that to relieve tension in the muscles they need to be used to obtain the balance between tension and relaxation.

By providing an explanation in this way, the patient will have an opportunity to ask questions and give feedback. This will help establish a shared understanding with the patient and will give you important feedback as to whether the patient understands and believes in the explanation.

PROVIDING REASSURANCE

Because patients normally worry about symptoms and fear serious disease, reassurance is a logical part of the first visit. Certainly, reassurance has been recommended for patients seeking care for back pain and is included as a major intervention in most guidelines. However, surprisingly little is known about how reassurance is actually employed in the clinic. Healthcare professionals appear to view reassurance as simply providing information. Nevertheless, reassurance is a complicated psychological process that involves two-way communication. For example, the patient's level of fear and worry may affect how well he or she listens to the information and it might also be central in determining the extent of the effect. Therefore, there is a real need to understand better how reassurance works and to practice skills that enhance effective reassurance.

Reassurance is one of the most often recommended methods for dealing with patients with low back pain. For example, reviews of advances in primary care research on low back pain concluded that reassurance is a vital method for management and the alteration of inappropriate beliefs patients may harbor (Borkan et al., 2002). As mentioned earlier, it is also recommended by virtually every expert group that has examined how back pain should be dealt with in the clinic. Waddell sums up the current view: "We must address our patients' fears and anxieties with firm, consistent and if necessary repeated *reassurance*. This is one of the major roles of the doctor in dealing with back pain—to provide reassurance that there is no serious disease. … We must avoid creating unnecessary worry" (Waddell, 1998, p. 185).

The basic idea with reassurance is quite compelling: patients with back or other types of pain are known to worry, which in itself may exacerbate the problem. Although back pain is almost never related to a serious injury (Waddell, 1998; Nachemson and Jonsson, 2000), patients nevertheless worry that their pain is caused by grave damage. Indeed, this worry is an important element in the fear-avoidance model of disability where fear and catastrophizing cause or catalyze the avoidance of movements which in turn propels disability (Vlaeyen and Linton, 2000). A good deal of research supports the idea that fears and worries are linked to catastrophizing thoughts and beliefs that in turn are related to the development of the so-called "disuse syndrome" (Crombez et al., 1996, 1998b, 1999; Vlaeyen and Linton, 2000; Sullivan et al., 2001). Based on this information, it has been suggested that dealing with fear and worry early on might be one method of preventing the development of persistent pain and functional problems (Waddell, 1998; Main and Spanswick, 2000; Linton, 2002a, 2002c). To be sure, providing reassurance is a logical method and it is easy to believe it would be particularly effective.

Nevertheless, there is reason for great concern because reassurance is often viewed as simply providing information. In this scenario, healthcare practitioners are assumed to provide effective reassurance because they are experts in the field providing essential information. However, because practitioners view reassurance as the imparting of information, the "reassurance" provided may *not* be particularly reassuring.

A psychological approach to reassurance suggests that it is a relatively complicated process. Rather than providing information, reassurance concerns the interaction between the patient and the caregiver. The evidence to date shows that simple information has little effect on health anxiety (Asmundson et al., 2001) or on the fears and anxieties of patients in general (Barlow, 2002).

A model for understanding the process of reassurance is provided in Fig. 11.2. The first step in the cognitive-behavioral model is the need to assess what (if) the patient is actually worried about. Since this may vary greatly, it is of obvious importance in gauging the reassurance. Not all patients are particularly worried and it is good to know the extent of the worry. Second, there is a need to identify the focus of the worry. In healthcare situations, the focus might involve a belief (e.g. what the cause of the pain is) or an expectation of the consequences (e.g. death or handicap). Thus, exploring the source of the worry is important in order to understand and deal with the fear involved.

Third, the healthcare provider needs to specifically address this worry or fear and help the patient to *disconfirm* it. Providing general information like "there is nothing to worry about" or "there is nothing serious wrong with you" has little effect if the patient is worried about a cancer tumor or of severing a nerve if bending too far forward. To relieve the fear and worry, two techniques are illustrated in the figure. The first involves providing an example that the patient can relate to as disconfirming evidence. For example, providing information from a previous patient's experiences may be especially beneficial (Lyons et al., 2002). *"A patient last week was quite concerned about resuming activities. However, to her surprise she found that resuming her jogging did not increase the pain, but actually seemed to be helpful."* The second disconfirmation technique is the so-called behavioral test. Here, the idea is to clearly identify the worry and then devise a test to see if the worry is actually credible. By experiencing that the feared outcome does not occur, the patient will experience a disconfirmation of their worry and thereby a reduction of the associated fear and worry (Barlow, 2002). The anxiety literature supports the idea of behavioral tests, as does the idea of exposure treatment for pain-related fear of movement (Vlaeyen et al., 2001; Barlow, 2002; Linton et al., 2002a; Boersma et al., 2004). According to my model, then, effective reassurance must specifically challenge the worry and actively disconfirm it (see Fig. 11.3).

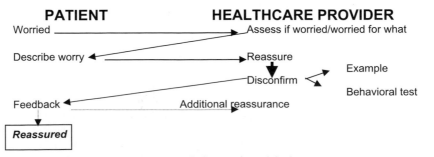

Figure 11.2 A cognitive-behavioral model of reassurance.

REASSURANCE MODEL

1. Worried?
2. About what?
3. Disconfirm (reassure)
   by experience e.g. a "behavioral test"
4. Reassured?

Figure 11.3 A simplified version of the reassurance model as a heuristic aid.

Once disconfirmation has been attempted, the fourth step involves getting feedback to evaluate if the worry has actually decreased, i.e. if reassurance has been achieved. If the patient continues to be quite worried, further efforts will need to be made to disconfirm the worry.

PAIN RELIEF

Although pain relief has been described above, it is underscored here again to emphasize its importance. Pain relief is one key to maintaining function and reducing worry and fear. Pharmacological methods may be used to help the patient maintain activities. This message will also reinforce the idea that hurt is *not* harm. In other words, the message is that activity is not harmful. Finally, nonpharmacological methods such as relaxation may be used to promote self-care (Linton, 1983; Main and Spanswick, 2000).

REACTIVATION

Because functional problems are frequent, maintaining or regaining function is vital. Although some patients may believe that maintaining daily activities is harmful, being active actually promotes healing and recovery. This does not mean that doing the activities is painless. It does mean that participating in daily activities despite some pain, or with the aid of pain-relieving techniques, is helpful for function. Indeed, relatively short periods of inactivity greatly reduce mobility, physical capacity and muscle strength. Consequently, it is important to encourage the patient to maintain daily activities even if they cause some pain.

An effective way to begin is to ask the patient whether function is or will be a problem. *"Are you having any problems doing your normal activities because of the pain?"* This will set the stage for a discussion. Typically, patients have questions regarding specific movements such as whether it is all right to bend to pick something from the floor, or whether it is good to continue walking when it hurts. Given that there are no red flags, the message to convey is that the pain, in

and of itself, is not harmful. It does not break or permanently damage anything. Instead, the movement is helpful to stretch out tense muscles, increase circulation (and thereby healing) and maintain mobility. Thus, the patient may perfectly well maintain everyday activities as best they can despite some pain. Having said this, certain movements may be extremely difficult to do during an acute bout of pain. However, the patient should try to resume these as best as possible. After the interview with the patient, you will also have information that will help you determine the tone of your advice. Those who are fearful may need clear encouragement to participate in activities, while those who tend to be "overdoers" may need to understand that the recommendation is for normal everyday activities.

If function is an issue, the first line of advice is for the patient *to maintain her or his normal, everyday activities.* The disruptions to everyday routines that the pain may cause may lead to a number of other problems. Indeed, as we have seen earlier, changes in daily routines and function are clearly linked to the process of chronification. Therefore, it is important to maintain daily routines as best as possible. Moreover, this will have a beneficial effect on healing time and it will be a central contribution to high quality of life.

Often, however, patients are already having problems with function when they come to the clinic. The rule here is to *regain activity level through gradual increases.* Because of the pain, patients may be having problems doing a variety of movements and activities. It is essential that normal movements and activities be regained to ensure a good quality of life and to prevent the development of long-term problems. It is not uncommon, however, that patients have an "all or none" approach to regaining activity. In other words, the particular activity is attempted (vacuuming) and it either works well or is stopped because of the pain. However, this is an unfair test. As pointed out above, we lose muscle tone, mobility and strength quickly when inactive. Thus, attempting to do an activity full out may lead to fatigue and pain simply because we are not in good condition. To overcome this trap, a gradual increase in the activity is recommended. For example, the patient may begin by vacuuming for a short amount of time, say three minutes. The main focus should be placed on succeeding with the activity rather than the pain. The time period can subsequently be increased gradually every day. This will help the patient to regain function and physical capacity.

A particular activity that should be included in the discussion is work. Patients may have difficulties performing certain aspects of their work routine because of the pain. However, an important message to convey is that working is helpful for recovery. It should either be maintained or regained just as with the everyday activities discussed above. Patients almost always associate their back or neck pain with work (Crombie et al., 1999). This issue may need to be dealt with. Again, given that no red flags are present, the message should be that working is normally good for your back.

Frequently, patients will have questions about doing specific work tasks. Because some work tasks are difficult to do with acute back pain, ways of modifying the work can be discussed. The patient may well be in a position to talk to her or his supervisor about accommodations at work that will enhance the patient's ability to do the job. If the patient is off work on sick leave, a return to work should be carefully planned. Here again a graded return to work is an excellent option. In this scheme the patient may begin by working short periods and gradually increase these. Although workplaces are often alleged to have the attitude that the worker should be 100% fit before returning, at the acute stage of the problem employers are normally quite willing to make accommodations. However, employers may not be aware of the necessity of these or of how best to be of help. Consequently, contact with the workplace may be of value. A telephone call, followed up by the patient visiting the supervisor, is a good method. Simple advice to employers is also available on the net (e.g. www.workingbacks-scotland.com).

Occasionally you may sense that a patient has real difficulty with the workplace. The patient may even be eager to be deemed unfit to work. This "sense" may well be picking up on an important issue. It should be addressed with open but direct questions such as *"How do you feel about working with this pain?"* or *"How is your employer responding to your back pain?"* These types of questions will open the door for a discussion about the patient's work situation. It will also help you to evaluate yellow flags that may be a barrier to recovery.

While most patients will only require a discussion and clear advice, consider making a more formal plan that can be monitored. This provides a clear method for the patient that is easy to remember. And it focuses on function and reinforces the gradual progress being made. Here are the basic steps. First, come to an agreement with the patient about the need for reactivation. Second, select target activities. These will be important everyday activities that the patient is having difficulties with and needs to increase. Third, establish the current level of the activity. Measure the activity in terms of length of participation time or number of repetitions. Fourth, set goals that require gradual increases. The increase should be a bit of a challenge, but yet be a gradual increase. Set the goal for several trials, e.g. three. Fifth, record results. A graph is ideal for presenting the goals as well as the actual results. Finally, provide reinforcement for improvements! This will be done indirectly by the graph and the natural consequences of being able to do more. However, it is also important that you, as a healthcare provider, give verbal praise for improvements. Setbacks may occur. These are natural as some days are better than others. Do not focus on these, but rather reset the goal level to accommodate the setback and continue!

SUMMARY

By providing excellent care during the first session, you will promote a speedy recovery and help prevent the development of long-term pain and disability problems. Employing good communication skills is a key to developing a working relationship with your patient. After conducting a physical examination that rules out the rare, but important, red flags, a series of steps will help provide the patient with the information and help they need most. Pain relief via pharmacological or nonpharmacological methods is a key to good practice. Further, assessing possible yellow flags is important, as is helping the patient to maintain or regain function. Above all, the first session is vital for establishing your relationship with the patient. It is a golden opportunity to educate and embrace the patient as a partner in whom self-care plays an imperative role.

CHAPTER 12

Early identification of patients at risk of developing persistent pain: screening

---

LEARNING OBJECTIVES

To understand:

- that early identification is important because usual practice may contribute to the chronification process;

- how psychological factors may be utilized to identify patients early on;

- the logic of screening: to focus resources on those most in need;

- skill to administer, score and employ a screening questionnaire in clinical practice.

In order to provide effective early interventions that may prevent the development of chronic problems, early identification is needed. Unfortunately, the healthcare system is designed to *diagnose and treat* patients and is often rather poor at early identification of patients at risk of developing persistent problems. Many professionals view musculoskeletal pain problems as "benign" problems. Most professionals decide to treat the patient with their usual methods first. If the patient does not improve, then the "dose" of the treatment is increased. Unfortunately, other factors, such as psychological variables, may not be considered until the usual treatment has failed. A consequent result is that the process of chronification has had a considerable amount of time to operate. At worst, the usual treatment may actually contribute to this process by reinforcing sick behavior, catastrophizing and fear-avoidance beliefs. There is a true need, then, to have methods available to help identify those relatively few patients who are at risk of developing long-term pain and disability problems. In this chapter we will explore the concept of screening and learn valuable skills for conducting screening in a primary care setting.

THE CASE FOR SCREENING

In order to identify the few patients who are at considerable risk of developing a persistent problem, screening may be essential for the elaboration of a successful prevention program. This is not an easy task. Consider that most people will suffer from spinal pain at some point and have recurrences (Crombie et al., 1999). Furthermore, only a relatively small number of these people (3–10%) are estimated to develop a long-term work absence after an acute bout of back pain (Reid et al., 1997). Given the large number of people who have back pain, the recurrent nature of the problem, and the relatively small number who actually develop persistent problems, it is a real challenge to identify "at risk" patients early on. Nevertheless, it is an important challenge as these patients suffer greatly and consume the majority of the resources (Waddell, 1996, 1998; Nachemson and Jonsson, 2000). Moreover, given the large numbers, it would be difficult to provide every person with back pain with a special preventive intervention.

The challenge of screening

Consider Fig. 12.1 which shows an example of the challenge of screening. Let us suppose that your clinic serves 1000 people in the community. Further, based on epidemiological studies, we would suspect that somewhere around 5 to 10 of these people may develop a long-term back pain problem during the course of a year. How might we locate these people? In the field of occupational medicine many attempts have been made, but with disappointing results. However, once the back pain problem has been signaled, identification is somewhat easier. Following the figure, approximately 100 people may seek some form of healthcare for back pain during the year. By focusing on this group we would have a better chance of isolating those who are at risk of developing chronic problems. Clinicians may feel that they can identify these patients by their "gut feeling". In part this is true. However, because only 5–10 of 100 patients actually develop a problem, most clinicians are aware that

help is needed. This is why screening tools have been developed.

The advantages of screening for psychosocial yellow flags

Screening offers many valuable advantages to the usual clinical assessment. Primarily it provides an opportunity to concentrate limited resources on those patients most in need of help. In addition, early screening may elucidate and direct attention to those psychosocial factors that are most pertinent. Since psychological factors are not normally included in clinical assessments of patients with acute or subacute pain in primary care facilities, it is valuable to develop relevant targets for intervention. Finally, screening might complement primary care facilities that often are not equipped or lack the resources for assessing psychosocial factors. Assessing the large number of identified psychosocial risk factors through an interview would, for instance, be time-consuming, especially considering the large number of individuals seeking care for musculoskeletal pain. Some healthcare professionals may find it difficult to address delicate psychosocial issues such as depression or anxiety and lack skills in how these issues should be handled.

The development of a screening questionnaire

Since psychological factors have been associated with the development of persistent pain problems, it is logical to explore the utility of such factors in screening. As described in Chapter 9, research has established a firm link between psychological factors and the development of a long-term pain problem (Turk, 1996a, 1997; Waddell, 1998; Turk and Flor, 1999; Linton, 2000c; Main and Spanswick, 2000; Vlaeyen and Linton, 2000). Psychosocial factors then might represent key factors that could be utilized in screening (Gatchel et al., 1995; Linton, 2000c).

A thorough review of screening procedures for back pain has concluded that screening is truly possible (Waddell et al., 2003). This report found numerous instruments that have been developed for screening purposes. Although these differ considerably, the most efficient identify about 85% of those who will develop a persistent back pain disability problem. The authors point out that while this is far above guessing, it still involves considerable imprecision in the clinic. Yet this is not unusual in clinical screening in a variety of medical areas even when biological tests are employed. Another important feature of screening questionnaires is that they may help to guide the content of the intervention.

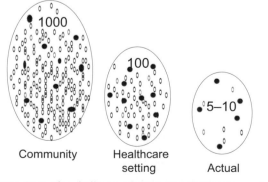

Community   Healthcare setting   Actual

Figure 12.1 The challenge of screening given a general population and an incidence rate of about 10 per 1000.

The purpose of screening

Screening procedures offer a rough assessment that helps to narrow down the number of patients who need to be assessed in more detail (Sheridan and Winogrond, 1987). The purpose of a psychosocial screening procedure for people with subacute or acute back pain problems is essentially threefold. First, it offers a rough estimation of the risk the patient runs of developing long-term disability. This is useful, for instance, in deciding the amount of treatment suitable. Second, it focuses attention on the patient's specific problem areas and is helpful in establishing goals. Third, it provides information about possible mechanisms and thus aids in matching the patient with the appropriate intervention. Identifying goals and possible mechanisms is of special value because the psychosocial aspects may be integrated with the medical findings. Accordingly, a screening procedure that can guide the initial assessment to those at risk and that can help focus on the most important psychological risk factors is beneficial.

While several instruments are available (Waddell et al., 2003), we have developed a special instrument for clinical use that provides an estimate of risk as well as information that is beneficial in developing an intervention strategy.

THE ÖREBRO MUSCULOSKELETAL PAIN SCREENING QUESTIONNAIRE

The Örebro Musculoskeletal Pain Screening Questionnaire (see Box 12.1 and Fig. 12.2) was developed as a tool for clinicians in the early identification of people at risk of developing long-term problems (Linton and Halldén, 1998; Boersma and Linton, 2002). The questionnaire contains 25 items covering a range of psychosocial variables that are related to long-term function; for example, work-related variables, coping, function, stress, mood and fear-avoidance beliefs.

BOX 12.1 AN OVERVIEW OF THE ITEMS IN THE ÖREBRO MUSCULOSKELETAL PAIN SCREENING QUESTIONNAIRE

Question	Variable name	Question	Variable name
1. What year were you born?	Age	14. How much have you been bothered by feeling depressed in the past week?	Depression
2. Are you a man/woman?	Gender		
3. Were you born in Sweden (country of study)?	Nationality	15. In your view, how large is the risk that your current pain may become persistent?	Expected outcome
4. What is your current employment status?	Employed	16. In your estimation, what are the chances that you will be able to work in 6 months?	Expected outcome
5. Where do you have pain	Pain site		
6. How many days of work have you missed (sick leave) because of pain during the past 12 months?	Sick leave	17. If you take into consideration your work routines, management, salary, promotion possibilities and workmates, how satisfied are you with your job?	Job satisfaction
7. How long have you had your current pain problem?	Pain duration		
8. Is your work heavy or monotonous?	Heavy work	18. Physical activity makes my pain worse.	Fear-avoidance belief
9. How would you rate the pain you have had during the past week?	Current pain	19. An increase in pain is an indication that I should stop what I am doing until the pain decreases.	Fear-avoidance belief
10. In the past 3 months, on the average, how intense was your pain?	Average pain		
11. How often would you say that you have experienced pain episodes, on the average, during the past 3 months?	Pain frequency	20. I should not do my normal work with my present pain.	Fear-avoidance belief
		21. I can do light work for an hour.	Function: work
		22. I can walk for an hour.	Function: walk
12. Based on all the things you do to cope, or deal with your pain, on an average day, how much are you able to decrease it?	Coping	23. I can do ordinary household chores.	Function: household work
		24. I can do the weekly shopping.	Function: shopping
13. How tense or anxious have you felt in the past week?	Stress	25. I can sleep at night.	Function: sleep

I.D. No: _____

ÖREBRO MUSCULOSKELETAL PAIN SCREENING
QUESTIONNAIRE (3)

Name: _____

Address: _____

_____

Telephone: _____ - _____

These questions and statements apply if you have aches or pains such as back, shoulder or neck pain. Please read and answer each question carefully. Do not take too long to answer the questions. However, it is important that you answer every question. There is always a response for your particular situation.

EXAMPLE:
Answer by circling one alternative.
I like oranges.

0	1	2	3	4	5	6	7	8	9	10
not at all										very much

Or check a box.
How many days per week do you exercise?

0–1 days ☐   2–3 days ☐   4–5 days ☐   6–7 days ☐

Figure 12.2 The Örebro Musculoskeletal Pain Screening Questionnaire. The questionnaire may be copied for nonprofit research or clinical use.

1. What year were you born?   19..........

2. Are you: male ☐   female ☐

3. Were you born in Sweden?

                          yes ☐   no ☐

4. What is your current employment situation?

       paid work ☐   studying ☐   unpaid work at home ☐
       unemployed ☐   retired ☐   other ☐: _____

5. Where do you have pain? Check the appropriate sites.   2*x

       neck ☐   shoulder ☐   upper back ☐   lower back ☐   leg ☐   ☐

6. How many days of work have you missed because of pain during **the past 12 months**? Check one.

       0 days ☐   1–2 days ☐   3–7 days ☐   8–14 days ☐   15–30 days ☐   ☐
       31–60 days ☐   61–90 days ☐   91–180 days ☐   181–365 days ☐   > 365 days ☐

7. How long have you had your current pain problem? Check one.

       0–1 weeks ☐   2–3 weeks ☐   4–5 weeks ☐   6–7 weeks ☐   8–9 weeks ☐   ☐
       10–11 weeks ☐   12–23 weeks ☐   24–35 weeks ☐   36–52 weeks ☐   > 52 weeks ☐

8. Is your work heavy or monotonous? Circle the best alternative.

       0   1   2   3   4   5   6   7   8   9   10   ☐
     not at all   extremely
                          not working ☐

9. How would you rate the pain that you have had during **the past week**? Circle one.

       0   1   2   3   4   5   6   7   8   9   10   ☐
     no pain   pain as bad as it could be

10. In the **past three months**, on the average, how intense was your pain on a 0–10 scale? Circle one.

       0   1   2   3   4   5   6   7   8   9   10   ☐
     no pain   pain as bad as it could be

11. How **often** would you say that you have experienced pain episodes, on the average,
    during **the past three months**? Circle one.

       0   1   2   3   4   5   6   7   8   9   10   ☐
     never   always

Figure 12.2 cont'd

12. Based on all the things you do to cope, or deal with your pain, on an average day, how much are you able to decrease it? Please circle the appropriate number.

| 0 | 1 | 2 | 3 | 4 | 5 | 6 | 7 | 8 | 9 | 10 |

can't decrease
it at all

can decrease
it completely

10–x

13. How tense or anxious have you felt in **the past week**? Circle one.

| 0 | 1 | 2 | 3 | 4 | 5 | 6 | 7 | 8 | 9 | 10 |

absolutely
calm and relaxed

as tense and anxious as
I've ever felt

14. How much have you been bothered by feeling depressed in **the past week**? Circle one.

| 0 | 1 | 2 | 3 | 4 | 5 | 6 | 7 | 8 | 9 | 10 |

not at all

extremely

15. In your view, how large is the risk that your current pain may become persistent? Circle one.

| 0 | 1 | 2 | 3 | 4 | 5 | 6 | 7 | 8 | 9 | 10 |

no risk

very large risk

16. In your estimation, what are the chances that you will be able to work in **six months**? Circle one.

| 0 | 1 | 2 | 3 | 4 | 5 | 6 | 7 | 8 | 9 | 10 |

no chance

very large chance

10–x

17. If you take into consideration your work routines, management, salary, promotion possibilities and workmates, how satisfied are you with your job? Circle one.

| 0 | 1 | 2 | 3 | 4 | 5 | 6 | 7 | 8 | 9 | 10 |

not at all
satisfied

completely
satisfied

10–x

not working ☐

*Here are some of the things which other patients have told us about their pain. For each statement please circle any number from 0 to 10 to say how much physical activities, such as bending, lifting, walking or driving, affect or would affect **your** back.*

18. Physical activity makes my pain worse.

| 0 | 1 | 2 | 3 | 4 | 5 | 6 | 7 | 8 | 9 | 10 |

completely
disagree

completely
agree

19. An increase in pain is an indication that I should stop what I am doing until the pain decreases.

| 0 | 1 | 2 | 3 | 4 | 5 | 6 | 7 | 8 | 9 | 10 |

completely
disagree

completely
agree

Figure 12.2 cont'd

20. I should not do my normal activities including work with my present pain.

| 0 | 1 | 2 | 3 | 4 | 5 | 6 | 7 | 8 | 9 | 10 |

completely
disagree

completely
agree

Here is a list of five activities. Please circle the number which best describes your current ability to participate in each of these activities.

21. I can do light work for an hour.

10–x

| 0 | 1 | 2 | 3 | 4 | 5 | 6 | 7 | 8 | 9 | 10 |

cannot do it
because of pain

can do it without
pain being a problem

22. I can walk for an hour.

10–x

| 0 | 1 | 2 | 3 | 4 | 5 | 6 | 7 | 8 | 9 | 10 |

cannot do it
because of pain

can do it without
pain being a problem

23. I can do ordinary household chores.

10–x

| 0 | 1 | 2 | 3 | 4 | 5 | 6 | 7 | 8 | 9 | 10 |

cannot do it
because of pain

can do it without
pain being a problem

24. I can do the weekly shopping.

10–x

| 0 | 1 | 2 | 3 | 4 | 5 | 6 | 7 | 8 | 9 | 10 |

cannot do it
because of pain

can do it without
pain being a problem

25. I can sleep at night.

10–x

| 0 | 1 | 2 | 3 | 4 | 5 | 6 | 7 | 8 | 9 | 10 |

cannot do it
because of pain

can do it without
pain being a problem

THANK YOU FOR YOUR COOPERATION!

Figure 12.2 cont'd

It provides an overall score from which risk may be judged as well as ratings on separate items. The total score is divided into three categories based on cut-off levels. These are high risk (definitely need to attend to this case), medium risk (may need special attention, continue to observe progress) and low risk (expect to get better). Several studies have shown the questionnaire to be reliable and valid (Hurley et al., 2000, 2001; Ektor-Andersen et al., 2002; Linton and Boersma, 2003). In the clinic, the estimate of the risk level is merely a small part of the assessment. The true value is in engaging the patient, identifying targets and building a potential intervention.

ADMINISTERING THE SCREENING QUESTIONNAIRE

The Örebro Musculoskeletal Pain Screening Questionnaire is designed to be a self-administered tool. This means that patients should ordinarily be able to understand the instructions and complete the questions by themselves. However, it does assume basic language skills and those with language deficits, e.g. the elderly or those with another native language, may need special assistance. It is also important to note that the questions are relevant to those suffering acute, subacute or recurrent musculoskeletal pain and who are seeking care.

Although the instrument is basically self-administered, several aspects of its administration need to be considered to ensure reliable results. Patients will undoubtedly expect an explanation as to the rationale for using the instrument. That is, they will be interested to know why they should complete the instrument and how it will be used in their assessment. The amount of time needed to fill in the questionnaire may also be a concern.

Providing a good rationale is extremely important as it should increase the patient's motivation to carefully complete the items. If patients are made to feel that this is a key part of their total assessment, this enhances completion of the items and ensures that care is taken in doing so. Here is a sample patient instruction:

"I would like you to complete this short questionnaire about your pain experience and the consequences it may have for you. It usually takes about 5 to 10 minutes to answer all of the items. This provides us with helpful information that we use as a complement to your physical examinations, clinical interview and other information in this assessment. We find that the information from this questionnaire helps us understand your problem better and it especially helps us evaluate the possible long-term consequences your pain may have.

It is important that you read each question carefully and answer it as best you can. There are no right or wrong answers. Please answer every question. If you have difficulty, select the answer option that best describes your situation. Please take a few minutes now to complete it while you are waiting."

The patient should complete the instrument without any help, such as from friends or relatives, in a relatively quiet environment. Ordinarily this is done while the patient waits. However, since answers ought to be confidential, waiting rooms may not be appropriate.

Time limit

Almost all patients will finish the instrument in 5 to 10 minutes (median time = 7 minutes). If the patient needs more time, this may be provided. However, if a patient has not completed the questionnaire in 15 minutes, this may be a sign of a problem. One problem may be language difficulty, that is, the patient does not understand the questions. This may be resolved by reading the questions to the patient. However, it is imperative that the clinician does not answer the questions for the patient. A second possible problem is that the patient considers the items too literally and therefore takes too much time to answer each question. A third possibility is that the patient is indecisive. The patient may be encouraged to provide "their best estimate" and reassured that the questions are interpreted in a general method.

Questions

Patients may sometimes have questions about an item in the questionnaire. This should be responded to by reading the question out loud to the patient. Then the patient should be told to answer the question as best as he or she can. Even if the patient may feel that the item is irrelevant, there is always an answer that should be appropriate, e.g. "no pain". Do not attempt to rephrase the item as this may easily change its meaning. Discussions about the true "meaning" of an item should be avoided as they tend to introduce bias into the measurement.

Patients not gainfully employed

Patients who are not currently working may express difficulty in completing the items that concern work. It is recommended, however, that the patient complete the items as best as they can using their latest job (if recently employed) or their current situation (e.g. if homemaker) to make the ratings. However, an alternative is provided in the questionnaire for those not working and who cannot complete these items (e.g. long-term unemployed, pensioned).

Compliance check

When the questionnaire is collected it should be checked to ensure that every item is answered properly. This provides an opportunity to have the patient answer any items that may have been missed. In addition, it demonstrates the importance of the information to the patient.

Provide positive feedback

When the questionnaire has been fully completed the patient may be praised for the good work. This will encourage their participation and show appreciation for the information being collected.

Scoring and interpretation

This questionnaire is designed to be relatively easy to score and interpret. With practice it may be scored in about one minute. However, as with all tests, care should be taken so that the interpretation is accurate. Moreover, as a screening instrument, the score only provides a rough guide and is to be seen as a starting point rather than an end point in the assessment and intervention routine.

Scoring

One result of the questionnaire is an overall score that may be used to estimate risk. The screening questionnaire in Figure 12.2 shows the items and the layout of the questionnaire. Each item has a maximum of 10 points and all but three items (pain site, duration and sick leave) have a minimum of 0 points. Scoring is based on having all questions oriented in the same direction so that *high scores indicate high risk*. In addition, since the first four questions (age, gender, nationality, employment) cannot be put on a rating scale, they are not included in the scoring. These items will nevertheless be of interest as background questions. Thus scores may range from 3 to 210 points.

Scoring is done by using the boxes provided to the right of each item. Scoring is straightforward for most items and is summarized in Box 12.2. The number circled is simply put in the box. Item number 5, concerning pain site, is an exception since it only has five categories. Consequently, the scoring box to the right indicates "2*x", so that the number of sites checked is multiplied by two. If a patient checks the boxes for neck and low back pain, then the two checks would be multiplied by two to produce 4 and this number would be placed in the scoring box.

Some items need to be inverted so that high scores indicate high risk. These items are marked with "10−x" which produces the inversion. Thus, if the patient circles 6 on one of these items, then the score would be "10−6", and a 4 would be put in the box.

Missing values

Each questionnaire should be checked to ensure that it has been properly completed when the patient turns it in. Moreover, items are designed so that all patients can answer all questions. Nevertheless, a patient may occasionally fail to complete an item. If a value is missing it is important to adjust the score as the risk estimate is based on the sum score. To adjust the score, calculate the patient's average rating on the other items and use it as an estimate for the missing item.

Missing values tend to reduce the validity of the questionnaire. Only a small number of missing items can therefore be accepted if we are to maintain good predictive power. Skipping over items may be a signal that the patient either does not understand the questions, or why answering them is important. It may also indicate that the patient does not see the questions as being relevant. Naturally, these issues need to be examined and resolved before proceeding with a risk estimate.

Not working

If a patient ticks the box for "not working" on the two relevant items, this is scored in the same manner as for a missing value.

Interpretation of scores

The question of interpretation may be illustrated by reiterating that of 100 patients seeking healthcare for acute musculoskeletal pain, only a small minority, say 10, will develop a long-term problem during the coming year. The question is of those seeking care, can we identify the 10 who risk developing the long-term problem?

BOX 12.3 ROUGH CUT-OFF POINTS FOR INTERPRETING SCORES FROM THE ÖREBRO MUSCULOSKELETAL PAIN SCREENING QUESTIONNAIRE. THESE ARE BASED ON A NONCHRONIC, PRIMARY CARE POPULATION.

- A score over 105 indicates a relatively high level of risk. Further assessment is warranted.

- A score of 90 to 105 indicates a medium risk and that practitioners may want to pay attention to these patients.

- A score under 90 suggests low risk and we would expect these patients to recover.

The screening questionnaire provides a sum score that is easily interpreted into rough risk estimates (Box 12.3).

Predictive accuracy

Predictive accuracy is how well the questionnaire actually identifies patients who will develop long-term problems. This has been investigated in several studies (Hurley et al., 2000, 2001; Ektor-Andersen et al., 2002; Linton and Boersma, 2003) that demonstrate that approximately 80–85% of those risking future sick leave may be identified. In this research, patients have been given the questionnaire and then followed for several months to determine whether they in fact develop a problem. For example, in our first study we followed patients for six months and defined being off work for back pain as a measure of outcome (Linton and Halldén, 1998). With the help of our screening questionnaire we were able to identify at the first visit 88% of those who went on to have problems working.

Consider Table 12.1 below, which illustrates accuracy. The concept of "hits" and "misses" may be helpful as are the terms "false positive" (an "at risk" score for a patient who in fact is not at risk) and "false negative" (a score indicating no risk when in fact the patient is at risk). If we refer again to the table, we see that a cut-off score of 105 correctly identifies (hits) 88% of those actually sick-listed more than 30 days. Thus it would incorrectly identify (misses) 12% as false positives, i.e. identified as at risk when in fact they did not develop such sick leave. On the other hand, the table shows that the 105 cut-off point correctly identifies 75% of those who do *not* need to be off work. This means that 25% would be false negatives, i.e. identified as not being at risk for taking sick leave, when in fact they actually take sick leave absence from work.

Consequently, the Örebro Musculoskeletal Pain Screening Questionnaire is helpful in identifying early on those patients who may develop persistent pain and disability problems.

Providing feedback

A notable part of screening is providing the patient with proper feedback. Typically, people are curious to know what the result of the screening is, particularly when they have invested the time and effort to complete a questionnaire. Thus, the patient may be concerned about their pain problem as well as the results of the assessment. To counteract this anxiety, a clear explanation is necessary that includes concrete information about how the patient may actively participate in treatment and prevention.

Table 12.1 Examples of the effect of various cut-off scores on prediction of prognosis ($N = 137$). The median score for the entire group is 104. Correct classification refers to specificity for the healthy group (0 days) and sensitivity for the other two groups (i.e. correctly classifying those with sick leave).

	% correctly classified		
Cut-off score	0 days (specificity)[a]	1–30 days (sensitivity)[b]	>30 days sick leave (sensitivity)[b]
90	48	90	96
100	64	90	92
105	75	86	88
110	79	62	79
120	88	38	54

[a]Percentage with indicated score and below; denotes specificity, i.e. correctly classified as healthy and not sick-listed.
[b]Percentage with indicated score and above; denotes sensitivity, i.e. correctly classified as being off work and sick-listed.

Providing feedback also represents an excellent opportunity to develop rapport with the patient, provide educational information and promote self-help behaviors. In providing feedback on the screening questionnaire results, an overview should be provided. A short summary that stresses the usefulness of the information, underscores some positive results and leads into detailed questions is ordinarily done at the beginning of the meeting. (A final summary is provided at the end of the session.) Although professionals often discuss patients in terms of "risk levels", I recommend avoiding this word, as it is often misunderstood. For patients, "risk" is often a dichotomous concept that indicates either a "normal" score or the terrible certainty of developing chronic disability. Instead, the discussion might focus on consequences of the pain and how the problem might best be dealt with to avoid future problems.

The communication skills outlined in Chapter 10 are an imperative aspect. Remember that we are collecting information and the individual patient is in a position to provide us with key features. Therefore, we need to communicate effectively with the patient in order to understand their concerns and pick up on important yellow flags.

Provide positive feedback

It is important to encourage the patient to continue with positive beliefs and behaviors by providing positive feedback. This provides for a significant balance to the possible "negative" factors where further discussion may be necessary.

"There are a number of positive aspects that are illustrated in the questionnaire. You seem to be able to manage your pain quite a bit as seen in question 12. [wait for response] Although the pain is fairly intense now, you have not been off work before and the duration of this episode is relatively short. Finally, you have been able to remain active in spite of the pain which is enormously helpful for recovery."

Identifying target behaviors

Screening seems to make sense only if it promotes a more effective way of proceeding with the case. Identification per se has no certain value. Indeed, using psychological screening to simply *identify* patients at risk would seem to be a waste of important information. Certainly, going a step further and using the information to develop ideas about goals for intervention as well as factors maintaining the problem would utilize the information more wisely and enhance the assessment. After all, the promise of screening is to appropriate resources to those patients most likely to benefit from them. Attention may therefore be turned to possible targets for intervention as well as

probable maintaining factors that in turn would help in tailoring the intervention to the individual's actual needs.

To identify targets in the clinical situation, I recommend using the answers to individual items on the Örebro Musculoskeletal Pain Screening Questionnaire as a basis for a discussion with the patient. After reinforcing positive behaviors, I ask open-ended questions about items that have atypical responses. Areas of concern such as a high score on a fear-avoidance or depression item can in this way be identified and assessed. For example, we may ask: *"I see that you have rated your mood with an 8, could you tell me more about this?"* This creates an opportunity to assess and understand the patient's beliefs about their problem and probable recovery.

As we proceed through the various items on the questionnaire, a picture should begin to emerge concerning potential targets. The patient's conception of the problem should become clearer. Moreover, barriers to recovery, e.g. workplace factors or fear, should become apparent. The patient's goals typically also come to the forefront. In short, the patient and practitioner develop a "shared understanding" of the problem and what the focus of the treatment should be on.

A preliminary analysis may be conducted in order to generate hypotheses about factors causing or maintaining the problem. This characteristically involves combining items on the questionnaire to get a picture of antecedents, behaviors, thoughts and beliefs, as well as consequences. For example, anticipated problems for a return to work may be enhanced by fear-avoidance beliefs. Specifically, the patient may believe that her or his work is harmful and should be avoided until after full physical recovery. Or, fear-avoidance beliefs may be pertinent even though some activities, say walking, are not affected, while others, such as household chores, are affected. An attempt to identify why the patient can walk but not do household chores could proceed, as the patient may believe that certain movements (bending, twisting, lifting) are harmful. Thus, the screening setting offers an opportunity for initiating an analysis of factors that maintain the problem.

Planning for treatment

A key feature of screening is that it provides an occasion for clear communication. To engage patients in early interventions, communication seems essential for providing an understanding of the problem and its treatment. The time pressures of the clinic make this a true challenge, but research indicates that poor communication contributes to the development of problems. Bear in mind that a recent study of chronic pain patients revealed that only 32% could provide an accurate cause of their problem, while 20% gave a cause that did not coincide with their actual diagnosis, and the remaining 48% could not report the cause at all (Geisser and Roth, 1998). Consider further that patients come to the clinic with expectations about the cause of the problem and treatment and these are relatively powerful predictors of future disability (Waddell et al., 1993; Linton and Halldén, 1998).

Once an understanding of the problem has been reached, potential interventions may emerge and be discussed. We may also evaluate the patient's interest in the various options for interventions available. For example, we may ask an open-ended question regarding how mood might be dealt with. At this point we may need to employ our own problem-solving skills to make decisions with the patient on what might be done and how we should proceed. Having established a shared understanding of the cause of the problem and the targets for intervention, it should be easier to establish an alliance with the patient to enhance cooperation. Although back and neck pain often remit undramatically, certain action may be warranted. Often this action will involve relatively simple measures such as information or further assessment. It may also involve advice, education or skills training. Fortunately, many patients may not need additional treatment as information and advice may be sufficient to enhance their own self-care skills.

When should the screening be conducted?

Because screening demands some resources, and because most patients recover, the question is when the screening should be conducted. Because patients often recover, one suggestion has been if the bout is not resolving within two to four weeks after the first visit (Kendall et al., 1997). The idea is that yellow flags would be assessed in the interview during the first session with a few questions. Those recovering would not require further assessment while those having continued problems would complete a screening. The problem is that many patients continue to have problems, but do not return. Further, busy clinics may have difficulties in establishing a routine for the screening.

I recommend using the screening questionnaire with every patient who seeks care for musculoskeletal pain problems. It is relatively inexpensive to use (takes only a minute to score) and provides a thorough ground from which to conduct the clinical interview. It can be a valuable aid in communication and the establishment of a shared understanding. Above all, by using this tool from the start, *focus will be put on early interventions.* Patients will not be "missed" by lack of routine or the belief that usual medical care will be successful.

CASE STUDY: HANK

Hank was asked to complete the screening questionnaire. Consequently, he spent a few minutes at the clinic and provided his answers. Look at the questionnaire over the next few pages and attempt to analyze the yellow flags present and how this might affect planning for further assessments or interventions.

Hank has a total score of 125 which clearly puts him above the high-risk cut-off zone. This means that if we do not intervene we would expect that Hank will develop long-term disability in the form of being off work for his back pain. It also means that we need to look further into the psychological "yellow flags" that may be operating. A perusal of Hank's answers provides a good start for understanding his situation and for obtaining more information about his problem.

The first few items deal mainly with the experience of pain. We see that Hank has been suffering for some time (item 7) and has been off work 31–60 days during the past year (item 6). Moreover, he experiences quite a lot of pain (6 on items 9 and 10) and he has the pain more or less the whole time (item 11). Furthermore, Hank does

not feel that he has the possibility to control or cope with the pain very well (item 12). Thus, one area of concern is Hank's experience of the pain. Discussion with Hank may well point to the need to have some targets with regard to pain management.

Some items deal with Hank's work. Since Hank is in construction, it is not surprising that his job is somewhat heavy and a bit monotonous (item 8). Yet he mainly enjoys his work (item 17). However, Hank is not at all certain that he can return to his work. This is important. On item 16 he related that he has little chance of returning to his work within 6 months and on item 15 he rates a rather large risk that his problem will develop into a persistent one. This opens the door for a discussion of why Hank believes this to be the case.

Hank does not seem to be suffering from anxiety or stress (item 13), but does signal a possible depressed mood (item 14). It would be worthwhile discussing with Hank how he feels and why.

Three items are concerned with fear-avoidance beliefs. On all three items (18–20) Hank has relatively high ratings. It is important to know why Hank believes this to be the case. Further, this discussion is an excellent

1. What year were you born?   19.60.....

2. Are you: male ☒   female ☐

3. Were you born in Sweden?

                    yes ☒   no ☐

4. What is your current employment situation?

    paid work ☒   studying ☐   unpaid work at home ☐
    unemployed ☐   retired ☐   other ☐: _____

5. Where do you have pain? Check the appropriate sites.

                                                                                        2*x

    neck ☒   shoulder ☒   upper back ☐   lower back ☒   leg ☐ | 6 |

6. How many days of work have you missed because of pain during **the past 12 months**? Check one.

    0 days ☐   1–2 days ☐   3–7 days ☐   8–14 days ☐   15–30 days ☐
    31–60 days ☒   61–90 days ☐   91–180 days ☐   181–365 days ☐   > 365 days ☐ | 6 |

7. How long have you had your current pain problem? Check one.

    0–1 weeks ☐   2–3 weeks ☐   4–5 weeks ☐   6–7 weeks ☐   8–9 weeks ☐
    10–11 weeks ☐   12–23 weeks ☐   24–35 weeks ☐   36–52 weeks ☐   > 52 weeks ☒ | 10 |

8. Is your work heavy or monotonous? Circle the best alternative.

    0   1   2   3   4   5   ⑥   7   8   9   10 | 6 |
    not at all   extremely
                    not working ☐

9. How would you rate the pain that you have had during **the past week**? Circle one.

    0   1   2   3   4   5   ⑥   7   8   9   10 | 6 |
    no pain   pain as bad as it could be

10. In the **past three months**, on the average, how intense was your pain on a 0–10 scale? Circle one.

    0   1   2   3   4   5   ⑥   7   8   9   10 | 6 |
    no pain   pain as bad as it could be

11. How **often** would you say that you have experienced pain episodes, on the average,
    during **the past three months**? Circle one.

    0   1   2   3   4   5   6   7   ⑧   9   10 | 8 |
    never   always

Continued

12. Based on all the things you do to cope, or deal with your pain, on an average day, how much are you able to decrease it? Please circle the appropriate number.

| 0 | 1 | 2 | 3 | ④ | 5 | 6 | 7 | 8 | 9 | 10 |

can't decrease
it at all

can decrease
it completely

10−x

6

13. How tense or anxious have you felt in **the past week**? Circle one.

| 0 | 1 | ② | 3 | 4 | 5 | 6 | 7 | 8 | 9 | 10 |

absolutely
calm and relaxed

as tense and anxious as
I've ever felt

2

14. How much have you been bothered by feeling depressed in **the past week**? Circle one.

| 0 | 1 | 2 | 3 | 4 | 5 | 6 | ⑦ | 8 | 9 | 10 |

not at all

extremely

7

15. In your view, how large is the risk that your current pain may become persistent? Circle one.

| 0 | 1 | 2 | 3 | 4 | 5 | 6 | ⑦ | 8 | 9 | 10 |

no risk

very large risk

7

16. In your estimation, what are the chances that you will be able to work in **six months**? Circle one.

| 0 | 1 | ② | 3 | 4 | 5 | 6 | 7 | 8 | 9 | 10 |

no chance

very large chance

10−x

8

17. If you take into consideration your work routines, management, salary, promotion possibilities and workmates, how satisfied are you with your job? Circle one.

| 0 | 1 | 2 | 3 | 4 | 5 | 6 | 7 | ⑧ | 9 | 10 |

not at all
satisfied

completely
satisfied

not working ☐

10−x

2

*Here are some of the things which other patients have told us about their pain. For each statement please circle any number from 0 to 10 to say how much physical activities, such as bending, lifting, walking or driving, affect or would affect **your** back.*

18. Physical activity makes my pain worse.

| 0 | 1 | 2 | 3 | 4 | 5 | 6 | 7 | 8 | ⑨ | 10 |

completely
disagree

completely
agree

9

19. An increase in pain is an indication that I should stop what I am doing until the pain decreases.

| 0 | 1 | 2 | 3 | 4 | 5 | 6 | 7 | ⑧ | 9 | 10 |

completely
disagree

completely
agree

8

20. I should not do my normal activities including work with my present pain.

0	1	2	3	4	5	6	7	8	⑨	10
completely disagree										completely agree

9

Here is a list of five activities. Please circle the number which best describes your current ability to participate in each of these activities.

21. I can do light work for an hour.

0	1	2	3	4	⑤	6	7	8	9	10
cannot do it because of pain										can do it without pain being a problem

10−x

5

22. I can walk for an hour.

0	1	2	3	4	5	6	7	⑧	9	10
cannot do it because of pain										can do it without pain being a problem

10−x

2

23. I can do ordinary household chores.

0	1	2	3	4	5	6	⑦	8	9	10
cannot do it because of pain										can do it without pain being a problem

10−x

3

24. I can do the weekly shopping.

0	1	2	3	4	5	⑥	7	8	9	10
cannot do it because of pain										can do it without pain being a problem

10−x

4

25. I can sleep at night.

0	1	2	3	4	⑤	6	7	8	9	10
cannot do it because of pain										can do it without pain being a problem

10−x

5

THANK YOU FOR YOUR COOPERATION!

125

Continued

opportunity to ask Hank why he believes he has the pain, i.e. what is wrong.

Finally, five items are designed to assess function. These are important since function is a common problem. Also, functional problems may be related to beliefs or fear. Indeed, Hank has a clear problem with everyday function. Compared to before the back pain began, Hank has a rather drastic reduction in function. Again, questioning might illuminate the extent of this and how Hank experiences this. Moreover, Hank reports some problems sleeping. Since sleep may enhance the pain and increase emotional irritability, follow-up questions might provide more information. For example, it would be of interest to know how often the sleeping problems occur, if Hank has problems falling asleep, if he wakes during the night with pain, and the like.

It is interesting to compare various questions within the screening questionnaire. For example, the items on fear-avoidance beliefs might be compared with the items on function and follow-up questions posed. (Do you believe you will injure your back if you do everyday activities?)

Because the physical examination showed no red flags or any organic problems that might be treated medically, other options were discussed with Hank. He was clear that he wanted to be able to function much better. This meant being able to do household duties, participate in sports as well as leisure activities with the family, and to return to work. Hank also wanted to manage his pain better, although he was aware that he could not get completely rid of it. Hank had already tried several painkillers, but he was not satisfied with the pain relief or the side-effects and therefore he wanted to learn other ways of dealing with the pain. As a result of Hank's goals and previous treatment history, he was asked if he was interested in participating in a pain management group. It was explained to Hank that the aim of this was to learn ways of managing the pain, but also of developing better function at home and at work so that he might improve his quality of life as well as his function. Further, it was stressed that the group focused on preventing the development of future problems. Hank said that he was interested and was therefore given the telephone number to call to apply for this intervention.

SUMMARY

Employing screening routines as a complement to other examinations may help to identify patients who may well develop chronic problems. Tools such as the Örebro Musculoskeletal Pain Screening Questionnaire are helpful in identifying those patients most in need of early interventions. These instruments not only help us to identify these patients, but they also provide a basis for communicating with the patient to develop targets and a plan for intervention. In order to provide early interventions that will prevent the development of persistent problems, early identification should be incorporated into routine practice.

CHAPTER 13

Early interventions: a cognitive-behavioral approach

LEARNING OBJECTIVES

To understand:

- when expert help is needed;

- the content of effective psychological early treatments;

- the essential strategies employed in cognitive-behavioral preventive interventions.

What should be done for patients who do not recover or are found to be at risk of developing chronic problems? Once we realize that a patient may well develop persistent pain, how should this be handled? In this chapter we will deal with how these problems might be tackled. This is a stimulating task as two key decisions are on line and the patient's future is at stake. First, we need to make the decision as to whether special interventions are necessary. In other words, will the patient benefit from an early, preventive intervention focusing on psychological factors? And second, we need to make the decision as to how this will be accomplished. Should the patient be referred to another professional or could this intervention be performed in your own clinic?

To be sure, early intervention is important. Delay and failed treatments not only provide time for the process of chronification to march forward, they may also feed the process by reinforcing passive behaviors, pain cognitions, fear, frustration and the like. The question then is not whether an intervention is needed, but what and how it should be achieved.

Providing patients with psychologically oriented interventions requires special skills. You may wish to obtain these skills yourself, work in a team with someone who is competent, or refer such patients to other competent professionals. However, identifying a patient at risk of developing persistent pain and disability is a point to mark because it implies that psychologically oriented help is warranted. Providing this help necessitates distinct training. In contrast to previous chapters where skills like communication and screening can be learned and improved upon by everyone, unique competence is needed to conduct psychologically oriented therapy. While the intervention described in this chapter is normally conducted by a trained psychologist, other healthcare professionals with proper training may wish to conduct such groups. In this chapter we will explore a specific program designed to provide early, preventive intervention that truly addresses the psychological aspects of the problem. This will provide a clear description of the content of a successful early intervention and may help you to decide how such an intervention might be made available. For those interested, a session by session description of the cognitive-behavioral group treatment is provided in the Appendix. Whether you want to provide the service yourself or through a team or a referral, it is important to underscore that the method of delivery and the content are important basic factors that surely are related to effectiveness.

THE NEED FOR COGNITIVE-BEHAVIORAL INTERVENTIONS

Although psychological factors are believed to be central in the development of a chronic back pain problem, there have been relatively few attempts to prevent chronic disability using psychological techniques. Still, if psychological risk factors enhance the development of a chronic problem (Kendall et al., 1998; Linton, 2000b, 2000c), then psychological interventions might be of real value. Moreover, because the model of pain perception and disability in Part I entails cognitive, emotional and behavioral aspects, an intervention encompassing these aspects is logical.

The utility of cognitive-behavioral interventions

A particularly salient reason for employing any intervention is effectiveness. We need to know whether the intervention is the best available according to scientific evaluations. Cognitive-behavioral (CBT) interventions have been used in the treatment of chronic pain for many years and several studies have examined their utility. Thus, when faced with building an early intervention, researchers naturally turned to what had previously been accomplished. Let us look at typical cognitive-behavioral programs and their success rate in part as important information for treating persistent pain problems, but above all as a background to understanding how the early psychological interventions were designed.

Content

Although cognitive-behavioral programs vary considerably in practice, there are several characteristics that unify them. Some of the basic aspects that define the approach are shown in Table 13.1. As may be seen in the table, there is a real emphasis on applying psychological knowhow to the treatment. Thus, the focus is on behaviors such as coping and function, cognitions

Table 13.1 Characteristics of cognitive-behavioral pain treatment programs.

Characteristic	Description
Learning-based	Apply learning principles to teach new behaviors and lifestyle
Coping-oriented	Patient is actively involved in treatment; stresses methods to deal with situation
Cognitive focus	Cognitive techniques are used to control pain and alter maladaptive pain beliefs
Goal setting	Clear goals are established with the patient and attainment is planned in small steps
Assessment	Psychological assessment included as a vital method for matching the treatment to the patient's actual needs
Multidimensional approach	Treatment includes a comprehensive program
Function	Function is in focus rather than pain
Homework	Patients practice between sessions
Everyday life	Goal is functioning in everyday life, thus this is a main focus
Follow-up/adherence	Long-term outcome is central. Generalization and adherence enhancement are incorporated from the start.

Based on Linton (1994).

and the application of learning principles to change these. There is also an emphasis on the here and now so that clear goals are established and a plan for step-wise achievement is made. Because functioning in everyday situations is viewed as vital, real prominence is placed on practicing newly learned skills and coping strategies at home and at work. Indeed, to obtain good long-term results, various procedures to ensure adherence and generalization of the techniques from the treatment setting to the everyday setting are incorporated.

Even though there are many factors that define cognitive-behavioral treatments, there is also great variety between different programs. In my review of the literature, I found that the exact content, duration and administration of the cognitive-behavioral programs varied enormously across clinics and studies (Linton, 2000d). The procedures ranged from the use of one technique like biofeedback to the use of a wide assortment of basic techniques ranging from applied relaxation and stress management to graded activity training and medication reduction. The duration of treatment also varied from a few hours to several weeks. In addition, the setting in which the treatment was provided ranged from outpatients to hospitalized patients treated individually or in groups. While most were administered in conjunction with other medical services such as a pain or rehabilitation clinic, others were given at spas or in nonmedical settings. Thus, the cognitive-behavioral programs have been adapted to a huge array of uses.

Utility for chronic pain

The usefulness of cognitive-behavioral programs in the treatment and management of persistent pain has been evaluated in many studies that have employed good scientific methodology. These studies have been reviewed by various experts in the field. Early reviews concluded that multidimensional pain programs that included cognitive-behavioral interventions were effective (Flor et al., 1992b; Cutler et al., 1994; Turk, 1996b). However, it was not always clear what the specific contribution of cognitive-behavioral treatments was. In Sweden, I was asked to review this material for the national agency responsible for evaluating healthcare (Swedish Council on Technology Assessment in Health Care, SBU). To accomplish this we searched the literature for studies that fulfilled certain vital criteria.

First, the study needed to isolate the effect of the cognitive-behavioral intervention. This is crucial because many clinics employ an integrated program that contains a variety of other treatment methods. While this is good clinical practice, it makes drawing specific conclusions about the cognitive-behavioral interventions impossible; you do not know what

aspects of the program have led to which results. Second, the patient population had to consist mainly of patients with back or neck pain. Third, the study needed to be a randomized, controlled trial (RCT). Randomized trials eliminate a large number of factors that can otherwise bias outcome such as selecting the "best" patients for the intervention. Several studies compared the cognitive-behavioral intervention to a waiting list control (WLC). This is a group waiting to receive the cognitive-behavioral treatment. Other studies used some form of alternative treatment such as a standard rehabilitation program. Twenty-nine articles fulfilled these criteria.

To judge the worth of the studies, key outcome domains were used. Thus, five domains were employed: *pain* (e.g. intensity ratings, descriptors), *psychological functioning* (e.g. fear, anxiety, depression, distress), *physical function* (e.g. activities of daily living), *medication* (e.g. painkillers) and *healthcare utilization* (e.g. number of visits). Since the various studies employed a great range of measurements, a criterion was developed to determine if the cognitive-behavioral treatment was effective. If the cognitive-behavioral treatment produced a statistically significant greater improvement on at least two domains, then it was classified as a "positive" outcome. However, if the comparison group was significantly better than the cognitive-behavioral group on any of the domains, it was classified as a "negative" outcome. Thus, a relatively stringent criterion was employed where the cognitive-behavioral group needed to produce clearly greater improvements than the groups to which it was compared.

Figure 13.1 illustrates the results of the review. In all, 16 investigations employed a WLC as the comparison group. As seen in the figure, nearly 90% of the studies showed the cognitive-behavioral intervention to be superior to the WLC. Although WLC groups serve an important role, they do not actually provide the patient with an intervention. Thus, patients may be affected by expectations for future treatment and any nonspecific effects of providing treatment (e.g. attention) are missed. However, 14 studies did include a comparison group that received another active treatment. As Fig. 13.1 shows, nearly 90% of these studies also demonstrated that the cognitive-behavioral intervention was superior. Finally, because of the recurrent nature of the problem, long-term results are of the utmost importance. In other words, whether treatment results are maintained is an imperative issue. In fact, 28 of the 29 studies provided some sort of follow-up data. Figure 13.1 shows that over 95% indicate that the results were maintained at follow-up. Thus, there was strong evidence that cognitive-behavioral interventions produced moderate to large

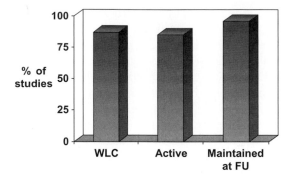

Figure 13.1 The percentage of studies where the cognitive-behavioral program had significantly better results on at least two of the four domains (pain, function, medication, psychological function) than a waiting list control (WLC), or active treatment (control group received another active treatment), and the percentage maintaining improvements at follow-up.

improvements on key outcomes as compared to WLC groups or other active treatment.

Additional reviews, conducted in slightly different ways, by different authors, have also drawn the conclusion that cognitive-behavioral methods are useful. For example, Flor (1997) examined some 80 studies and pooled the data. She concluded that the additional benefits of adding such psychological treatment were quite large, such as improving ability to return to work by 43%, reducing healthcare costs by 35% and increasing physical activity by 53%. Two so-called systematic reviews are also interesting. This type of review is probably the most stringent evaluation of the literature. For example, in one systematic review it was found that cognitive-behavioral procedures produced "moderate" improvements on a variety of outcome domains and concluded that this was a very worthwhile outcome when compared to other treatments or other chronic problems (Morley et al., 1999). Finally, the second systematic review was conducted within the framework of the Cochrane Back Review Group (van Tulder et al., 2000). Positive effects were found for pain, function and behavioral outcomes. The conclusion was that "Behavioral treatment seems to be an effective treatment for patients with chronic low back pain…". Thus, there is considerable evidence that cognitive-behavioral programs are helpful in managing or treating long-term pain problems. The next step was to utilize this information in developing interventions that could be administered at an earlier point in time.

Early interventions

Using cognitive-behavioral methods early on seems logical, but how should these methods be adapted for earlier use? Patients with acute or recurrent pain may not have the same needs as those with persistent problems. A perusal of the early literature showed that only two studies had used such methods with nonchronic populations. Fordyce and his team (1986) used a behavioral program for patients seeking care for an acute bout of low back pain less than 10 days in duration. The results, however, were not outstanding. The behavioral elements produced some differences on function, but still the differences appeared to be relatively small. In another study with subacute patients, Lindström and associates (1992) used a graded activity program, a back school and a workplace visit as early interventions. Compared to a group receiving traditional care, the results showed significantly better function and return to work. This study, however, used only one specific behavioral technique and it was embedded in a program with other elements.

Based on a psychological analysis of the problems patients face early on, strategies were developed for providing cognitive-behavioral interventions as an early, secondary preventive intervention (Linton and Bradley, 1996). These are summarized in Table 13.2. The strategies have similarities to the multidimensional management programs reviewed above, but they also reflect important aspects concerning communication (Chapter 10) and getting the therapeutic management right from the beginning (Chapter 11). These may be considered in conjunction with other components of a multidimensional program. It is important, for example, to have consistency in these programs so that all treatments are provided in a "psychologically sound" manner in order to maintain focus on the goals and enhance results by applying learning principles.

A fundamental prerequisite for prevention is good communication with the patient, as was argued in Chapter 10. Although the time pressures of the clinic make this a real challenge, research indicates that good communication contributes to effective outcome results and greater sastisfaction. A strategy that is sometimes taken for granted is pain relief (Dworkin, 1997; Linton, 1997b). While it is quite difficult to significantly reduce chronic pain, an earlier approach might have a better opportunity to relieve pain. Traditionally, the goal is total pain relief and it is achieved with drugs until healing occurs. However, with many types of pain such as musculoskeletal pain, it is important to address the patient's expectations (as total pain relief may not occur), as well as exploring other avenues for *controlling* the pain. Accordingly, this provides a brilliant occasion to introduce and emphasize the use of self-care skills. Another strategy is dealing with the patient's expectations. Patients come to the clinic with a host of expectations and beliefs about

Table 13.2 Characteristics of a cognitive-behavioral approach to early intervention.

Strategy	Description
1. Early	Time is a central aspect, intervention should be initiated before disruption of lifestyle, etc.
2. Facilitate communication	Patients may not understand the problem and may have anxiety or fear. Good communication is essential in promoting self-care and alleviating fear avoidance.
3. Engage patient as partner	Problem cannot be "cured" and intervention requires patient to change behaviors, therefore patient participation is necessary.
4. Clear behavioral goals, maintain activities	Focus on health and behaviors and what patient should do rather than on medical, etc., variables. Recommend maintaining daily activity, some training and return to work.
5. Defuse negative emotions	Anxiety, fear, anger, guilt and frustration are common feelings which may disrupt recovery or promote disability. Apply available techniques.
6. Promote coping strategies	Dysfunctional beliefs and thought patterns may limit progress. Probe patient's expectations. Apply psychological techniques to develop self-efficacy.
7. Coordinate	Workplace, family, insurance carriers, other medical facilities, etc., are instrumental in enhancing or hindering recovery. Therefore it is important that there is clear communication as well as coordination of services.
8. Follow-up, maintenance	Pain is recurrent and behavioral change is often difficult to maintain. Thus, follow-up is of value in evaluating results and adjusting the program to meet the patient's needs.

Based on Linton and Bradley (1996).

the cause of their problem, but also about the examination, treatment and consequences of the problem. It is important to probe and deal with expectations concerning diagnostics, appropriate treatment, work and the role of self-help.

Assisting the patient in maintaining everyday activities and lifestyle patterns is a cornerstone of early intervention. Many people are surprised to learn that it can be therapeutic to participate in ordinary everyday activities. Maintaining normal routines ought to reduce the disruption of the pain problem and enhance quality of life. It also would prevent the gradual lifestyle changes that may occur in the chronification process described in Chapter 9. If there are any exceptions to this rule, they would need to be very specifically defined and written down (e.g. "Do not lift more than 20 kg during the next 7 days").

Promoting self-care skills is important for establishing a working relationship and self-efficacy. The patient may be helped to incorporate a number of coping strategies to manage the pain problem and potential disability. This should reinforce the patients' belief that they can influence their own situation and health. Patients may be taught to discriminate when

they can deal with the problem themselves as opposed to when healthcare services should be sought. To maintain the right focus it is wise to use interventions that incorporate the patient as an active partner and are health behavior oriented. Because programs for early, secondary intervention require the patient to adhere to advice by engaging in various self-care behaviors, the patient must be a central part of the process. For example, the patient should be integral in defining the problem, setting goals, selecting interventions and following through with them. This will help to ensure adherence with the program by greatly increasing the patient's commitment. Furthermore, this should reinforce a belief in the utility of the program and, specifically, self-care.

Anxiety, distress and fear avoidance should be addressed, for example by providing reassurance and activity training (Chapter 11). Information and instructions should be provided about specific behaviors that ought to be performed and what the expected results may be ("Maintain your daily activity routines; this will not hurt you although you may expect to experience some pain while practicing during the coming week(s)"). Informing patients that it is advantageous to the healing process to return to work relatively soon may be helpful in relieving uncertainty. Self-care skills such as relaxation and finding momentary pain-relieving rest positions may also be helpful. Health behaviors should be systematically reinforced.

Engaging the cooperation and coordination of efforts of all involved parties and services is a challenge that becomes increasingly important with time. The interaction between the patient, his family, workplace, insurance carrier, government agencies and healthcare providers appears to be vital for ensuring recovery and especially a return to work. As an illustration, a patient who believes that the workplace or insurance carrier are not interested in their case may be more likely to pursue litigation (Philips and Grant, 1991). Contact between the involved parties should increase the probability of identifying important obstacles to a full recovery and provide support in administering the prevention programs.

Empirical evidence

To test an early intervention, our clinic offered nursing personnel with a history of back pain problems a cognitive-behavioral program that included exercise, ergonomics, limited physical therapy and group cognitive-behavioral therapy aimed at improving coping and returning to work (Linton et al., 1989). Although participants were not yet deemed to have chronic problems, they did have a considerable history of back pain problems and had been off work several months when entering the study. Relative to a "treatment as usual" group, the intervention group improved significantly on a variety of variables at the 6-month follow-up and maintained improvements at an 18-month follow-up (Linton and Bradley, 1992).

Providing occupationally oriented services for patients relatively early was also successfully executed in a population of workers with upper extremity pain (Feuerstein et al., 1993). All patients were work disabled for a minimum of 3 months (the average was about 9 months) and consequently were at about the point where the problem can become chronic. The mulitmodal program included physical and work training, pain and stress management, ergonomic consultation and vocational counseling. Although this is not a randomized study, the results clearly demonstrated that the early multimodal intervention returned 74% back to work while the usual care group returned 40%. The study shows the potential value of an early, preventive intervention and demonstrates how a psychological perspective may be combined with a broader intervention package.

An intervention designed to reduce fear and maintain normal activities provided patients off work for 12 weeks with an average of four consultations (Indahl et al., 1995), where the patient was examined, radiographs taken, and a great deal of information on self-care and activity was supplied (Indahl et al., 1995). Every other patient was assigned to the treatment group ($n = 463$) or to a conventional treatment control group ($n = 512$). Treated patients were provided with a model of why they hurt and told that moderate activity would improve their condition by increasing blood flow. Results indicated that the intervention group had about half as many days off work as the control group and were more than twice as likely to return to work.

A clear application of psychological knowledge to early treatment is the Pain-Disability Prevention Program which has been run in Canada (Sullivan and Stanish, 2003). This program was developed specifically to help people off work with occupational low back pain to reestablish activity patterns and reduce psychological barriers to activity. Patients participate in the program during a 10-week period. The program contains five basic components: an activity log, activity scheduling, a walking program, graded activity, and coping to overcome psychological obstacles to activity involvement. The activity phase was designed to regain capacity but also to challenge fear and negative thinking. In the coping phase, the focus is on skills to overcome fears of reinjury and learning to monitor and modify self-defeating catastrophic thinking. A study was conducted on 104 patients off work for 6 weeks because of a back pain problem and who had at least one "yellow flag" indicating a psychological risk factor. Patients were recruited through the Novia Scotia Worker's Compensation Board. The program was quite effective. For example, it boasts a 60% success rate that may be compared to a base rate of 18% for a matched group at the Worker's Compensation Board. Moreover, initial scores on fear, catastrophizing and depression correctly identified outcome for 92% of the patients. This indicates that the intervention did indeed yield reductions in psychological risk factors and that these in turn were highly related to a successful outcome.

Early cognitive-behavioral intervention in primary care

Because repeated studies show that cognitive-behavioral techniques produce good results for pain patients and because the first attempts at early, secondary prevention appeared to produce good results, an early intervention for use in primary care was developed. The knowledge and experience gained from earlier studies was of tremendous value. However, we also focused on the risk factors identified in the screening assessment and the developmental process described in Chapter 9. Thus, from the beginning this intervention has uniquely focused on the prevention of persistent pain and disability and not merely on the treatment of pain intensity. The intervention encompasses a six-session structured program where participants meet in groups of 6 to 10 people, six times, once a week for 2 hours. The intervention attempts to address the psychological factors identified and thus assists patients in making changes that will enhance their ability to deal with the problem.

THE COGNITIVE-BEHAVIORAL INTERVENTION

The cognitive-behavioral program that we use has several features that directly address the psychosocial yellow flags thought to be propelling the development of a chronic problem (Linton, 1996, 1997a, 1999a, 2000a, 2000d). Below is a rather detailed description of the ideas behind the groups. In addition, the strategies for enhancing behavioral and cognitive changes are described. This section is written as a guide for setting up such groups and therefore is directed toward the group leader. However, the section is oriented to all healthcare professionals because it presents the nuts and bolts of providing a cognitive-behavioral intervention. By reading this section you will gain important insight into how a cognitive-behavioral intervention is delivered in clinical practice.

Goals

The course has several goals, but the overriding aim is for each person to develop her or his own coping program. We ask that all skills presented during the program be tried and tested so that participants can develop a tailored program that best suits each person's needs.

From a provider's point of view we hope to prevent pain-related disability and the need for healthcare services, in addition to improving quality of life. In short, the aim is to prevent pain-related absenteeism and the need for back pain-related healthcare. A natural goal is to improve the patient's quality of life so that they feel and function better. This includes factors like pain intensity, stress levels and participating in everyday activities. We realize that back pain is recurrent and therefore we do not intend to eliminate all back pain, but rather to decrease recurrences and reduce their impact.

A distinctive goal is that each member should have fun! Learning should be enjoyable and, as will be seen below, considerable effort is extended so that participants are truly engaged. Humor is used and even homework assignments are given to tickle the funny bone. The social aspect of participating in a group

is utilized. Managed wisely, this provides camaraderie and the experience that participating in the group is rewarding. Finally, since improvements are often made in very small steps and since *preventing* pain is not as dramatic as relieving it, special efforts need to be made to underscore progress, reinforce it, and ensure that the individual builds reinforcement into his or her own program.

Strategies for behavioral change

The interventions we offer participants involve coping that in turn requires the person to alter current cognitions and behaviors. Plainly put, the preventive intervention is based on changing beliefs and behavior. For example, beliefs about the relationship between pain and activity (*"The more I do, the more it will hurt"*) or beliefs about stress (*"I must do everything asked of me and exactly on time"*) may need to be revised. Likewise, behaviors may need to be changed, e.g. increasing activity levels or being able to say "no" to certain demands. The question becomes *how* this might be accomplished; we have employed several strategies.

First, the program is designed to actively engage the participant. Rather than a passive "school" approach, active participation is prompted and then reinforced. Discussions, for example, involve *every* patient in roundtable fashion. Problem-solving exercises are done in pairs to promote discussion and the results are reported by each pair. In the skills training module, each participant is encouraged to learn each skill and then apply it at home or at work during the week. Homework assignments are individualized to accommodate idiosyncrasies. Above all, each person is given the charge of developing his or her own personal coping program.

Second, restricted amounts of information are used to prime behavioral changes. It appears that information may have an impact in certain situations since it challenges beliefs (Burton and Waddell, 2002). However, health information is normally a rather weak method for modifying behavior. Thus, while we use modern information, we severely limit this part of the session so that more potent behavioral change methods will have precedence.

A third strategy is behavioral tests. We examined this concept earlier in developing reassurance routines. In this case, a patient's negative or inappropriate belief is examined and then a test is performed to see if the belief is actually true. For patients we conceptualize this as learning through experience. Thus, we ask patients to "test" each skill they learn to assess its possible value for them. This is one basis for participants to select the skills for their personal coping program.

Problem-solving is a fourth strategy utilized throughout to promote engagement and enhance maintenance.

It is the first skill taught! Further, this skill is honed in a special problem-based learning module where pairs of patients are asked to read a case study and then to solve various "problems" the patient is having.

Fifth, the group leader is taught to shape new thoughts and behaviors by reinforcing successive approximations of good coping behavior. Positive reinforcement, e.g. in the form of encouragement, is contingently provided when participants correctly approximate a goal behavior. Thus, gradual change is encouraged.

To maximize engagement and maintenance, another strategy is to enhance each patient's self-efficacy, that is, the patient's belief that he or she can impact on their pain and its course. This is logical since many patients have low self-efficacy levels and as the participant, in fact, is changing his or her health behavior. While therapists are facilitators, it is *not* the therapist that causes the change. For example, we might ask a person who has successfully completed a homework assignment (e.g. practiced relaxation resulting in decreased pain) to tell the entire group how he or she has accomplished this, to share the "secret" of their success.

Finally, as mentioned above, enjoyment is utilized to enhance learning, engagement, maintenance and pleasure. It is an important strategy to ensure that every participant feels that he or she has learned something during each session. People should have the opportunity to laugh and to receive social support. Not least, encouragement should be contingently delivered on a rich schedule so that participants may feel good about their accomplishments.

Targets

From the healthcare provider's perspective this early, preventive intervention has a number of targets. These are:

- Preventing new episodes of pain.
- Reducing the impact of new episodes.
- Maintaining/improving quality of life despite pain.
- Preventing or reducing the number of healthcare visits required.
- Preventing or reducing the number of days the participant is unable to work because of pain.

Objectives

In order to achieve the goals of the program and produce the desired changes in the targets, several objectives have been developed. The detailed objectives of the program are to:

1. Provide each individual with an understanding of their pain problem and its management.
2. Prevent (or extinguish) the development of excessive fear-avoidance responses.

3. Teach coping skills in the control and management of pain.
4. Promote health behaviors including physical and social activities.
5. Promote the application of skills in everyday life.
6. Provide a framework for long-term benefit through adherence and reanalyses of the problem.

Therefore we work with the following methods in the program:

1. *Knowledge/assessment.* Theory and other types of information where the individual is encouraged to use the information to analyze his or her own situation. Each person will be active in identifying problems as well as *solutions.*
2. *Fear avoidance.* Fear-avoidance problems will be controlled by (a) pain reduction, e.g. via relaxation, pause gymnastics; (b) exercise and activity prescriptions provided on a *time* (not pain) basis; (c) maintaining everyday activity routines by prescription.
3. *Coping.* Individualized methods of dealing with pain problems, stressing that the "big picture" will be used. This approach will incorporate a selection of skills to improve health, e.g. relaxation, self-statements, mini-pauses, stretching and flare-up control.
4. *Promote health behaviors.* Coincides with 3, but includes behaviors associated with general health and well-being. Stress management and the need for physical, social and personal activities.
5. *Application.* Match skills to needs. For example, monitoring may be used to identify when and where a special skill might be employed. Training in home or work situation. Use "life planning" and "scheduling" techniques.
6. *Long-term framework.* The program should be stressed as a method of analyzing the musculo-skeletal pain (MSP) problem and developing skills. Therefore, it may be utilized in the future to meet new demands and as the individual's situation changes. Address adherence by identifying which behaviors are effective in maintaining a healthy back and then working with relapse prevention and the health behavior model.

What every participant should get from each session

Participants ought to look forward to coming to sessions even though some sessions may contain frank discussions of problem areas. In order to ensure this, every session should be rewarding for the participant. This may, in part, be achieved by having participants list what they have gotten out of the session, e.g. what they have learned, improved or enjoyed. Alternatively, a description of suggestions for future sessions may be obtained from the participants.

When the participants leave, it should be clear (maybe used as a summary method to underscore this) specifically what the participant has gained:

1. What new information or facts have been learned?
2. What skill has been acquired, renewed or improved?
3. How information or skill may be applied; relevance, feedback.
4. What "insight" was gained, i.e. application to person's own situation.

In addition, each meeting should provide for:

5. Giving and/or getting emotional support.
6. Social interaction (coffee time, discussions, etc.).
7. Pleasure. The course should be fun! Hopefully everyone will have an opportunity to laugh.

Therapy content

Treatment is typically provided in groups of up to 10 or 12 participants. We have found that groups of about 8 work optimally. However, with groups of this size, the therapist will need to make special efforts so that each person has an opportunity to actively participate. In addition, measures need to be taken to encourage friendship and a sense of being at ease within the group.

The group sessions meet for two hours on six occasions. A follow-up session may be scheduled approximately three months after the last session if the group is in favor of this. A break during the session may be provided, but participants will need to organize their own coffee and snacks. One way of letting the group get to know each other is to have them organize this! In fact, as you will see in session 1, this provides an excellent opportunity to practice problem-solving skills.

Another important aspect that challenges the group leader is to make the material relevant for each individual. Discussions may be more general in nature, but the analyses and homework assignments should be relevant for the individual. In addition, participants should be reinforced for sharing their experiences (but not forced or "judged") within the group.

An important consideration is the confidentiality of the discussions in the group. Depending on your setting, members of the group may or may not know each other. In addition, some members may come from the same workplace. Consequently, it is important to come to an agreement about confidentiality. Some groups may suggest not having confidentiality, as it may nevertheless be difficult to maintain. This need

not cause difficulty since most of the discussions can still be successfully conducted.

You will need to use your comments and encouragement to reinforce a supportive and healthy atmosphere in the group. Remember that your views and comments carry considerable weight. Thus, they should be used *contingently* to encourage a positive feeling as well as to support the behavioral goals set.

Problem-based learning

Difficulties with participants who lack motivation may be avoided by using a problem-based learning approach. This teaching technique is based on presenting students with a problem that they are to solve themselves rather than simply "pumping" them with information. The teacher is therefore a resource person and advisor. In the therapy situation, problem-based learning may be incorporated by defining problems with the group and subsequently using these problems as the basis for exercises where participants will seek solutions.

Typical groups need a fairly large amount of structure. Problem-based learning provides a basic structure. Yet using a problem-based learning approach also enhances interest and "motivation". Moreover, with guidance, the participants ought to identify problems that we, as therapists, would ordinarily have included in the therapy. In fact, they often cite problems and goals that we would *not* have identified as therapists. Thus, active participation actually may improve results. The fact that participants have actively worked with identifying problems and finding their solution also has important therapeutic consequences as it increases integration and adherence.

The therapist

Administering these pain groups requires several skills. This is why the description of the sessions in the Appendix presumes knowledge of basic psychological skills and behavior therapy techniques.

In order to form successful groups, the therapist will need to selectively reinforce positive participation. This involves shaping members' behavior so that they contribute to the group and learn to deal better with their pain problem. Creating a positive atmosphere to a great extent depends on the therapist's skills in promoting constructive discussion that allows people to talk and develop their own skills. Humor is an excellent way of reducing anxiety and increasing interest. In fact, we try to present fun cartoons or tell short stories that can create laughter but also illustrate a point. It is important to remember, however, that the story should poke fun at the therapist or a neutral person, but *never* a member of the group. Another method is to encourage members to reinforce each other's behavior by providing constructive comments.

In addition to proficiency in creating a positive group atmosphere, the therapist will need to understand basic cognitive-behavioral techniques. During the course you will be required to teach participants several different skills. Moreover, given the time limit and number of skills presented, most of the methods are presented in abbreviated form. Consequently, a fundamental working ability to teach each skill is required. Literature concerning the skills is provided in the reference section for those who wish to brush up on their clinical skills.

Basic knowledge about pain and cognitive-behavioral treatments for pain is central as the course underscores coping with pain. It is not necessary to have worked with chronic pain patients, although this will provide valuable experience. In addition, it is important that the course focuses on prevention, i.e. preventing the development of disabling persistent pain problems.

Although a formal behavior analysis is not conducted during the course, each person will analyze his or her pain problem. Behavior analysis is an excellent clinical tool for psychologists, but it is beyond the scope of this course for participants to conduct a formal one.

Given the group format, it is difficult for the therapist to conduct such an analysis for each member (and this would also contradict the "self-help" rule of the course). Rather, by working with case studies and themes, each participant will make an "informal" analysis of his or her problem. By actively applying each of the coping skills, members will also empirically test the value of each skill.

Leading groups should be a very rewarding endeavor! Most groups make good progress and it is satisfying to experience this development. In addition, members often make considerable contributions and provide reinforcement.

OUTLINE OF EACH SESSION

Ideally each session should provide each participant with the opportunity to gain knowledge ("insight"), learn a skill, and obtain emotional release and social support, as well as to receive homework and some pleasure. Almost everyone enjoys talking and sharing experiences. This provides tremendous opportunities for learning!

To achieve these goals, each session is divided into several parts. As shown in Table 13.3, each session focuses on a particular area of relevance and participants develop a personal coping program.

Table 13.3 An overview of the content of the CBT intervention.

Session	Focus	Skills
1	Causes of pain and the prevention of chronic problems	Problem solving Applied relaxation Learning and pain
2	Managing your pain	Activities, maintain daily routines Scheduling activities Relaxation training
3	Promoting good health, controlling stress at home and at work	Warning signals Cognitive appraisal Beliefs
4	Adapting for leisure and work	Communication skills Assertiveness Risk situations Applying relaxation
5	Controlling flare-ups	Plan for coping with flare-ups Coping skills review Applied relaxation Own program
6	Maintaining and improving results	Risk analysis Plan for adherence Own program finalized

First, the *introduction* will provide a welcome, and set the tone for the session. Important aspects include a review of assigned homework and dealing with practical questions. It is crucial that *every* individual be asked about his or her experience with the homework. Completing homework and going through it during the session should be viewed as an adventure. The therapist should not act as though he or she expects participants to complete the homework, especially without any problems. This should help to create a "no fault" atmosphere where people are free to describe how much homework they have completed as well as how much success they experienced. Reinforce people who have attempted to complete their homework! Ask them how they managed to fit it into their busy schedule as well as what benefits they experienced. Be sure to help people feel that benefits are their own achievement (rather than the therapist's or someone else's). Discussing possible hindrances may help participants who have not completed the homework. A helpful technique is to gain the help of members who have successfully done the homework. If a person does not find the skill helpful, accept this. Not all skills will be valuable for all participants. Be aware, however, that some people do not employ the skill properly and may need some help in fine-tuning their skills.

The introduction should put participants at ease and make them feel an important part of the group. This is why it is imperative that everyone has an opportunity to briefly describe his or her "weekly adventure". The introduction ordinarily takes about 15 minutes.

Second, a short *"lecture" period* is designed to provide knowledge and "insight". The main purpose is to stimulate participants' thinking and introduce them to the topic for the session. Consequently, the "lecture" will contain information about the topic such as facts about the problem and known ways of dealing with it. In addition to the facts, the lecture will help people to relate the topic matter to the discussion, skills exercises and homework so that each person may learn the knowledge and how to apply it in their own situation (insight). The lecture will set the stage for the next part of the session. Although most of us may be tempted to expand the lecture, it is absolutely necessary to restrict it to a maximum of 15 minutes.

The third part of the session is *problem-solving* employing a case study. Members of the group work in pairs to maximize participation. A case study (see below) is read and each pair is asked to solve one or more problems. These problems have direct relevance for the theme of the session. The purpose of using a case study is to allow members to discuss a "neutral" third person rather than themselves. However, as participants become comfortable with the group, they typically begin to relate the case study to their own situation. This should be encouraged.

CASE STUDY: LENA, FOR USE IN CBT GROUP INTERVENTION

Below is an example of the case studies we use in the cognitive-behavioral group intervention. Participants read the case study, which is designed to be a typical case, and they are then asked to solve various "problems". By doing this participants are able to begin to analyze their own situation as well as to practice skills. Case studies are used in every session and participants work in pairs to solve specific problems for the given session.

Lena is a 38-year-old secretary who is married and has two children. She is an active woman and her health is comparable to other women in her age group.

One day Lena woke up with a stiff, aching neck. Although she hadn't been involved in any accident or trauma, she had been working intensively at the computer during the past several days. Her neck was stiff, with pain and sore muscles all the way out to her shoulders. When she got out of bed she felt like she was getting a bad headache. It was difficult for Lena to move her head normally and even small movements hurt.

Nevertheless, Lena saw the children off to school and got ready for work. This was troublesome since

she had so much pain. She had difficulty thinking about anything else. Lena decided that she should go to her doctor. She also went to work.

The doctor examined Lena and was not surprised by the symptoms she reported. Her muscles were tense and there were tender points that appeared to be inflamed. She described her pain as stiffness and tenderness with a particular spot that felt like a knife being stuck into her neck. The doctor determined that there was no serious injury or disease, but that the pain was caused by muscle contractions and inflammation. He advised Lena to rest a few days at home and subsequently to work less intensively with the computer since this put extra load on the neck and shoulder muscles. The doctor provided a prescription for some painkillers that also contained a muscle relaxant.

At home, Lena had problems keeping up with her chores. Rather than cooking the usual meals, Lena bought convenience foods. She asked her husband to help more with cleaning and buying groceries. As her husband was quite concerned about Lena's health, he was very willing to do this. Lena also had difficulty playing with her children as usual. It simply didn't seem possible to continue with their regular playtime after supper. At work people were also concerned about Lena. She is a well-respected, efficient worker and everyone wants her to get better so she can return to work.

Gradually, Lena gets better and she only needed to be away from work a few days.

Three months later Lena had a relapse. This time she felt so much neck pain that she could hardly get out of bed. She knew that she had to do something about this. Consequently, she called in sick and visited her doctor again. The doctor examined Lena briefly and said that this was the same sort of problem as before: muscle tension. The doctor completed a sick leave certificate and he advised Lena to rest. Lena thought that this was wise since she felt that the pain was worse when she worked. She decided she would take it easy at home as well. An additional prescription was provided.

Unfortunately, the pain did not disappear. Although Lena improved slightly, her neck pain continued to bother her considerably. It was arduous for Lena to keep up with her work as the company was in an intensive, stressful period. Lena tried to make up for this by resting more at home. However, she feels guilty that she has not been able to participate in activities with her children and husband and that they have to do her work. In addition, she wonders why she doesn't get better. "Is there a serious injury the doctor missed? It hurts every time I move too much or a certain way, there must be a reason. Should I wait until the injury is completely healed; can I hurt myself more by working?" Lena had many questions and thoughts.

Lena went back to work, but soon developed a pain problem again. This time the pain gradually gets worse.

She decides to get to the bottom of the problem and to really take care of herself, as she is afraid the pain may become permanent or is caused by a dangerous injury. Lena goes to her doctor and receives another sick leave certificate and prescription. These tablets are stronger and help some even though Lena feels dizzy and tired when she takes them.

Still the pain persists. After three weeks at home, Lena has a follow-up visit with her doctor. Lena thinks a lot about her pain and why she doesn't get better. She wonders if she will ever be able to go back to work and take responsibility again for her family. Lena feels tired and blue; the pain has stolen Lena's vitality. Despite the fact that Lena rests a good deal she feels grumpy and irritable. The doctor says there is nothing more he can do and refers Lena to a physical therapist for treatment. Lena is happy about this and goes to therapy twice a week. Although she improves some, her neck is still stiff and painful after weeks of therapy. Moreover, Lena has also begun to have problems with her back. This in turn has made it difficult for her to sleep. The family's routines at home have changed considerably now and Lena feels that she cannot manage the social life they once had.

After another three weeks at home, the insurance case manager calls Lena. The case manager wonders when Lena will be able to go back to work. This upsets Lena greatly; it is as though they do not believe that Lena is actually sick. It's easy for a healthy case manager to talk about the benefits of going back to work; she doesn't have to put up with a stressful job, tight schedules, and a boss who is never satisfied with a worker with neck pain!

Participants are given roughly 15–20 minutes to read the case study and solve the problems for the session. Subsequently, the group meets again and each pair presents its solution. Discussion is encouraged and focuses on identifying the reasons for the "problem" the case portrays as well as coping strategies for solving it.

The fourth part of the session is *skills training*. New skills are presented in each session. The particular skill will be new for most people, but some may have experience with some of the skills. People with experience may be called upon to help teach others. In addition, they may wish to improve their skill. The technique should be taught and ample opportunity for practice provided. The techniques provided serve as a base for developing a coping strategy program. Thus, the relevance of each person learning and applying the basic technique is highlighted. Since the methods are directly aimed at addressing the problems that are isolated in the case study, the relevance of the method is clear. Discussion may be directed to the appropriate

use of the technique as well as how it might be incorporated into daily living.

Finally, the session is rounded off with *homework assignments and a résumé* of the session. Examples of homework are provided for each session. However, the therapist will need to explain the importance of practicing skills in everyday life so that participants clearly understand that some skills will be very relevant and others less relevant. To get an accurate feel for which techniques may work for them, members must apply them. Thus, the therapist may ask the group *why* the skill should be practiced to ensure that every participant understands. Homework should be individualized. Consequently, after presenting a "general" description of the homework, each person should verbally and in writing describe what he or she will be doing for homework. In addition, each person should note when and where the homework will be done. Homework should be fun and therefore I recommend presenting it as "the weekly adventure"! To minimize pressure, you may want to tell participants that they cannot expect perfect results on the first try. Instead, practice will improve results.

Feedback for the session is obtained with a formal summary of the day. Each person is asked to briefly state what they have learned and what the positive and negative aspects of the session have been. This gives members an opportunity to reinforce the therapist. It also provides feedback to members and serves as a ruler for judging the overall success of the session. Not least, having each person make a statement helps them to integrate the new information and skills. If negative aspects are brought up, the therapist need not defend him or herself. Instead, a plan should be initiated to rectify the problem. Fortunately, most feedback is very positive and the occasional negative points are relatively easy to deal with.

Enjoying the experience

Each session should be enjoyable. People enjoy talking, socializing and learning. Thus, the program is designed to bring forward active participation. Self-control, coping and learning are fun! There is no need to take the task too seriously either, a good laugh may enhance active participation and encourage patients to attempt cognitive and behavioral changes that might otherwise be difficult. At the end of a session, members should feel good about the group and the achievements they have made.

Adherence and maintenance

A major concern is that progress made during the course is continued in the future. A major threat is that participants will fail to adhere to their coping program, and thereby compromise the maintenance of the results. Compliance enhancement techniques such as relapse prevention, risk assessment and the health behavior model will be used. By promoting active participation where the participant develops his or her own package, we hope to ensure good adherence. Nevertheless, the last two sessions will deal specifically with this question. Please bear in mind that the base for maintenance will be planted early on in the course and reinforced throughout.

To enhance adherence and maintenance, this course uses a novel approach based on choice. A typical approach to maintenance is a lecture on individual responsibility and the need for a long-term view. However, this often is of little help. Rather than cajoling or making participants feel guilty, this program concentrates on planned behavior. In essence, participants are challenged to make conscious choices about the content of their coping program. Since needs may change with time, reevaluation of the program is encouraged. Participants may choose to add or eliminate

techniques as required. However, this should be a conscious choice and not something that simply "happened" unplanned. As described later, a "road map" will also be used to identify factors that are associated with success as well as failure to adhere to the program.

Emotional and social support

Opportunities for emotional and social support need to be provided. This may include discussions, relaxation exercises, group training and the like. Participants should be helped (and help each other) to feel good about themselves. Successful behaviors, for example, may be highlighted, e.g. when someone in the group has helped another, disclosed something important, controlled their pain or improved a coping skill.

RESEARCH RESULTS

This cognitive-behavioral group intervention has been applied in various settings and evaluated. In fact, four randomized, controlled trials focusing on its preventive effects have been reported in the literature (Linton and Andersson, 2000; Linton and Ryberg, 2001; Marhold et al., 2001; Linton et al., in press). In addition, several other researchers have shown that cognitive-behavioral early interventions can be quite successful in preventing future disability (Loisel et al., 1997; Von Korff et al., 1998; Moore et al., 2000; Sullivan and Stanish, 2003).

First trial with high-risk participants

Since the intervention was designed as secondary prevention for those at risk for developing a persistent problem, our first study investigated the utility of this approach for participants with high scores on the Örebro Musculoskeletal Pain Screening Questionnaire (Linton and Andersson, 2000). We envisioned that participants might be representative of patients seeking care at a primary care service, but although these patients had higher scores on the Örebro Pain Screening Questionnaire, they nevertheless were at an early stage as none had long-term sick absenteeism, and healthcare utilization at baseline was low. To assess outcome in a randomized trial, we compared people receiving our program with two other groups. These comparison groups received "treatment as usual" and, in addition, modern written advice about dealing with their back pain.

Participants were recruited via primary care facilities and an advertisement in a local newspaper. To be eligible, applicants had to be suffering pain from the spinal area, aged 18–60, and have less than 3 months of cumulative sick leave during the past year. Exclusion criteria were being retired or having another medical condition that contradicted participation.

Participants were then randomized to one of the three groups according to a block randomization procedure. The mean score on the Örebro Musculoskeletal Pain Screening Questionnaire for participants was 106. The results summarized here are based on those completing the study: 107 participants in the CBT group, 70 in the pamphlet group and 66 in the information package group.

Participants received a secondary preventive intervention according to a protocol, and all participants also were free to pursue ordinary treatment as usual. One group received a previously evaluated pamphlet (Symonds et al., 1995) that provides straightforward advice about how to best cope with back pain by remaining active and thinking positively. The reader is clearly encouraged to confront rather than avoid activities that may be associated with pain.

The second comparison group also received information, but in the form of a packet once a week for six weeks. The number and timing of the packages therefore matched the number of sessions the CBT group received. This material utilized more traditional sources of information and was based on a back school approach. Each package contained advice and illustrations of how one might cope with or prevent spinal pain such as by lifting properly and maintaining good posture. The information also encouraged participants to maintain their usual activities to speed recovery.

Finally, the experimental group received the cognitive-behavioral group treatment described above. Groups were run periodically and those randomized were asked to join.

Results

The results were analyzed for a broad spectrum of variables including the key outcome variables of function and healthcare utilization (Linton and Andersson, 2000). First, it should be underscored that since the patients selected suffered from acute or subacute bouts of back pain, considerable improvements would be expected according to the natural course of the problem. Indeed, for a number of variables such as pain intensity, mood and activity levels, all three groups experienced improvements, but the difference between the groups was not significant. However, a noteworthy finding concerning patient satisfaction was found. Patients rated how satisfied they were with the treatment received in terms of how helpful they found it to be. The cognitive-behavioral group rated the intervention as significantly more helpful than did either of the two information groups. Second, the key variables of sick absenteeism and healthcare utilization were selected since they are directly tied to long-term disability and costs.

For the key outcome variable of healthcare utilization, the main result was that while the cognitive-behavioral group *decreased* their number of visits from pretest to follow-up, both of the information groups reported *increases*. The cognitive-behavioral group, relative to the two comparison groups, had a significantly lower level of utilization with regard to doctor's visits as well as visits to a physical therapist.

As various forms of compensation payments account for about 90% of the costs for back pain, the second key variable was sick absenteeism. Figure 13.2 shows that while the comparison groups increased their average sick leave levels, the cognitive-behavioral treatment prevented this from happening. To examine the main question concerning the development of long-term sick absenteeism, we calculated the risk of developing sick leave of more than 30 days during the follow-up period. To accomplish this we compared the cognitive-behavioral group with the combined two information groups. This analysis showed that participants in the cognitive-behavioral groups had a 9-fold decreased risk of being on long-term sick leave as compared to the information groups (OR = 9.3; 95% CI = 1.2–70.8)!

Five-year follow-up

Recently, we conducted an additional follow-up to ascertain the very long-term results. Figure 13.3 shows the five-year results in terms of the percentage of participants who needed to be off work on sick leave for their back pain more than 15 days during the past year. As the figure illustrates, none of the participants had that much sick leave during the baseline year (this was a selection criterion). We have already examined the one-year results showing a clear advantage for the cognitive-behavioral group. The five-year follow-up demonstrates that dramatic differences are still visible and of roughly the same magnitude as at the one-year follow-up.

The results from this trial demonstrated that the cognitive-behavioral group intervention resulted in significantly less disability and healthcare utilization than did the control groups. This was true even at the five-year follow-up. Interestingly, these participants had high scores on the screening instrument, which suggests that psychological factors were quite relevant. Thus, the current intervention with its focuses on psychological aspects of the problem seemed well gauged for these participants as a preventive intervention.

Trial in primary care setting

In a second study we attempted to incorporate the cognitive-behavioral groups into a primary care setting

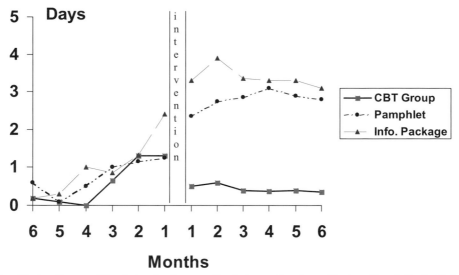

Figure 13.2 The effects of a cognitive-behavioral preventive intervention for patients with relatively high levels of "yellow flags". The mean number of sick days for back pain six months before the intervention and at the one-year follow-up demonstrated a significant preventive effect for the CBT group. (Based on data from Linton and Andersson, 2000.)

(Linton et al., in press). To compare various levels of intervention we randomized participants to one of three groups. The first received a standardized examination to rule out red flags and guideline-based advice where patients were given the message that it is important to maintain/regain normal activities including work. The second group received this care plus the cognitive-behavioral group intervention, while the third group received the same plus preventive physical therapy oriented toward regaining function and physical exercise. Figure 13.4 shows the preventive effect for sick leave one year later in terms of the percentage of participants in each group with more than 15 days'

sick leave over the past year. As the figure shows, the minimal intervention group experienced a dramatic increase during the follow-up while the groups receiving the cognitive-behavioral group intervention with or without physical therapy did considerably better. In fact, the two groups receiving the cognitive-behavioral intervention had a 5.3 times lower risk of developing long-term sick leave. Improvements were also seen in terms of decreases in healthcare utilization and patient satisfaction.

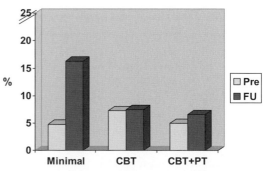

Figure 13.4 Percentage on long-term sick leave (>15 days) during one year before and after intervention for back pain in a primary care setting. The comparison group received an evidence-based "minimal treatment" regime. The second group received that plus a cognitive-behavioral intervention (CBT), while the third group received the minimal treatment, the CBT and a form of preventive physical therapy. The two groups receiving the CBT intervention reduced their risk by 5.3-fold as compared to the comparison group. (Based on Linton et al., in press.)

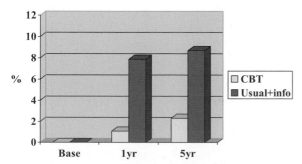

Figure 13.3 The percentage of participants in the cognitive-behavioral group treatment as well as the comparison group on long-term sick leave for back pain at a five-year follow-up. The cognitive-behavioral group had reduced the risk of developing such long-term sick leave by more than 3-fold at the one-year follow-up. (Based on data from Linton and Nordin, submitted.)

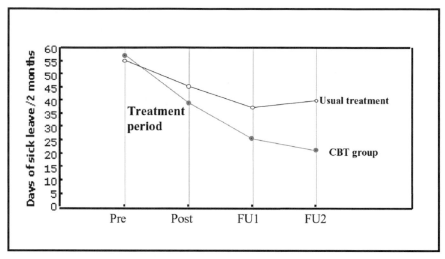

Figure 13.5 The average number of days off work for back pain before and after two different interventions. One group received an early cognitive-behavioral intervention, while the comparison group received treatment as usual. The CBT group had significantly fewer days off work. (Based on Marhold et al., 2001.)

Trial focusing on return to work

A third trial converged on return to work for those already on sick leave (Marhold et al., 2001). One effect of our previous studies was that the patient's function and work ability were enhanced. It seemed that this might be utilized even for patients off work for their back pain. At the same time, we reckoned from the literature and clinical experience that patients off work may need to learn certain skills in order to successfully return to work. Thus, a 12-session intervention was developed where the first six sessions consisted of the cognitive-behavioral treatment described above and where the last six sessions dealt specifically with return-to-work issues. The intention was that patients should make gradual steps to return to work. These sessions dealt with generalizing coping skills to the work setting, e.g. coping with repetitive movements, heavy lifts, stress due to time urgency and insecurity about how to perform work tasks. Patients were taught skills for dealing with difficulties that might arise when returning to work, such as increased pain, fatigue or social anxiety. A plan was made and patients did homework between the sessions for taking successive steps toward a return to work. Examples of these include contacting a supervisor, visiting the workplace and modified work.

The effects of the above-described program were tested in a randomized study that included patients with either short- or long-term work absence due to musculoskeletal pain (Marhold et al., 2001). To examine the effects of the length of the problem, patients had either long-term (>12 months, mean = 26 months) or short-term (2–6 months, mean = 3 months) sick leave. These patients were randomly assigned to either

the cognitive-behavioral return-to-work program or a "treatment as usual" comparison group. The most common treatments for the comparison group were visits to a doctor or physical therapist.

To evaluate outcome, patients were followed for one year. An overview of the results is shown in Fig. 13.5. Here the number of days per two-month period are shown for the two main groups. The analyses confirmed what is demonstrated in the figure, namely that the cognitive-behavioral program was more effective than treatment as usual in reducing the number of days on sick leave for patients with *short-term* sick leave. In addition, the treatment program, relative to the comparison group, helped these patients to increase their activity level and gain control over their pain. However, there was no significant difference between the groups on any variable for the patients with *long-term* sick leave. These results underscore the need for an early return-to-work program that focuses on the skills needed to actually make the return. The study suggests that intervening at the right time point with this intervention is crucial for obtaining good results.

CASE STUDY: HANK

Because Hank had a relatively high score on the screening questionnaire and the further assessment isolated several risk factors, an early intervention became relevant. A discussion with Hank isolated some relevant goals. Hank wanted to regain his confidence and get control over his life. Specifically, Hank wanted to be able to function effectively at home and at work. Thus, goals were developed for a return to work as well as for resuming household chores and social activities with the family. Hank also wanted to be able to deal with stress and the pain better. He looked forward to the day he could enjoy leisure activities again.

Because of the risk profile, Hank was recommended to participate in a cognitive-behavioral early intervention group. Here, goals were developed and techniques to meet the goals practiced. Furthermore, Hank was put in command of developing his own coping strategy program for meeting his goals and maintaining good quality of life even in the future.

Although the doctor was a bit skeptical about recommending the group, Hank was actually pleased to have the opportunity for this intervention. It offered a concrete way of moving forward and Hank realized that this was very important.

SUMMARY

When a patient is identified who risks developing long-term disability because of the presence of yellow flags, psychologically oriented interventions are a logical consideration. This chapter has presented and described a cognitive-behavioral intervention program for early intervention that requires some special skills to operate. A particular advantage of the program is that it keys on the psychological risk factors identified. As a result it provides a method for dealing with risk factors that traditional healthcare facilities may lack and it provides an alternative to merely providing larger doses of traditional treatment when a persistent problem is imminent. The results in four randomized trials are promising as all four demonstrate advantages as compared to usual treatment. Cognitive-behavioral interventions are one feasible option for preventing the development of persistent pain and disability. The healthcare professional will have to decide whether such interventions are necessary and whether this can be accomplished in one's own practice, in a team, or whether it should be done externally via a referral.

CHAPTER 14

The way forward: Implementing a psychological perspective in the clinic

LEARNING OBJECTIVES

To understand:

- there is a dire need for applying a psychological perspective of pain in the clinic;

- individual clinicians may apply it;

- system changes may be initiated to augment application.

This book has focused on the incredible contribution that the psychology of pain can make to the understanding, assessment, treatment and prevention of pain and disability. Unfortunately, there is still a need to work actively to incorporate this approach into clinical practice. The implementation of this knowledge lags sadly far behind the production of new knowledge and techniques. Understanding the psychological processes involved in pain perception makes such a unique and valuable contribution that it deserves to be applied. It helps us, for example, to unite a broad range of knowledge into a picture of the experience where such factors as biological, sociological, behavioral, cognitive and emotional aspects are integrated. Humans are marvelously equipped to perceive pain and use these signals to develop coping strategies that help us survive. By understanding the psychology of pain, and specifically how pain problems may develop into persistent problems, we may utilize these factors to provide better care. In this final chapter, we shall scrutinize how we might move forward by promoting the clinical application of this knowledge as well as continued research.

Application is a key to better care. A clear move forward is to utilize the knowledge we have in the clinic. At first glance this may seem to be an easy task. However, considerable evidence suggests that it is not.

The evidence suggests that a considerable decrease in the devastating effects of musculoskeletal pain could be achieved if only healthcare providers would implement currently available knowledge (Grimshaw, 2002; van Tulder, 2002). The latest evidence shows that incorporating psychological factors into clinical

A RECAPITULATION OF THE MAIN POINTS OF PAIN FROM A PSYCHOLOGICAL PERSPECTIVE

- Understanding the psychology of pain adds a crucial dimension to the field of pain.

- A psychological perspective helps us to understand the experience of pain, but also the *consequences* of the pain.

- The development of persistent pain is characterized by psychological processes.

- Psychological variables (yellow flags) may be successfully employed to identify patients at risk of developing chronic problems.

- Good communication skills help to fulfill the psychological needs for a patient in pain. Good communication helps to meet patient expectations, develop a shared understanding of the problem and enlist the patient as an active partner in treatment.

- The first visit provides a unique opportunity to address the psychological aspects of a pain problem such as expectations, worry and functional problems.

- Early cognitive-behavioral interventions are effective in preventing the further development of pain and disability.

practice could reduce the risk for long-term pain-related disability significantly. Yet changes in clinical routines lag far behind research findings. As the scientific literature expands by leaps and bounds, primary care facilities have struggled with staff shortages and shrinking resources. This has created an indisputable hurdle for busy clinicians to find, read, understand and incorporate the latest findings. Nevertheless, there is good reason to believe that implementing the latest findings would very significantly reduce the burden of musculoskeletal pain.

THE PROBLEM OF RESEARCH TRANSFER

Researchers and educators are familiar with the gap between the production of knowledge and its application. This may be especially apparent in musculoskeletal pain, because pain is a multifaceted problem and a variety of healthcare professionals may be involved. As an example, Koetting O'Byrne et al. (1997) found that while 87% of healthcare units were using an ineffective procedure, only a minority employed methods

known to be effective for reducing pain in children. Similarly, we found that primary care doctors and physical therapists did not adequately follow the most recent recommendations on how to best treat back and neck pain (Linton et al., 2002b). As an illustration, over 25% of doctors and physical therapists said that sick leave was an effective treatment, although the evidence shows that it is neither a treatment per se nor is it effective.

Several explanations have been put forward to explain this problem. First, professionals have limited time for reading the latest results. A survey in the UK, for instance, showed that 75% of doctors had not read any scientific information during the past week (Sackett et al., 1997). A second explanation is a lack of program evaluation. The reasoning is that as most clinics are never formally evaluated, there is little motivation for change and those attempting to incorporate new methods may find considerable resistance. Finally, there is often a gap between obtaining knowledge and the skill needed to apply it clinically. The newer or more complicated the procedure, the more need for learning the skill.

Whatever the reason, the gap between current knowledge, with psychological aspects being underscored, and actual practice is huge. In fact, one conference (the Fourth International Forum on Low Back Pain Research in Primary Care) focused entirely on getting research into practice. Why? Because investigations unmistakably show that despite clear evidence indicating that certain strategies are successful, they are still not being implemented (Davis et al., 1995). As an example, a study in the UK followed 200 patients with back pain to ascertain how well guidelines were being applied (Armstrong et al., 2003). They found that the guidelines were seldom properly employed. Although x-rays are not recommended in the guidelines, patients were frequently referred for these. Despite clear recommendations that the assessment include psychological "yellow flags", this was seldom done. Most troubling, they concluded that the guidelines had little influence on practice decisions. Thus, even though the guidelines highlight effective methods, these were not employed. Worse still, methods shown to have few, no or negative effects were often used instead. Another example concerns an attempt to provide primary care doctors with an educational package meant to enhance their implementation of a biopsychosocial approach to back pain (Cherkin et al., 1991). It included guideline-driven principles. Despite the perceived benefits the doctors believed they had obtained, it had little impact on practice or patient outcomes. A clear conclusion, then, is that there is a dire need for proper

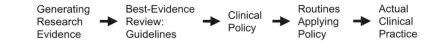

Figure 14.1 An overview of the process of implementing psychological knowledge into practice.

implementation of new knowledge (Grimshaw, 2002; van Tulder, 2002) (Fig. 14.1).

THE INFORMATION DEFICIT FALLACY

Even if a variety of specific reasons may be given to explain the lack of clinical implementation, the most frequent view is that clinicians lack the proper information. According to this information deficit model (Marteau et al., 2002), knowledge changes practice behavior. The healthcare system has many examples of this model in action. For instance, medical students become practitioners through the learning of knowledge, and one subsequently becomes a specialist through even more accumulation of knowledge. Accordingly, the remedy to the problem of implementation would be providing more information.

However, there are several theoretical and empirical reasons that fail to support the information deficit model. On a theoretical level, the informational model assumes that we learn by passive assimilation of information. In this view, all one needs to do is to read about a particular technique, and then one could directly apply this into practice. However, a newer view is that we learn, just as this book has emphasized that patients learn new coping strategies, by active participation (Marteau et al., 2002). This theoretical model suggests that implementation would be best served by emphasizing direct involvement, problem-solving, reflection and self-assessment. Indeed, this mirrors the approach to the cognitive-behavioral groups in Chapter 13 where behavioral tests, active participation and the like are employed to stimulate cognitive and behavioral changes.

Besides theoretical doubts about the information deficit model, the scientific evidence clearly does not support it. Various scientific articles conclude that passive dissemination of information is ineffective (Davis et al., 1995). Based on exhaustive literature reviews, there is a consensus that passive approaches such as sending articles to clinicians, or attending a lecture, are ineffective in changing clinical practice (Davis et al., 1995; Grimshaw, 2002; Marteau et al., 2002). However, techniques that actively engaged the clinician were often effective such as outreach programs, reminders and workshops. Moreover, programs that used multiple interventions were more successful than those using only one. One-shot efforts, then, are not particularly effective. An example study will help

to illustrate these findings. In one study, primary care doctors were randomly assigned to a group receiving a continuing education program or a group waiting to receive such instruction (Sibley et al., 1982). The program had explicit objectives and used modern educational techniques including audiovisuals. Doctors were then followed and specific aspects of care were evaluated through records. The startling results were that it had virtually no effect on clinical care. Even though the knowledge of the doctors receiving the continuing education program improved, it did not transfer into changes in actual clinical practice.

It is obvious, then, that a program to implement the psychology of pain into practice will involve an active multifaceted approach that engages the various stakeholders. More passive educational programs appear to be necessary, but not enough to ensure that this valuable new knowledge is applied in the clinic.

System factors

A particular problem for incorporating psychological factors into clinical practice appears to be the organization of the healthcare and other systems (Nicholas, 2002). The current system is normally based on a medical model of disease. Consequently, the service is organized in order to provide a diagnosis of a disease. A correct diagnosis is then assumed to automatically ensure that the right treatment is initiated. This seems to work wonderfully for many types of disorders such as infections. However, as this book has repeatedly underscored, pain is not a disease but a symptom that is influenced by a broad range of variables. Thus, the medical model approach does not always work adequately. Moreover, the medical model is aimed at treating a disease rather than prevention. As a consequence, the system is not particularly designed to accomplish tasks such as early identification. For example, we recently intiated a service to provide the cognitive-behavioral group intervention in several primary care practices. Although the local National Insurance Authority had identified virtually hundreds of people with musculoskeletal pain being off work, few patients were initially referred to the service. The reason? The primary care centers were not organized to identify candidates for this early, preventive intervention. Indeed, there was no routine or system for identifying such patients as the current system is organized around computerized journals that focus on the diagnosis. As a result, system changes are often needed in order to ensure that the newest psychological knowledge is incorporated into practice.

Changing policy and routines

A first step in attuning the healthcare setting with the implementation of psychological knowledge is developing appropriate policies. Although changing policies will not ensure that changes are actually made in clinical practice, it does provide a framework for support. Policy statements will reflect on the goals the unit has. For example, having a policy that every patient with back pain will be screened to identify possible barriers to recovery provides support for these efforts and reflects the goal of early identification and prevention. Other policy statements may focus on early interventions such as providing such services for patients who have been off work for more than a specified time (for example three weeks). Such policy sets a clear course for clinical action. Finally, some clinics have policy statements regarding the use of evidence-based medicine; that is, the policy states that the latest methods with documented scientific results should be incorporated into clinical practice. Again, while this does not ensure that this will automatically happen, it does provide a clear statement of the goal.

Once the policy is in order, a next step is to specify clinical routines to fulfill the policy. This is probably the most difficult aspect of changing systems. Generally speaking, systems, and the people in them, are resistant to change. The normal reaction is to find difficulties with the new routine. Yet providing new routines is essential to improving healthcare. The exact content of the new routines will be particular to the setting and the needs of the patients. Some examples from my experience in consulting with primary care clinics can, however, be given. In one clinic, a routine was developed so that all patients seeking care for neck, shoulder or back pain completed a screening questionnaire as a complement to the other examinations. To be clear, this was done with *every* patient and the questionnaire was entered into the patient's journal for reference. In this way, the routine ensured that screening would not be "missed" and that these important psychological data would be available to all clinicians who may be involved in the case.

Another clinic developed the following routine. Here journal records were examined to identify patients at the primary care facility who were off work for their pain (of any type) for more than four weeks. A case conference was then held to examine the patient's case and develop plans for an (early) intervention. The conference was attended by a variety of professionals including a nurse, doctor, physical therapist and psychologist. In this manner, the routine ensured that cases in need of possible early interventions were attended to. It also provided a format for examining these cases since some may be reasonable (a hip fracture) while others need attention (e.g. nonspecific back pain).

By developing policies and routines, individual professionals are encouraged to apply the latest knowledge in clinical practice.

Team approach

A team of professionals appears to be in a better position to incorporate psychological knowledge into clinical practice. This is because the team normally provides support for the individual members to follow the new routines. Further, the team together can provide vital feedback and troubleshooting when the inevitable problem arises. Often the team will have discussions to solve problems and to synthesize the approach. Team members will naturally have different views about what the current knowledge is and how to best apply it. Therefore, the team may function as a springboard for implementation and the development of best-practice routines.

Utilizing a team also has advantages since it reflects the multimodal nature of the pain problem. Having various professionals as members of the team provides a unique opportunity to capitalize on a multidimensional approach. This does not mean that every team member will meet every patient. It does mean that each team member may learn from the other team members. It also means that team members may seek guidance from other team members in applying the program. Further, it means that other experts are available for the patient to consult should it be deemed appropriate.

The importance of education and outreach programs

Educational efforts are necessary, if not sufficent, in order to achieve changes in practice. A program that incorporates a series of workshops is likely to be more effective than a one-time conference. This allows for learning, reflection and discussion. The workshops, in addition, may be focused on active participation and the practicing of skills. This provides a crucial opportunity for participants to attempt the new techniques in a nonthreatening situation. It allows for practice and the honing of skills as well as feedback and reflection. In short, it provides repeated opportunities for learning important new methods.

An outreach program is especially valuable. Outreach programs involve having a professional colleague experienced in the techniques come to the clinic to demonstrate, and provide clinical guidance. This is a sort of on-the-job training where a person with clinical expertise helps another clinician to learn and execute the new method. The reviews mentioned above bear out that outreach programs are particularly effective for implementation. They have the advantage of engaging the "learner" because they work with real patients. Moreover, they are extremely relevant since they work with current, real-life, problems and their solutions. The outreach expert can also provide immediate feedback and help shape the new skills.

PROFESSIONALS' BELIEFS AS BARRIERS TO IMPLEMENTATION

Just as the beliefs and emotions that a patient have may create barriers for patients, they may also form obstacles for us in the implementation of a psychological perspective in the clinic. In point of fact, so-called professional compliance, that is, how well professionals follow recommendations, is about the same as patient adherence. Patients, but also professionals, frequently do not follow the advice provided. In this section we will explore some common beliefs that healthcare professionals harbor that may create barriers for implementation. As with many cognitive "errors", such as those examined in Chapter 6, there is often a grain of truth in the belief. However, the belief may be generalized in an absurd manner or catastrophic thinking may make it impossibly negative. Let us carefully examine these common beliefs since they may affect you or a member of your team. We have recently formulated a list of common beliefs that may hinder the implementation of working with psychological factors in healthcare (Linton and Boersma, 2002).

Someone else's responsibility

The belief

Perhaps the most common reason clinicians give for *not* working with psychological factors is that it is *not their responsibility*. This belief entails the idea that because one is not a trained psychologist specializing in this area, then one cannot possibly be charged with the duty of working with these factors. Of course, training is an important issue and clinicians should not delve into areas or techniques where they do not have competence. The devastating aspect of this belief is that it closes the door on an open discussion and buries yellow flags. As a consequence, even clear indications that psychological aspects are important will not be taken into consideration.

Is it true?

There are many reasons to conclude that this assertion is not true. First, as healthcare providers we have a responsibility to provide the best possible care. This truly means taking the whole patient into consideration. Second, even if other professions or other professionals may be somewhat better at working with these questions, it is appropriate to work with them. This is because a psychological perspective infiltrates many aspects of the contact we have with patients such as basic communication and how we enlist the patient's help in treatment. Clearly, we have a responsibility to see that patients receive the best possible opportunities to recover. Good practice, then, normally means including a psychological perspective. Third, assessing yellow flags, even at a simple level, will help us to make proper decisions. The patient may need to see another professional for further assessment, for example. However, by ignoring the yellow flags you may be doing the patient a great disservice as an important aspect of the problem is not taken into account.

Takes too much time

The belief

A belief that causes great concern is that including psychological factors will take enormous amounts of time. The situation may be viewed with fear as asking a question about psychological factors opens the door for an endless outpour. Further, by taking valuable time to listen to the patient's description of their psychological problems, less time will be available for dealing with the somatic problem. An associated assumption is that the time is actually being wasted.

To be truthful, including a psychological perspective can take time. Discussing depressed mood or sexual problems related to the pain are not always simple matters. Because the issues are often emotionally charged, it may also take time for the patient to express concerns.

Is it true?

We have seen in Chapter 10 that effective communication leads to better outcome and more satisfied patients. A key to this communication is including a psychological perspective. Dealing with these factors does take time, but should be worth the investment. In part, taking time early on can save time at a later date when the problem has evolved into a major predicament. By understanding the patient and providing interventions that are better tailored to the patient's needs, the necessity for future interventions can be reduced. Finally, employing time management techniques (described in Chapter 10) is effective in controlling the length of visits and maintaining your clinical schedule.

Too uncomfortable to ask

The belief

A belief tied to our own emotional state is the idea that bringing up psychologically oriented topics will make us very uncomfortable. In this belief, we may worry that we will feel distinctly nervous about dealing with such issues. In addition, there is the worry that this will result in embarrassing situations such as having your face turn red or clumsily asking a question ("Do you have pain because you don't like your work?"). Further, the belief suggests that bringing such topics up is a breach of the patient's private life. This may trigger fears that the patient will question why such topics are being pursued and indirectly may question our competence.

Is it true?

Some issues are sensitive. Avoiding them, however, always involves drawing a border. The question is, where do you draw the line? In many other disorders, clinicians are also faced with issues that can be sensitive, from lifestyle matters (do you exercise enough/eat the right foods?) to sexual behavior and death itself. Thus, the idea that because an issue causes us to be uncomfortable is reason to avoid it does not seem to be logical. In addition, psychologists would argue that an issue that seems to make you uncomfortable may be doing so precisely because it *is an important issue*. Asking how family members are responding to the patient's pain problem may be quite sensitive, if this is a serious problem for the patient. Contemplate futher about how sensitive issues might be dealt with. Professionals who deal with sexually transmitted diseases are typically quite skilled in bringing up even the most sensitive issues concerning the patient's sexual behavior. Thus, discomfort may be related to how skillful one is, and skills may be learned. Lastly, many behaviors that we are not used to performing may cause us to feel uncomfortable. Hence, this feeling may also be related to the fact that you are not in the habit of discussing such topics. Practice will make this easier.

Asking about psychological aspects upsets the patient

The belief

Closely related to the belief that dealing with psychological issues is too uncomfortable is the belief that doing so will genuinely upset the patient. Bringing up any issue that is not directly related to the somatic complaints is therefore seen to be beyond the scope of the healthcare visit. Embedded in this belief is the suggestion that something terrible will happen if the patient becomes at all upset. The barrier then is that avoiding such issues will prevent the patient from becoming upset, and in turn prevent a catastrophe from occurring. A further implication is that if the patient becomes upset, they may do things such as cry or ask questions that will be difficult to deal with.

Is it true?

Although patients sometimes become upset, this is rare. And becoming upset is not necessarily strictly negative. Patients usually report greater satisfaction when clinicians include psychological aspects in the consultation (see Chapter 10). For example, in our work with the Örebro Musculoskeletal Pain Screening Questionnaire we have found that most patients find these aspects of the problem to be relevant. After all, the consequences of their pain impact on their emotions, cognitions, function, family and work. In fact, patients frequently comment that they appreciate these aspects being considered. In a practice that has now administered over 3000 screening questionnaires, the experience has been very positive.

Even though patients who become upset may find the experience to be distressing, we cannot assume that expressing emotions is always bad. On the contrary, expressing the emotional aspects of a problem may be an appropriate response that underscores the weight of the issue.

Having the proper skills to deal with potentially sensitive issues will also reduce any "unnecessary" distress. In point of fact, how such issues are addressed is highly related to how upsetting they may be. Learning to ask open-ended questions, for example, that open doors, rather than placing someone in a corner, is quite helpful. Rather than asking a pointed, yes/no question ("Is your pain related to not liking your job?") that may be interpreted as an accusation instead of a question, open-ended questions open the area for discussion ("Could you tell me how your work is affecting your pain problem?"). In research studies we have routinely asked patients about their experiences of any physical or sexual abuse. Although this represents an extremely sensitive issue, the clinical experience has shown that patients normally deal with the question quite well. An occasional patient cried or showed other signs of distress, but none questioned our motives or commented that we were out of line in asking such delicate questions.

Must have a solution

The belief

This belief asserts that before allowing psychological aspects to be brought up, you, as a healthcare provider, must have a solution to all such problems. The worst possible scenario from this perspective is asking a patient whether he or she is depressed and the reply being "yes". In this case we would be at a loss to know what to do. Moreover, an implication is that we are not fully competent. Moreover, we might well feel inadequate. By avoiding such topics, one might also avoid these embarrassing situations.

Is it true?

Healthcare providers can never be assumed to have solutions for all problems. This is true of whatever ailment we may examine. In fact, it is relatively common in medicine to make a diagnosis, but to lack adequate treatment methods. Diabetes, many cardiovascular problems, cancer and the like may all be diagnosed with precision, but cures are typically not available.

Dealing with new factors such as psychological aspects naturally creates some uncertainty. Skills and experience are needed here as in any other aspect of patient care. However, avoiding the problem because an immediate solution is not available may actually lead to overlooking important aspects of the problem.

A related fallacy is that all problems mentioned by a patient must be "treated". This is very rarely the case. Patients commonly report psychological aspects such as feeling depressed or stressed as a result of the problem, but do not expect immediate or direct treatment. In addition, patients often have ideas about how such aspects of the problem might be dealt with. This opens the door to reinforce self-help skills and to encourage the patient to engage in problem-solving.

Always try usual care first

The belief

A good way to determine if psychological factors may be relevant is to try your usual arsenal of treatment first. If there is no improvement, then it would be appropriate to start looking for other factors. Thus, those holding this belief will provide a package of physical therapy, injections, surgery, exercises, manipulations or other techniques before considering psychological aspects. The assumption is that if the patient responds then you have provided a valuable service. In contrast, if the patient does not respond, then you know that the problem is due to something else.

Is it true?

This belief appears to be quite common. It is also quite destructive. Providing unnecessary treatments is not only costly, it creates certain risks as well. For example, it results in "one more" failed treatment that has negative psychological consequences for the patient. The patient gets the message that something is wrong and if we could only find out what, it could be cured. Above all, each failed treatment takes time and this contributes to the chronification process. Thus, one or two such treatments may put the patient at considerable risk for developing persistent pain and disability.

Moreover, whether a patient responds to a given treatment may have little to do with psychological aspects. Certainly, there is little truth in assuming that a problem is of a psychological nature simply because the patient did not respond to a particular treatment. Nor does identifying psychological aspects necessarily rule out other types of treatment such as medical ones. As we have seen, psychologically oriented methods may be included in treatment delivery such as in communication and first visit programs. Further, psychologically oriented techniques are normally coordinated with other types of treatments.

Ignore the psychological factor; it will get better spontaneously

The belief

According to this belief, people always have psychological problems if you look sufficiently. However, these fluctuate from problem to problem and they get better or worse. Consequently, if one simply ignores the factor and waits it out, it will get better. As an example, people sometimes feel depressed or blue. However, this usually doesn't last very long and the person feels better.

Is it true?

There is a big difference between normal swings in mood and psychological risk factors. Although people do have good and bad days, and ups and downs in joy, stress or happiness, this is not the same as the psychological perspective described in this book. Although some risk factors will get better on their own, ignoring such a factor may have dire consequences. We would not dream of ignoring high blood pressure, for example, even though it may well go down on its own.

Acknowledging psychological consequences of pain is a clear step in attaining a shared understanding with your patient. Ignoring such factors will communicate a lack of interest in the patient and provide a message that such aspects are not relevant—that a cure can be provided medically.

Ignoring psychological factors also usurps the proper assessment of the factor. A signal that the patient is fearful may need to be followed up. However, by ignoring this signal there is no chance of determining whether it is a serious risk factor or a natural reaction to the pain.

Treat each new complaint as a new case

The belief

Here, each complaint the patient presents with is seen as a separate problem. Each time the patient describes a new complaint, this is then treated as a new problem. Thus, if the original back pain seems better, but the patient now complains of shoulder ache, a new assessment and treatment program would be initiated. This is deemed necessary because each complaint may be caused by a specific and separate disease process.

Is it true?

We function as a whole being. The musculoskeletal system is particularly well coordinated. Separating various symptoms and treating them like completely different problems is therefore untenable. It may also reinforce the patient for bringing up new symptoms and changing the focus of what the main problem is. Providing in-depth new assessments for each symptom also give the message that each may be a serious new problem.

Most seriously, jumping from symptom to symptom delays a proper analysis of the problem and the development of an intervention that will focus on secondary prevention and self-help skills.

Psychological factors are not really that important

The belief

In this attitude a psychological perspective is viewed as being highly overrated. Admittedly, patients may experience psychological consequences of their pain. However, psychological factors do not cause the problem. Therefore, these factors will not have impact on remediating the pain. In the end, psychological factors are not that important and they detract from a good physical assessment.

Is it true?

The main conclusion of modern pain research is that it is a multidimensional process. To a great degree, pain is a psychological perception and experience. As we have seen previously, psychological factors have considerable relevance and are truly inseparable from physical factors. There is clear evidence that psychological factors are related to the development of persistent pain problems (see Chapter 9).

What if I miss the true cause?

The belief

Working with psychological factors is fine, but what if there really is something else wrong? In this attitude it is assumed that one must therefore exclude every other possible cause before dealing with psychological factors. This is based on a worry that focusing on psychological factors may lead to missing a physical factor. An implication is that patients or the authorities may find the clinician to be incompetent if such a situation occurred.

Is it true?

Dealing with psychological variables in no way rules out other examinations. Missing a psychological risk factor may be just as important as missing a medical one! Since psychological and medical factors are linked in the same person, it is absurd to believe that these factors can be completely distinguished. Developing good clinical routines is central so that no key risk factors are overlooked.

A waste of time since no psychological service is available

The belief

Even though I may identify patients where psychological factors are important, this has no value since we do not have a psychological service available. Many healthcare settings have a lack of psychologically oriented services. Moreover, the ones available have not incorporated the latest techniques described in the literature. As a result, there is little use in working with these factors, since appropriate interventions will not be available anyway.

Is it true?

In many areas of the world, there are shortages of proper psychological services for pain problems. However, this is no different from any other advancement being made in medicine. New techniques, based on new apparatus or medications, are constantly being introduced. These are subsequently incorporated into practice despite the often considerable cost involved. In other words, when techniques provide better care, we normally attempt to obtain that service. Thus, there may be a need to request or develop such services.

However, as this book is meant to illustrate, a sizable amount of this work can be accomplished with the current personnel. It is a matter of developing the skills and a program for delivery. Thus, you and the team you may well wish to work with can implement many aspects of this approach. Including a competent psychologist on the team is beneficial.

Modernizing services to include the methods borne out by the latest evidence is a continuing process. Although some services may not include the latest methods, requests for specific techniques is a glorious way of encouraging their development. As an example, one healthcare clinic I have worked with specified the service that they wanted including such things as assessment of fear-avoidance beliefs and the availability of cognitive-behavioral treatment techniques. Although no local service currently had such things available, several began developing these in direct response to this request. Demanding modern interventions is a good way to ensure quality care.

Challenging beliefs, changing behavior

Thus, the beliefs that healthcare providers harbor may influence how readily new routines are initiated or adapted. Just as with pain, cognitions, emotions and behaviors are important for healthcare providers. Implementing a psychological perspective into clinical practice involves making behavioral changes and these are coupled to emotional and cognitive factors. Being aware of the beliefs clinicians may have will help to identify possible problems and to employ problem-solving skills to move forward in implementing a modern approach to pain problems.

PROGRAM EVALUATION AND TESTING

Program evaluation and testing are integral links in changing attitudes as well as practice behavior. In fact, they are the key to program development. Without evaluation it is difficult to motivate program changes, and moreover it is tricky to pinpoint which parts of the program need to be developed further. Perhaps most important is that evaluation allows you to see what progress is being made. Since many pain conditions heal over time, it is often hard to know whether improvements depend on the intervention or simply normal healing. We saw earlier, for example, that most people with back pain get better over the course of a few weeks. How do we decide, then, if our interventions are optimal? Program evaluations and testing are the keys.

Behavioral tests

The use of behavioral tests was advocated to help patients make appropriate changes in their cognitions and behaviors (see Chapter 13). They are also suitable for testing new routines in the clinic. Rather than changing an entire program in one go, elements of the program may be evaluated with one or more patients. Thus, employing open-ended questions might be attempted with patients over the course of a few days and then evaluated. This is particularly effective if the expected results are written down before the behavioral test takes place.

Thus, gradual implementation, using behavioral tests as a guide, can propel program development.

Outcome evaluation

Programs should be accountable and progressive. Outcome evaluation is a good method for revealing how effective the program actually is. It may also form a base from which to judge how the content might be improved. Although it is beyond the scope of this book, such evaluation should be properly done using modern methods. Such information is also useful for audits and for program reports.

RESEARCH IS THE WAY FORWARD

The role of research in stimulating the development of viable, effective interventions is difficult to underestimate. During the past ten years we have seen incredible breakthroughs that have opened the door for a revolution in intervention and prevention. This includes a better understanding of how biological, cognitive, emotional and behavioral aspects are integrated into a surprising system for pain perception. The role of psychological variables in pain perception has become evident. So, too, has the role of psychosocial yellow flags in the development of persistent pain and disability. This research has led to new ideas about treatment and early, preventive interventions. For patients seeking care this has meant a new variety of intervention possibilities. It has also meant the availability of much more effective methods.

The next ten years will be crucial to the further development of the psychology of pain. I envision the development of better techniques so that most cases of persistent disability due to pain problems such as back and neck pain are eliminated. This does not mean that people will not suffer from musculoskeletal or other pains. However, the methods we employ to treat the pain will be better, and the procedures we use to *prevent* the disability will be more effective. This will have a great impact on how we in healthcare work. It will also have a huge impact for patients, healthcare services, workplaces and society at large.

Future research will need to solve some particular riddles to make these advancements. Although we have now managed to identify the psychological variables involved, we have just scratched the surface of how these variables actually operate. In other words, we have insight into which variables are involved in persistent pain and disability, but our understanding of the *development* of these problems is in its infancy. Moreover, the research to date has mainly involved groups and how psychological factors affect the "average patient". Yet there is an awareness that the road to persistent problems is unique to the person. Therefore, future research will need to solve the puzzle of what affects specific individuals. For example, why does one patient have a particular problem with fear, while for another distress or workplace factors appear to be prominent? This research has the potential to vastly improve our understanding of the psychology of pain, but also to revolutionize treatment. This is because such information could be utilized to tailor intervention programs to the individual.

Finally, future research will undoubtably make unexpected discoveries. Some of the models we hold today will surely be revised, while others may be discarded. Still, the basic psychology of pain will remain. New discoveries may well change the practices we employ. Some practices may disappear and others improved upon. Ten years ago, advice to rest was routinely given to many patients with back pain while today that same routine calls for advice to remain active. Even though many practices will without doubt change, other aspects will remain as the basis of good clinical practice. Take good communication skills as an example. In the future we may learn better practice methods, but good communication will certainly remain as an important foundation to good patient care.

SUMMARY

Implementation and research are ways that we may bring pain from a psychological perspective forward. At the moment we have an extensive body of knowledge. This has resulted in a new and better approach to the management and early intervention of pain problems. Indeed, this approach has the promise of the prevention of persistent pain and disability. However, the transfer of this knowledge into clinical practice has lagged far behind the research. The modern practices that research show to be effective are not yet incorporated into the clinic. For this reason, one way forward is to concentrate efforts on the implementation of these programs into clinical practice.

Although, comparatively speaking, we have a great deal of knowledge, new discoveries await us. The development of knowledge is an ongoing process and we should not make the mistake of believing we have the final answer. Instead, we need to understand better how the psychology of pain actually works. The integration of biological, emotional, cognitive and behavioral factors may lead us forward to understand how pain problems develop over time. This will have significant implications for future clinical practice. We may strive to see the day that patients receive such superior care that the risk for developing persistent problems is virtually eliminated. As a consequence, research is also a vital way to move clinical practice as well as pain from a psychological perspective forward.

APPENDIX

Session manual for therapists:
Cognitive-behavioral early intervention for groups

This manual is designed to help therapists lead the cognitive-behavioral groups described in Chapter 13. It consists of a session-by-session description of the content. It is designed to be used as a complement to the strategies and framework for the groups described in Chapter 13. A background in cognitive-behavioral therapy is necessary because the specific techniques are named but not described in detail. Reading this appendix will provide a more in-depth understanding of how the groups work. It also provides the detailed information needed if you wish to conduct such groups. The manual is written as a direct instruction to group leaders.

SESSION ONE
The causes of MSP and how to prevent it from becoming chronic

Objectives
1. To bring the group together and create a positive atmosphere.
2. To relate information about the causes of pain and factors that may influence it.
3. To relate information about the risk of developing *chronic* problems.
4. To help members work with identifying relevant factors concerning their own pain problem, thereby obtaining "insight".
5. To provide stimulation and interest for participating in the next five sessions.
6. To start with "skills training": problem-solving and "letting go" as relaxation (to be used as coping later).
7. To teach pain control techniques.

Introduction

Welcome the participants. Conduct a "getting to know you" exercise, e.g. letting each person say a few words about themselves. Another technique is to have members interview their neighbor and describe that person for the rest of the group.

Provide information about the purpose and structure of the groups stressing problem-solving, a coping approach, "help to self-help", and support from the group and guidance from you as a group leader.

A fun task is to have the group organize the refreshment (coffee) break inadvertently using the problem-solving technique. This sets a positive tone for the course, is fun, and underscores the fact that participants will be actively working during the course rather than having a group leader who solves problems.

Education: theory and discussion

(*Use a case study and participants' own experiences*)
The theory in this session centers around the question "Why are you here?" Therefore, you may describe the various causes of pain problems, e.g.

(a) structural and soft tissue injuries
(b) gate-control theory
(c) self-control
(d) difference between "hurt" and "harm"
(e) the consequences of pain (e.g. psychosocial, emotional depression, self-blame, anxiety, etc.)
(f) family
(g) work, disuse of physical capacity, etc.

Next, *shift the focus from pain to function*. Underscore the fact that many pain problems involve much more than pain. Typically, people are just as concerned with being able to function properly at work, during leisure and at home. Moreover, suffering as well as function is influenced by a variety of variables. Many of these variables may be altered or controlled, in whole or in part, ourselves.

The risk of developing chronic problems is highlighted as an introduction to prevention. Provide recent statistics, e.g.

1. About 85% of adults seek help for back pain during their working career.
2. The pain tends to recur periodically.
3. It is possible to influence pain intensity.
4. It is possible to minimize the consequences of the pain (e.g. activities, mood).
5. A small number (5–10%) develop persistent problems.
6. This usually happens very gradually and the person may not be aware of the development until it is "too late".
7. Work, family and psychological factors are related to the development of persistent, disabling pain.
8. Thus, it is not only possible but highly desirable to *prevent the development of a chronic problem*.

You may wish to illustrate this part of the presentation with examples of how chronic pain develops. Be sure to underscore the gradual change in lifestyle that occurs. Moreover, point out that these attempts at coping are often beneficial in the short term, but are problematic in the long run.

Problems to solve

Ask members to work in groups of two or three. Provide them with instructions to:

1. Read through the case study "Lena" (see pages 133–134 above).
2. Solve the problems listed below:
   - Why did Lena develop chronic problems? Individual factors (e.g. she was weak, obese, low pain tolerance), environmental factors (heavy work, family gave too much support), medical factors (worn-out disk, injury).
   - What do you believe Lena should do/should have done to prevent the pain from getting worse, i.e. becoming chronic?
   - Why do you believe you have pain?
   - What is your risk for developing chronic pain?
   - What do you feel might be done about this, i.e. what factors should be dealt with? (Be specific, define in terms of behavior.)
3. Be prepared to present your results informally to the rest of the group.
4. Do not expect to solve all problems completely today. However, by considering these problems we hope to start a process that can be used in the future.

These small groups are allowed to work for about 10–15 minutes at a time and then asked to report to the larger group for discussion.

Allow each group to briefly present their results. Each group should present something even if they feel it is basically the same solution as another group presented. Surprisingly, this often leads to additions. Moreover, it provides an opportunity for reinforcement, integration, etc.

The discussion should center on defining preliminary goals or areas that should be covered in the course. Attempt to formulate these areas or goals in the terms we have outlined for the coming sessions, e.g. pain control, activity training, etc.

If areas not included in this program come up, you will need to deal with that, e.g. allowing them to seek the proper information or help. Alternatively, some aspects may be added especially if they focus on a particular technique such as sleep problems or headaches.

Skills

One skill being practiced above is analyzing the problem and developing a strategy for coping with it. This is important since it is the basic approach we have.

Problem-solving. This skill may be presented and information used to illustrate its use. Our technique includes an operational definition of the problem. Then, brainstorming is employed to come up with as many possible solutions as possible *regardless of their consequences.* Each suggestion is then evaluated for positive and negative aspects. Finally, the best solution is chosen. The technique highlights that no problem has a solution that only has positive aspects (otherwise it wouldn't be a problem!).

Pain control. Several techniques may be used. To introduce the skills you may illustrate that we indeed can control our perceptions by doing an exercise together. Ensure that it is quiet. Ask people to close their eyes and relax. Instruct them to concentrate on how it feels in their body and to note all internal sensations. Continue this demonstration for 2–4 minutes. Discuss what people felt and how this compares to what they ordinarily feel. Some will feel pain or other sensations that they ordinarily do not "feel", i.e. are not aware of. Others may find that their pain increases (did they concentrate on it, become anxious, etc?) while others may note a decrease (did they relax, etc?). *The point is that what we do and think (cognition and behavior) influences how we feel and how much pain we experience. This is true even when there is a clear injury and pain signals are being sent in the nerve system.*

We employ brief written instructions for a variety of techniques. As a result, the skills can be demonstrated and briefly tried by participants.

Given the large number of techniques available, groups may be asked to select the techniques in which they are most interested. We attempt to teach a wide variety of techniques as long as they promote *self-help.* The program has selected certain techniques on offer based on the latest evidence.

Simple massage may be taught as a method of pain control. It is presented as a self-help method. We do this by emphasizing the advantages of massage when done within the family (friends).

We also briefly teach cognitive methods, e.g. distraction and reinterpretation. The use of positive self-statements is also presented.

Rest positions that reduce load on the back are also shown.

An important coping strategy for pain is applied relaxation. Explain that this technique will be practiced throughout the course. The goal is to be able to relax quickly in a variety of situations so that the relaxation may be "applied" to situations where it is most needed. Short periods of application during the day provide for an active method of coping with pain. In addition, longer periods of relaxation may reduce current pain levels. Finally, relaxation may be beneficial to help people unwind after stressful events or work. In this program we use the "letting go" technique. (Traditional muscle relaxation has not been shown to be more beneficial, provokes pain for some people, and takes considerably more time to learn.)

The "letting go" relaxation exercise:

1. Do not "try" to relax.
2. Find a comfortable position.
3. Take two deep breaths, hold them (about 15–20 seconds), exhale.
4. Focus your mind on something repetitive (mantra!) when giving instructions: use breathing (slow and steady) plus thoughts "calm and confident", etc.
5. "Let go" when exhaling. *Imagine and concentrate on breathing, not on relaxing.*

This *relaxation response* (Benson, 1975) may be relatively quickly achieved. Typically, a first trial will take 10–15 minutes plus the time needed for a short discussion afterwards.

Homework

Be specific: what, when, where, why. Alternatives:

* 1. Practice problem-solving skills by applying it to one important area identified during the session.
  2. Monitor pain/pain-free situations, e.g. during one day.
  3. Reading information, e.g. patient information booklets (the Back Book).
**4. Relaxation: Letting go. Provide written instructions above.

**Should assign.
*May assign.
Others are optional.

SESSION TWO
Managing your pain to maintain quality of life: activities and the prevention of pain

Objectives

1. To create a positive group atmosphere.
2. To provide information about the relationship between activity and MSP.
3. To help participants learn about fear avoidance and how attitudes and behaviors may influence the problem in the long run. Underscore the idea that normal levels of activity do not need to provoke pain.

4. To teach participants how to identify goals for a satisfying activity level.

5. To teach participants activity management skills, e.g. scheduling, pacing and graded increases.

6. To teach participants how they may cognitively work with beliefs/thoughts to minimize problems with activities (coping, e.g. self-statements).

7. To introduce stress and stress management.

Introduction

Welcome the group members. After introductory pleasantries go through the homework assignments. Ask each and every individual to briefly summarize his or her experience with the homework during the week. *Reinforce positive behaviors such as attempts at completing the homework.* Remember that each *participant's behavior needs to be shaped.* Consequently, even approximations of "correct" behavior should be specially reinforced. Problems and questions should be addressed. Engage other members of the group in evaluating problems or providing comments. All members should be involved in the discussion. They should optimally provide support for other members as well as help in improving.

Provide an overview of the session's activities and ask for comments. You may wish to see if the organization of the break agreed upon in session 1 has functioned.

Education: theory and discussion

This session concentrates on activity levels. First, the relationship of pain and activity needs to be examined as most people will experience pain in association with specific movements or activities. Then, the development of chronic pain needs to be underscored, i.e. that healing may take place, but activity problems persist. The emotional reaction as well as the consequences needs to be highlighted. Activity is central in how we feel and determines to a large extent our quality of life. Consequently, it appears to be an extremely important part of our life that needs to be considered if pain is a problem. Important questions to pose during the talk are: Why does it hurt when we move? Is movement dangerous? Stress that "hurt" does not usually mean harm!

Go through the idea of fear avoidance as a natural way of responding to such pain problems. A natural reaction to acute pain is anxiety, fear and muscle tension. However, these reactions may be conditioned to other stimuli and thereby set the stage for avoidance. These behaviors usually are oriented toward avoiding particular movements that are associated with pain. They are reinforced by a reduction of the anxiety and fear. Avoidance is typically self-propelled. This is because when we avoid a movement we lose the opportunity to see what actually happens. In this case we do not have a chance of experiencing that we actually are capable of doing the activity with little or no more pain. This behavior may be compared to phobic behavior of other sorts. Since avoidance behavior is self-propelled by strong emotions, it often becomes a serious problem (compare to other phobias). (Phobias and fear-avoidance behavior can be treated! We will address this below.) Therefore, it is important to prevent the development of fear-avoidance behaviors.

Another common problem concerning MSP is our activity pattern. Pacing refers to our natural predisposition to adjust and vary the rate of our activities. Typically, this involves taking short pauses periodically as well as changing the tempo of the work. This provides for healthy variation. However, when we experience MSP, the natural pattern of behaviors may be disrupted. Pain behaviors, e.g. guarding and bracing, may occur which temporarily reduce pain but disrupt the natural activity pattern. While this is appropriate in the short term, it may create a problem in the long run. Again, it is important to prevent this.

Problems with pacing may also occur as the result of stress or attitudes (cognitions). Some people may reason that they want to "get the activity done" so that they can rest later. Others feel so stressed that they do not believe they have time for rest or pacing. The end result is monotonous work that may actually enhance the pain. In fact, research shows that you accomplish more by taking short pauses and varying tempo relative to continuous, monotonous work. To underscore the value of pacing, you may make a comparison to a long-distance runner and the need for finding the right pace. In addition, an illustration using the fable of the race between the rabbit and the turtle may be helpful. Pacing is therefore an important method in stress management.

Pacing also raises the question of priorities. Time is the same for everyone; there are 24 hours in each day. How we use the time concerns priorities. Thus, developing clear goals may help us to set priorities. This in turn is valuable for selecting activities as well as for pacing them at the right tempo.

Attitudes and the way we interpret bodily sensations are also important. The brain processes all of our sensations and this allows for interpretation. Sometimes this interpretation may influence whether we experience a sensation as "painful", "negative", "an injury" or as normal feedback. When we move, if we pay attention, we get feedback from soft tissues, e.g. muscles.

If we do too much, we may feel stiff and sore the next day. If we twist or move suddenly we may feel a "jolt" as well. It may be difficult, after a back or neck pain episode, to discriminate whether these signals are normal or "red flags" telling us to stop. The problem is not the signal (you really do feel something, and this is important) but it may be difficult to judge the meaning of it. This in turn may cause uncertainty and contribute to the fear avoidance above. In fact, some people have rather negative interpretations and catastrophize. Catastrophizing blows the true meaning of the sensation out of proportion. They also tend to start a vicious circle that leads to more and greater negative thoughts. In the end, this affects not only our perception of the pain, but our behavior. We may become inactive and depressed. Therefore, it is important to prevent the development of negative attitudes and thoughts that enhance the development of vicious circles.

Treatments may be mentioned as an introduction to skills training. Talk about exposure training for phobias which translates to "graded activity" for movements/exercises. Mention scheduling as an important way of actually identifying and overcoming obstacles, as well as ensuring maintenance. Stress that individuals can significantly influence a pain problem, and above all prevent the development of persistent pain and disability.

Finally, the above is vital since it opens the door for pain control. A number of techniques may be used to control pain levels while increasing activity levels. This should result in improved quality of life.

Problems to solve

Use the case study. Let participants work in groups of two or three. However, make sure that there is rotation so that the same people do not work together on the problem-solving in every session.

The problems to be solved are:

1. Why did Lena's activity pattern change?
2. What could she (herself) do/have done to prevent this?
3. What should she do to improve her quality of life?

Instruct people to be as specific and concrete in solving the problems as possible.

During the group discussion that follows, have participants relate their analysis to everyday life, e.g. their own situation.

Skills

The skills for this session include selecting activity goals and then fulfilling them employing various methods. Problem-solving is used from session 1 and the group will continue with relaxation exercises.

In addition, graded activity and scheduling should be taught as skills for making activity plans actually come true! Note that there will not be enough time for thorough training in all of the skills. Instead an introduction and basic instructions may be given. Additional practice will be done in the homework assignments.

For those interested, a written program for simple exercises is provided. This presents a short series of movements and exercises that are not only safe, but promote a strong back:

1. Identify goals with your activity level/quality of life. Do something fun! For yourself, or include the family!
   Which activities do you want/need to learn to do?
   Which activities do you want/need to increase?
   Which activities do you want/need to decrease?
2. Teach pacing and graded activity.
   Be sure to include long-term vs. short-term goals.
3. Use problem-solving to overcome obstacles.
4. Use scheduling as a tool to really make sure you are able to participate in the activity.
5. Letting-go relaxation should be practiced again.

Homework

Participants will need to practice and apply the skills from this session:

1. Activity program. Write down your own activity goals. Try to include a fun activity and/or a new activity.
2. Use scheduling to "book" a time and place for this activity.
3. Write down how pacing might be applied to one or more of your activities.
4. Follow through! Do the activity you have chosen.
5. Letting-go relaxation. Continue practicing daily.

Don't forget to get feedback from every person concerning what has been learned, the negative and positive aspects of the session!

SESSION THREE
Self-care and the promotion of health: or how to prevent relapse

Objectives

1. To maintain a positive group atmosphere.
2. To provide information on how pain problems may be prevented.

3. To provide information on how thoughts and behaviors may be utilized to enhance preventive efforts.

4. To teach participants how various skills such as relaxation, activity management, beliefs, pauses, etc., may be applied as *coping*.

5. To help participants identify targets for developing coping strategies that may be applied in everyday life.

6. To specifically teach participants *applied relaxation as a coping strategy*.

Introduction

Welcome group members to another exciting session. Review homework assignments and any particular problems or successes that may have occurred. *Reinforce positive behaviors!*

Provide an overview of this session's activities and organize the refreshment break.

Education: theory and discussion

This session focuses on the idea of coping as self-care. Consequently, the development of coping strategies for a problem will be highlighted as a method of dealing with pain problems in everyday life. This will combine information and skills that participants have already worked with concerning problem-solving and management skills such as relaxation and activity management. This session will help students learn how to apply these skills to develop an individualized coping program. Applied relaxation will be focused on as an example of a coping strategy and self-statements will be added as an example of how several strategies may be combined.

In addition, this session should introduce the concept of how beliefs may influence behavior and the pain problem. One aspect is to present information on why we may interpret our body's signals as "harm" when they may actually be saying "hurt". Reiterating information (from session 1) on how thoughts may influence experience and behavior should be included. A specific example of how thoughts may influence the experience of pain should be given. One example is the "no pain no gain" concept in sports. Another is the exercise described in session 1, where participants are asked to concentrate on bodily sensations for a couple of minutes (with their eyes closed, in a quiet room). Finally, changes in pain perception during relaxation practice may also be used as a pertinent example.

Thoughts, beliefs, cognitions, etc., may then be connected to *self-statements*. This is important since a skill exercise will focus on self-statements. You may describe how self-statements both reflect and influence such things as self-confidence (the person who always says to him/herself "I can't do this" as opposed to the one who says "Now's my chance to show how well I can do this"). Another relevant example is from performers (athletes, music, theater) since they often rehearse with imagery, but definitely include positive self-statements ("This will be a great performance, I'm in top shape for this event, Now is my chance to be center-stage", etc.).

You may also wish to discuss the power of positive thinking as opposed to automatic negative thoughts. An example might be: "Our thoughts can have a profound effect upon our behavior and physiological function. For example, thinking about stressful situations that create frustration or anger in truth increase our heart rate and blood pressure and lower our immune defense. Likewise, negative thoughts can adversely affect a pain problem (give some examples)."

Interestingly, negative thoughts and emotions that are disruptive are often based on notions that simply are not true. Indeed, there are many myths about pain that almost everyone has believed at one time or another. Once these thoughts occur they may be maintained by so-called "cognitive errors" that we make. Fortunately, devastating negative thoughts can be altered.

By identifying your negative thoughts you are well on your way to changing them. By producing positive thoughts you will find your evaluation of the situation becomes more accurate. Moreover, this will help reduce the disappointment and anxiety that surrounds the problem and it will promote recovery.

A key to changing negative thoughts is recognizing that they are not accurate. Many people make what psychologists call *cognitive errors*. This means that we develop a tendency for negative thoughts that tends to distort the problem. There are at least two special ways that this occurs: overgeneralization and catastrophizing.

Overgeneralization involves taking a statement that is true and grossly applying it to a wide range of situations. "When I have pain, no one can stand me!" "I'll never hold a job because I will never get over this pain." These are examples of overgeneralization. If you examine these statements closely, you will see that they may contain a grain of truth. Irritable people with pain are more difficult to get along with. Yet the statements above make absurd generalizations. While none of us may be a pearl of charm when in pain or irritated, the idea that "no one can stand me" goes far beyond the truth. And although we may feel that we do not work efficiently when in pain, we nevertheless most certainly can make valuable contributions. Overgeneralization, like other negative thoughts, often serves to fire a vicious circle and paralyze coping.

Catastrophizing is the tendency to draw the worst possible conclusions when confronted with pain (or some other problem). "With this pain, I won't be able to sleep." "That sharp pain must be related to a serious disk disease." These statements, like overgeneralization, draw conclusions that go far, far beyond the logical truth. Like other negative thoughts they trigger a vicious circle of thoughts that produce a negative mood and cripple our ability to deal with the problem.

To alter your pattern of thoughts you first need to identify your negative thoughts, and then attempt to rephrase them more accurately. You will need to identify negative thoughts in the coming days as you become more and more aware of them.

In order to modify your negative thoughts, you need to ask two central questions:

1. Are these thoughts accurate?
2. What effect would it have if I altered this thought to a more positive and accurate one?

The idea of *coping* should be introduced. Most people will have attempted various coping strategies, but few will probably be familiar with the term and the way we use it to mean how you deal with pain. Examples of coping representing both cognitive aspects (which ties into beliefs and self-statements above) as well as behavioral aspects will help to explain the idea to participants. It is important to stress that *coping strategies may be developed to deal with troublesome problems.* In fact, we naturally develop coping strategies although we seldom actually think about this (e.g. how to deal with pain at the dentist; when we receive an injection or other potentially painful treatment; removing a Band-Aid, etc.).

Coping as prevention involves *employing the strategies at the proper time and place.* That is, usually we try to identify a problem situation and employ the technique at the crucial moment to prevent a bout of pain from occurring or becoming worse. Judging when the strategy should be used is based on knowledge provided by the external environment (e.g. place, activity, etc.) or from one's own body (internal signals). You may want to use the example of migraine headaches where patients often report various physiological "warning signals" such as stomach churning, flashes, dizziness, etc., before the onset of a headache. Employing relaxation at an early point has been found to be an effective method of preventing these headaches.

Other coping techniques may include activity management and pauses. Activity management includes *pacing*, which was introduced in session 2. The idea in this context is that certain, specific activities may be employed to cope with pain or to prevent its onset. Exercise, to keep the muscles fit, may be one example. Another is going for a walk (e.g. to relax, get fresh air, or think about something else) to prevent, i.e. cope with, pain when a warning signal has been identified. Pauses may be used in various forms. These include pause gymnastics, mini-pauses, etc. Pauses may be used to disrupt the development of a bout of pain or as a method of minimizing pain sensations. One particular form that may be used as coping is *applied relaxation*. The concept is to employ relaxation in short breaks to prevent, disrupt or minimize pain.

Self-care may also entail other types of behaviors more directly related to the pain problem. These may include massage, taking hot baths, stretching, etc. In this course, we do not have specific recommendations about which of these may be effective. Instead, the guideline is that self-care and coping may be one and the same. Thus, *they entail empowering the participant with skills.* The exact behavior may be different for different participants; however, it should involve behaviors that the person does which *increases their self-efficacy.* Consequently, passive methods, e.g. taking medicines, receiving treatments and so on, would not fit into this concept.

Some important aspects of employing self-care as coping include identifying the problem in terms of behavior, knowing when self-care is appropriate (compared to when I need a doctor), as well as knowing when and what should be self-administered. These points may be exemplified and discussed if time permits. Underlying this discussion will be questions of why pain may recur or get worse as well as how one may learn to identify warning signals.

Problem to solve

This section will need to be fairly short as we focus more on practicing skills during this session! Again, participants will work in twos or threes and be sure to have them rotate so that new pairs are formed.

1. What could Lena do to cope with her pain problem in a better way? When should she employ these techniques?
2. Relate to your everyday life.
   How may we learn to identify warning signals? Can we develop coping strategies for specific problem situations?
   How may we know when a problem needs professional medical attention and when it doesn't? (optional)

During discussion, remember that people will learn from experience. Highlight the fact that monitoring is important so that "warning" factors will be made visible. Likewise, trying simple techniques, one at a time, to evaluate how well they work for the individual may be a good way of developing a coping strategy. People are very different and consequently effective coping strategies may also differ greatly from person to person.

Skills

Skills training in this session will include identifying warning signals, applied relaxation (combining pauses, relaxation and coping) and self-statements (thoughts/beliefs). In addition, it builds on relaxation training started earlier as well as activity management (as a possible coping strategy) introduced in session 2.

1. Identify *warning signals*, i.e. situations and bodily feelings that signal pain. This may be done by analyzing past experience and writing down "suspected" warning signals. In addition, monitoring may be used to identify warning signals.
2. *Applied relaxation*. This skill will be introduced in theory as a potent coping strategy. It links warning signals with an effective method of disrupting the development of pain. It may also be used in association with activities where fear is an issue. Training today should focus on *rapid relaxation*. In the following sessions, relaxation may be linked to the warning situation in skill 1 above.
3. *Positive self-statements*. How to identify negative statements. How to reformulate as positive statements. Scheduling positive self-statements. Employing positive self-statements as a coping strategy. These positive self-statements may be linked to actually employing rapid relaxation in particular "risk" situations (this will be practiced in a later session).

Homework

1. Identify warning signals, for instance a particular problem (e.g. pain or stress) or in general (how I feel at the moment) via monitoring.
2. Practice rapid relaxation.
3. Identify negative thoughts.
4. Practice reframing negative thoughts to more accurate positive ones.
5. Practice using positive self-statements; that is, schedule positive statements at least three times during the week or in one specific situation that occurs more than once. The use of positive statements does not necessarily need to be practiced in conjunction with a "pain situation".

Finally, review the session to identify what participants have learned as well as the strengths and weaknesses.

SESSION FOUR

Getting the most out of your work and leisure time: coping with work and family

Objectives

1. To maintain a positive group atmosphere and provide opportunities for members to receive reinforcement for correct "coping" approximations.
2. To provide information about how the workplace and family may be influenced by the participant's pain problem (empathy).
3. To provide information and coping strategies concerning how the workplace and family may influence the participant's perception of their pain, their cognitive-behavioral reactions to the pain problem.
4. To teach assertiveness. Participants should understand how to apply these techniques in making their needs clear, yet be able to compromise. This includes being able to say "no" when necessary.
5. To help participants identify the kinds of reactions and behaviors, from others, which are most helpful in supporting the participant's "health behaviors" in the long run.
6. To teach participants to prompt the behaviors identified in 5 above in order to prevent others from feeling guilty as well as promoting positive relationships with family and friends.
7. To teach participants how to apply rapid relaxation to risk situations.
8. To teach participants how to employ several techniques, including 4, 5, 6 and 7, as coping in social situations. Among other things this should reduce feelings of guilt and promote healthy relationships.
9. To begin to plan a personal coping program.

Introduction

Tell participants how nice it is to see them again. Review homework and the most pertinent points from the last session. Provide an overview of the activities for this session. Keep shaping positive behavioral changes!

Education: theory and discussion

Today's "lecture" is quite broad and therefore will not be as in-depth as in previous sessions. Moreover, it is probably the most difficult session given the time limits and large number of objectives. So be sure to plan your time and remember that there will be additional time during sessions 5 and 6 to review (or continue) should it be needed. An especially important aspect of this lecture is that these effects are bilateral: the person's pain influences family and friends just as these important others influence how we perceive, react to and deal with pain.

Work, family and leisure-time activities are probably the most important aspects of your participants' lives. At the same time that they provide us with great enjoyment and rewards, they can also be a source of stress. Socially, psychologically and even physically, work, family and leisure shape a person's lifestyle. Thus, what happens in the work and family situation may have important implications for pain and how well it is dealt with. The effects are bilateral, that is, these situations, and the people in them, influence us, but we also influence them.

One example is how parents influence their children through modeling. Just as with other behaviors, there is a tendency for children to deal with ill-health in similar ways to their parents. In fact, a child reared in a family where a parent has a chronic disease has twice the risk of suffering chronic benign pain as compared to children in other families. Since most health-related behaviors are learned, children may use methods of dealing with pain—e.g. whether to seek a doctor, confront or avoid pain, take medication, rest—which are similar to their parents. This issue is also relevant for participants in that they may have children and thus are a model for their children.

A natural reaction of family members when we complain of pain is sympathy and a desire "to help". Consequently, family and friends may show concern and attempt to help out in various ways which they believe are appropriate. For example, we may express sympathy verbally and we may assist someone in pain by doing their chores or arranging for an appointment for the doctor. Generally speaking, many of us may feel an obligation to respond with "help" when a significant other complains of pain. While this is very normal and natural in the short term, it may have adverse effects in the long term. Social interactions, for instance, may become "pain-based". Family and friends may feel that their leisure activities are being hampered by constantly needing to take consideration of another person's pain. Family and friends may feel guilty since, in the long run, they no longer know what to do to help, but nevertheless believe that the pain sufferer expects them to "do something". Or they may feel guilty because they would rather not "help out" but view the pain complaint as a cue to do so.

Consider the wife who comes home after work and asks her husband how his day was and receives a long description of how difficult it was and how much pain he has. Even though it may be the husband's responsibility to cook supper and do the clean-up that day, the wife may feel "obligated" to do this, despite previous plans for enjoying a movie. Although chronic pain patients, for instance, often believe that they "hide" their pain from others, research shows that friends and relatives are quite good at detecting when these patients are suffering from pain.

People with MSP may also feel guilty because they do not want to or cannot participate in activities they previously have shared with family or friends. Children, for example, may want to play ball or play on the floor—activities that may be difficult if one is currently in pain. Telling the child that one cannot participate may generate guilt.

One important aspect of changes in the family or with friends is that they occur slowly over relatively long periods of time. Thus, major changes in routines and lifestyle may not be recognized as they are occurring. As an illustration, a father may play with his small child on the floor every evening after supper. This playtime may be fairly short, say 10 minutes, but happens every day. When the father suffers an episode of back pain, however, he may decline to participate. After just a few days the child may stop asking to play (the response is extinguished) and it may be weeks or even months later before the father realizes that he has lost a small but important part of his quality of life. One or two of these small changes may certainly be tolerable; the problem is that many such "small changes" may be occurring which together translate into a rather large, and very negative, change in lifestyle.

The way family and friends react to our pain may even influence how we perceive the pain and how we deal with it. Receiving attention (or sympathy) may be pleasant just as being "pampered" may be quite rewarding. After all, these are the basic ingredients in good hotels, restaurants, airlines and other services. But especially if few opportunities are available for other kinds of positive interactions, this may be devastating for a normal relationship in the long term. Furthermore, attention and pampering contingent on so-called sick behavior (e.g. complaining or showing pain behaviors) may actually reinforce (increase) these behaviors. Just as children or students may sometimes increase disobedient behavior to obtain "attention", so may people with pain begin to maintain sick behaviors because it results in attention, pampering, etc. *This usually is not a conscious act; many times it happens so gradually that the person is not fully aware of the change.* However, the negative aspect is that the person's lifestyle may change gradually and dramatically toward a passive lifestyle with a high degree of dependence on others.

Moreover, as people with pain base more and more of their interaction with others on pain, they become less interesting to socialize with since they become boring. So, in the long run family and friends may lose interest in the person, making the situation even worse.

On the other hand, family and friends (at work or otherwise) may be vital in giving support provided it is of the correct type. During the recovery period after an episode of pain, friends and family may provide support that is essential for the pain sufferer to make it through the difficult period of recovery. These friends and family may provide emotional understanding and yet encourage self-care, independence and active coping.

Family and friends may be encouraged to provide proper support with prompting and one may help decrease feelings of guilt too. First, it is possible to behave in ways so that others will not feel guilty. A person may make it clear, for example, that they do not expect/want help or sympathy. Or one might suggest a fun alternative to a suggested activity that one cannot participate in. Second, one may be assertive in making one's own needs clear and yet be flexible for compromise. In response to a request at work to do a particular task (which I believe I cannot do) I might say: "No, I'm sorry, I can't load the 25 sacks of grain today. They are really heavy and have to be lifted from the floor which is difficult and uncomfortable. Perhaps someone could help me or we could order the smaller size sacks. I'd be happy to organize this."

Third, appropriate support may be *prompted*. Briefly, this entails providing a clear stimulus to the other person which sets the stage for the appropriate supportive response. An obvious example of this is the person with new clothes or hairstyle who says: "Look, do you notice anything different?" This prompts a response from the other person and a probable positive comment such as: "Let's see, you have new pants. They're really stylish!"

Finally, coping, e.g. *applied relaxation*, pacing, etc., may be used to actually *confront* the activity in question. Ordinarily, normal activities are not harmful (in fact beneficial), although they may sometimes be painful. In other words, one may use coping strategies in order to participate in an activity that we may feel hesitant about doing. By confronting the situation one may actually learn to manage the situation better and thereby maintain good social and physical capabilities.

The physical environment at work and at home may also be important. Heavy work, bending, twisting, monotonous work, vibrations and the like have all been found to be significant risk factors for MSP. This is why, during an acute episode of MSP, doctors and physical therapists may recommend "taking it easy" for a couple of days. This may also be why recommendations for change in your work or workplace may be provided. Often, however, social aspects at home and work may be involved which steer the possibility of making such changes.

In addition, how well we like our job, how much we feel needed, how well we get along with workmates and supervisors may influence how much we are willing to sacrifice to go to work. If we really enjoy our work and feel needed and liked, we may work despite pain. On the other hand, stress and a poor "atmosphere" at work may actually exacerbate the pain. Another important aspect is how much support we may receive when attempting to return to work (or remain at work) after an episode of pain. Just as with family and friends, some workmates and supervisors may help in very appropriate ways while others do not. Similarly, the techniques mentioned above may sometimes be used to improve the situation (prompting, assertiveness, confronting the activity, etc.). Expectations that family and workmates have may also need to be actively addressed. For example, some supervisors may believe that a person with pain must be 100% well before returning to work. Since recovery is often very gradual in cases of MSP, this would mean waiting long periods of time which in turn increases the probability of chronic problems. A clear dialogue may be helpful, again using the techniques described.

Finally, pain problems may limit a person's leisure activities in undesired ways. Some activities may simply be difficult to participate in when in pain. Coping strategies, however, may be employed to help solve these problems and confront rather than avoid the situation. One may, as suggested above, need to use applied relaxation. Another example is positive self-statements to overcome fears that "I might not be able to do this activity".

Finally, one may need to do some sort of analysis of which leisure activities are important and why. Most often an activity that simply becomes impossible to do may be replaced by other equally fun things. Rather than participating in a sport, for example, one may become a coach. Rather than doing an individual activity, e.g. painting (art), one might participate in an activity with the family, e.g. a game, a walk, an outing. (Problem-solving may be used here.) The idea is that most of us have a rich variety of leisure activities that we would like to participate in. *Thus, real difficulties in participating in one particular activity need not mean* a decrease in activity level or quality of life. In the first place, coping may be employed to participate despite the pain. Second, a deep look at our family and leisure activities may provide us with the opportunity to analyze what we are doing and thereby maximize the possibility of planning to participate in the activities we really want to be doing.

Managing stress and pain often involves setting clear priorities. The coping strategies described may help us develop our priorities, communicate them to others, and follow through on them.

Problem to solve

This section will be fairly brief as skills training will take a considerable amount of time in this session.

Employ a case study as in previous sessions. Be sure that participants rotate. Problems to be solved are:

1. What problems does Lena have concerning her family and work situation?
2. Why have these problems developed? What maintains them?
3. What might be done to improve them?
4. What factors at work and home have important influence on your own pain?

Skills

1. Giving others positive reinforcement (compliments). The context is providing positive reinforcement so that assertive behavior will be effective. The rule of thumb is four positive compliments for each criticism or assertive behavior. This will also make life more pleasant and enhance positive relationships.
2. Prompting appropriate responses (identify appropriate response needed, learn to provide a discriminative stimulus to set the stage). "How do you think I'm doing, considering I've had trouble doing this (activity) before?" "Do you think one person can lift this all right?" *It is vital that this technique not be confused with guilt-inducing "hints" or verbal pain behaviors!! ("A real friend would help out." "I don't know how I will manage to do X with this much back pain, do you?")*
3. Assertiveness: How to say no without feeling guilty. Clearly presenting your need, want or opinion. Be prepared to compromise.
   Employ prompting and problem-solving to provide alternatives.
   Say no when appropriate!

Be prepared for positive reactions (reinforce!) as well as negative reactions. A typical negative reaction is to attempt to instill guilt, e.g. "A real friend would help out." "This person/event/thing really needs your help." "How can you let all of those children down?"

This may be defused by (a) knowing and expecting this tactic as a method of manipulation, (b) by counteracting it with relaxation and positive self-statements, (c) by offering a compromise.

4. Applied relaxation. Coupling risk situations with relaxation (based on monitoring and rapid relaxation). You may use an example for practice, e.g. sitting during a long period, lifting or getting up in the morning (if they provoke the pain).
5. Combine 1–4 as coping strategies for family, workplace and leisure activity planning. Participants may also use previously learned skills, e.g. scheduling, problem-solving.

Homework

1. Give compliments to at least three different people. Do it contingently, i.e. when the other person does something you like/admire. The three or more compliments should be given in situations where you ordinarily would *not* have given a compliment. Observe the reaction you get!
2. Say "no" and provide an alternative in a predetermined or other situation at least twice. Start with a relatively easy situation, but one that you nevertheless may have previously said "yes" to even though you wanted to say "no". Do this exercise if you have problems saying no, or formulating a compromise.
3. Practice applied relaxation in one specified situation every day.
4. Employ a prompt at least three times to attempt to obtain a supportive response.

This is a considerable amount of homework. However, 1, 2 and 4 do not take very much time, although participants may need help in remembering to do these. Applied relaxation is a bit more time-consuming, but still does not require a lot of time in that it is a short exercise being repeated a considerable number of times.

Remember to review the session!!

SESSION FIVE
Applying coping strategies in everyday life including flare-ups and maintenance

Objectives

1. To maintain a positive group atmosphere and provide opportunities for the reinforcement of correct coping approximations.

2. To provide information about flare-ups.

3. To provide information about maintenance.

4. To teach participants how to use applied relaxation as coping.

5. To teach participants how to apply their skills to cope with flare-ups.

6. To work on developing a personalized coping program.

7. To develop a strategy for self-care that is so successful it may reduce the need for healthcare visits.

Introduction

Welcome participants and review homework. Be sure to check on progress and attempt to deal with any problems people may have had with their homework. Reinforce approximations of coping behavior. The homework may well have produced some fun; utilize this to stress that coping can be a wonderful experience. Saying no, etc., may have produced anxiety or negative feedback. Help participants to deal with this, e.g. by defusing the guilt that may have been aroused. Provide an overview of this session's activities.

Education: theory and discussion

Today we will be working with developing a personalized coping program for the short term, but also for the long term. Most people can learn to master a number of coping techniques. However, the difference between success and failure in the long run is whether the person actually is able to *apply these skills in everyday life*. In addition, continual practice may be necessary to maintain certain skills at an optimal level. This session focuses on developing coping strategies to deal with everyday pain problems. It also looks at possible obstacles to applying coping strategies. Finally, the case of flare-ups is used as an example of a problem that may require special applications of skills.

Neither pain nor life is constant; our situation changes with time. Thus, we need to be able to alter our coping strategies in order to deal with new situations. Throughout this course we have worked with developing coping strategies to deal with problem situations. In addition, we have tried to identify some situations that currently are a problem so that one or more techniques could be used to deal with the situation. The question today is how we will deal with future problems that may arise.

One example is flare-ups. The natural course of MSP is cyclic variation. Thus, almost all people who

suffer pain will at some point have a relapse of some sort. For many this will be a period of more pain and discomfort, but not a condition that requires medical attention or sick leave. For others it will mean severe pain and functional problems. Unfortunately, people may "give up" trying to use coping strategies when a flare-up occurs. They may believe that their strategies have not been effective or they may not be prepared to deal actively with it.

Neither of these beliefs is correct. The strategies used may in fact have been very effective in preventing problems. Nevertheless, flare-ups, etc., may occur as a natural part of the nature of MSP. And few people have a 100% effective coping program. Thus, some future problems may be expected. Although the pain may feel different when a flare-up occurs, new coping strategies may be developed to help cope with the problem.

Thus, it is important to have a strategy for coping with flare-ups that may be initiated at the proper time. Usually this will involve a number of skills and even levels, i.e. what one may try first, second and so on.

One specific aspect of flare-ups is determining when to seek professional healthcare. Since most forms of back pain are not harmful, many visits will provide information or possibly pain relief, but not a cure. A typical visit will allow a doctor or physical therapist to tell you what you don't have (a tumor, disk disease, neurological damage, etc.), but they may not be able to specifically diagnose your problem. As for treatment, symptom relief is the goal of most of these. Consequently, you will need to weigh the possible benefits of seeking professional care, with the time, energy and costs involved. (A short list of signs that may signal the need for medical care may be given; see current guidelines. These usually include severe pain, pain that is not reduced by lying down, fever, problems controlling urination or defecation.)

Other new problems may also arise. This is why problem-solving and a "coping skills" approach is so vital. These skills may be applied to develop new coping strategies as they become needed in everyday life.

However, in order to be able to use many of the skills taught in this course, a certain amount of practice may be required. Relaxation, physical training, etc., may need to be trained regularly to retain the skill at a significant level.

Consequently, another problem is maintaining coping skills. There are a number of obstacles. Some of these, such as conflicts of interest with other family members (I need to practice, they need to do something else), lack of time planning, etc., have been brought up earlier, in terms of fulfilling homework assignments.

One of the greatest problems in the long run, however, is maintaining a skill which is preventive. Since successful prevention means we may not experience a problem with MSP, there is a natural tendency to perceive the training as less important (until the pain is experienced again!). Thus, there is a need to identify those skills that are vital, and develop a program for maintaining the skill at an optimum.

In the next session, maintenance and an analysis of risk for relapse will be addressed.

Problem to solve

Return to the case study and work as in previous sessions. This section will again need to be kept relatively short to provide enough time for the skills training.

Today participants should develop a coping strategy package for Lena:

1. How should she deal with her various problems? Be as specific as possible.
2. How might she deal with flare-ups?
3. Document the program briefly with a text or summary of the package.

Skills

1. Applied relaxation. Continue with the application phase. Participants should select at least one relevant situation to work with during the session.
2. Develop a program for flare-ups. This should be individualized. It ought to include various skills and levels, e.g. immediate reaction, more long-term plans. Stress the importance of a positive attitude in spite of the flare-up, coupled with planned coping strategies.
3. Review and polish any other skills that may be needed or that you did not have time to do properly in earlier sessions.
4. Begin planning the personalized coping program.

Homework

1. Practice applied relaxation in specified situations, or for advanced students in "all" situations.
2. Document your plan for dealing with flare-ups.
3. Identify necessary skills that need to be practiced and list possible obstacles.
4. *Develop and write down a personalized coping program!*
5. Apply other skills that participant believes are important which there has not been time to employ during the other homework assignments.

Review the session as described in session 1!

SESSION SIX
Maintaining and improving treatment gains: adherence and risk analysis

Objectives
1. To reinforce appropriate coping behaviors and provide support.
2. To provide information about maintenance and adherence and the analysis of risk for relapse.
3. To teach participants how to do a risk analysis.
4. To teach participants how to enhance adherence.
5. To teach participants about enhancing and fine-tuning their program.
6. To evaluate the course, and the participants' progress.

Introduction

Welcome everyone to this last session! Check homework assignments, providing the usual feedback and reinforcement for appropriate approximations. Provide an overview of the session.

Education: theory and discussion

Maintaining progress for people suffering MSP may be difficult since it often requires the individual to continue practicing a host of coping strategies. In fact, most patients attending a multidimensional treatment for chronic pain improve substantially. However, they lose an average of 50% of the gains over the course of a few months. One reason appears to be a failure to continue to apply coping skills in the home and work environment. Another reason may be that the skills are no longer practiced and thus lose their effect. A third reason may be a failure to have anticipated obstacles or relapse and "giving up". Other explanations are of course possible, but note that few patients will actually suffer an accident or other physical injury that will require medical attention; almost all cases involve flare-ups of previous soft tissue "injuries".

The modified health behavior model (Fig. 10.3, see page 94 above) may be presented to help participants understand why people may continue to adhere to their program as well as why they may quit. Emphasize the right-hand side of the model (since they have already started doing the behavior) which includes the situation and reinforcement for participating. This model may be used to help plan training programs for such things as relaxation, exercise, etc.

Relapse prevention theory may also be presented to help participants understand how one may better deal with relapse to previous behaviors (e.g. failure to exercise or practice relaxation) or symptoms, above all flare-ups. By analyzing the situation and planning for these events, one may prevent the "giving up" syndrome ("I've started drinking/smoking again, I might as well continue"). Furthermore, it provides steps to actively deal with the problem as it develops (the last step usually being: contact your professional to get a booster).

The above two methods are extremely helpful in identifying obstacles to application and maintenance. Once again, success is closely tied in with *the application of coping skills in everyday life*.

Having to practice relaxation or exercise may be experienced as negative by some. However, the program presented here is flexible and based on the self-care principle. Consequently, skills learned, but not currently employed in the individual package, may be activated at a later time. New skills may also be learned and applied! Not least, if an individual does not experience a benefit from employing a particular skill, *this is a signal that the program should be changed, i.e. enhanced*. So, rather than feel that one must continue certain skills or exercises for the rest of their lives, this approach is pragmatic. Problem-solving skills may be used to analyze the situation and provide a new program. Some aspects of the program may eventually need to be altered. In addition, some skills may need to be "brushed up" so that they may be employed once again.

However, whether a person participates in a coping program or practices certain skills or exercises should be a conscious choice. What we need to prevent is the subtle change of a successful program, to a state that it either is no longer applied or is done so in such an irregular way that it is not effective. The usual problem with maintenance of behavioral change is that it gradually reverts to the previous "inappropriate" behavior. You may wish to use the example of exercising to illustrate how this occurs.

Problem to solve

1. What obstacles might Lena face in maintaining an active coping program?
2. What might be done to ensure maintenance of those behaviors, i.e. a coping program one wants to continue with?
3. How might a change in the coping program actually enhance its effectiveness?

Skills

1. Use the "compliance road map" exercise to initiate a risk analysis. In short, this method uses the analogy of driving a car. On the right-hand side of the map is Hollywood gleaming with stars. On the left-hand side is Relapse City stinking with garbage. The objective is to construct a road map of how each individual may get to these destinations. What are the crucial events that "steer" or guide us there?
2. Relapse prevention. Use the risk analysis above as a base for developing a relapse prevention plan. Think specifically about the situations where a relapse probably might occur and subsequently develop specific strategies for coping with this.
3. Enhancing adherence. Using the road map to Hollywood, develop a plan for maximizing the positive events that help a person to get there! Demonstrate and work with how specifying the behavior, the situation and programming reinforcement may help to improve adherence. Underscore bridging the gap between naturally occurring reinforcement and the richer schedule of reinforcement needed to shape and bring the behavior to a steady state. In addition to programmed reinforcement, underscore the need for naturally occurring reinforcement, e.g. it is fun or provides relief for maintaining the behavior in the long run.
4. Schedule evaluations of your program. To avoid inadvertently altering the program, book a "planned choice" evaluation in your calendar. This will only take about 5 minutes, but may make a world of difference for long-term results. The following questions may be used as a guide: (a) Have I executed each aspect of the program as planned (e.g. applied relaxation, exercise, saying "no" to overtime)? (b) What effect(s) have I experienced? (Is the pain better, same, worse? Do I feel better, same, worse? Quality of life?) (c) Is there any part of the program that I want to change? If so, what? (d) If I haven't applied the program as planned, why not? Do I want to return to this plan or change the plan?

Homework

1. Apply your coping program to prevent MSP, stress and related problems!
2. Organize booster sessions yourself if you feel it would be beneficial.
3. Schedule your progress "planned choice" checks. Reinforce yourself for advances; plan any needed changes.

Session review

The session review today will be short since a course evaluation will be conducted. At this time it may be determined if the participants desire a formal follow-up session. It is not necessary that groups have a formal follow-up, but at the therapist's discretion this may be discussed and organized.

Course evaluation

At this time a review of the entire course is appropriate. Allow each person to provide a verbal evaluation. We also use written evaluations that ask a few key questions and also provide space for written comments.

Good luck!

FOLLOW-UP SESSION
Troubleshooting to enhance gains

Objectives

1. To assess treatment gains and possible relapse.
2. To determine adherence to individual programs.
3. To determine causes of adherence as well as consequences of compliance/noncompliance.
4. To revise individual programs to more appropriately deal with current status, e.g. to add or subtract components, change strategy.
5. To identify which skills may need to be "revived", i.e. need additional practice.
6. To revise plan for adherence and risk analysis.

Introduction

Participants should be warmly welcomed back to the group and attendance underscored. *It is extremely important to reinforce any progress that has been made. The question of how life would be had each person NOT attempted these programs should be kept in mind.* After a general introduction, a short round to assess how each person has done during the follow-up should focus on: (1) how well they feel; (2) how well they are coping with their pain problem; (3) adherence to the program they had designed; and (4) the relationship between adherence and outcome.

Reinforce well behavior and success!

Education

This section must be kept short during this session. A review of the material concerning long-term outcome (sessions 5 and 6) may be briefly presented. The essential points are the process of selecting and applying skills and the difficulties that may be encountered in the long run.

It should be pointed out that while success is golden, the general rule is a certain amount of setbacks. *Flare-ups and relapse are not uncommon and definitely do not mean that the program has been a failure!* Instead, each incident of problems may be used as a learning experience to find what is most helpful—a fine-tuning of the program.

Help participants to recall that life is not constant and this may necessitate (the continual) modification of the program. Since each person has learned the various skills in these group sessions, each skill is still relatively accessible. A comparison may be made with learning a foreign language: reviving an earlier "mastered" language is much easier and less time-consuming than starting from scratch.

The problem areas covered in the course may be reviewed together with the skills practiced! This should emphasize how much they have actually accomplished and how many possibilities they have for developing coping strategies.

Problem to solve

The problem to solve involves identifying progress (and reinforcing it) as well as troubleshooting for improving results. This exercise may be done in groups of two or three people:

1. How would life have been had the changes initiated in this group *not* taken place?
2. With the help of your partner make a written list of (a) your positive progress, (b) any setbacks encountered.
3. In brief outline form, *list ways of modifying* your personal coping program in order to improve outcome. Use problem-solving skills! Seek help from each other. If no problems have been encountered, use the time to (a) reinforce yourself/each other!, (b) further develop the program, and/or (c) to determine why the program has worked so well.

Subsequently, each group may very briefly report their results. The lists may be copied so that the group leader retains a copy as well as the individual participant.

Skills

No new skills are introduced in this booster session. Rather individuals should, on the basis of the problem-based practice above,

1. Modify their program, if necessary, for future use. This should be done in written form and will

probably be similar to the problem-solving exercise above. The idea is to do it specifically for each individual.

2. Recycle the risk analysis/adherence program (even if the program is working!).
3. Schedule program checks in calendar. (Is this program working? Am I complying with my goals?)
4. Identify skills that need to be practiced more frequently. If questions arise, some skills may be reviewed.
5. Develop a strategy for continued follow-up. Should the group, on its own, meet again?

Conclusion

Review session. Reinforce progress and idea that participants can control a pain problem.

Ask for feedback on session by underscoring progress made, program modification, etc. What have they learned? How do they feel about treatment?

Other comments.

Wish them good luck!

References

Abraham, C. and Sheeran, P., Cognitive representations and preventive health behaviour: A review. In: K.J. Petrie and J.A. Weinman (Eds.), Perceptions of health and illness, Harwood Academic Publishers, Amsterdam, 1997, pp. 213–240.

Aldrich, S., Eccleston, C. and Crombez, G., Worrying about chronic pain: Vigilance to threat and misdirected problem solving, Behavior Research and Therapy, 38 (2000) 457–470.

Al-Obaidi, S.M., Nelson, R.M., Al-Awadhi, S. and Al-Shuwaie, M., The role of anticipation and fear of pain in the persistence of avoidance behavior in patients with chronic low back pain, Spine, 25 (2000) 1126–1131.

Armstrong, M.P., McDonough, S. and Baxter, G., Clinical guidelines versus clinical practice in the management of low back pain, International Journal of Clinical Practice, 57 (2003) 9–13.

Arntz, A. and Peters, M., Chronic low back pain and inaccurate predictions of pain: Is being too tough a risk factor for the development and maintenance of chronic pain?, Behavior Research and Therapy, 33 (1995) 49–53.

Arntz, A., Van Eck, M. and Heijmans, M., Predictions of dental pain: The fear of any expected evil is worse than the evil itself, Behavior Research and Therapy, 28 (1990) 29–34.

Arntz, A., Dreesen, L. and De Jong, P., The influence of anxiety on pain: Attentional and attributional mediators, Pain, 56 (1994) 307–314.

Asmundson, G.J.G. and Larsen, D.K., Pain Anxiety Symptoms Scale. In: J. Maltby, C.A. Lewis and A. Hill (Eds.), Commissioned reviews of 250 psychological tests, Edwin Mellen Press, Lampeter, UK, 2000, pp. 607–612.

Asmundson, G.J., Norton, P.J. and Norton, G.R., Beyond pain: The role of fear and avoidance in chronicity, Clinical Psychology Review, 19 (1999) 97–119.

Asmundson, G.J.G., Taylor, S. and Cox, B.J., Health anxiety, John Wiley, Chichester, 2001, 415 pp.

Asmundson, G.J., Vlaeyen, J.W.S. and Crombez, G., Understanding and treating fear of pain, Oxford University Press, Oxford, England, 2004.

Atkinson, J.H., Slater, M.A., Patterson, T.L., Grant, I. and Garfin, S.R., Prevalence, onset, and risk of psychiatric disorders in men with chronic low back pain: A controlled study, Pain, 45 (1991) 111–121.

Bandura, A., Self-efficacy mechanisms in physiological activation and health promoting behavior. In: J. Madden (Ed.), Neurobiology of learning, emotion and affect, Raven Press, New York, 1991, pp. 229–269.

Banks, S.M. and Kerns, R.D., Explaining high rates of depression in chronic pain: A diathesis-stress framework, Psychological Bulletin, 199 (1996) 95–110.

Barlow, D.H., Anxiety and its disorders: The nature and treatment of anxiety and panic, Guilford Press, London, 2002, 704 pp.

Barsky, A.J., Fama, J.M., Bailey, E.D. and Ahern, D.K., A prospective 4- to 5-year study of DSM-III-R hypochondriasis, Archives of General Psychiatry, 55 (1998) 737–744.

Beckman, H.B. and Frankel, R.M., The effect of physician behavior on the collection of data, Annals of Internal Medicine, 101 (1984) 692–696.

Beecher, H.K., Measurement of subjective responses: Quantitative effects of drugs, Oxford University Press, New York, 1959.

Benedetti, F., How the doctor's words affect the patient's brain, Evaluation of Health Professionals, 25 (2002) 369–386.

Benedetti, F., Toward a neurobiological understanding of the therapist–patient interaction. In: E. Kalso, A.M. Estlander and M. Klockars (Eds.), Psyche, soma and pain, The Signe and Ane Gyllenbergs Foundation, Helsinki, 2003, pp. 132–141.

Benson, H., The relaxation response, McGraw-Hill, New York, 1975.

Biering-Sörensen, F., A prospective study of low back pain in the general population: I. Occurrence, recurrence and etiology, Scandinavian Journal of Rehabilitation Medicine, 15 (1983) 71–80.

Boersma, K. and Linton, S.J., Early assessment of psychological factors: The Örebro Screening Questionnaire for Pain. In: S.J. Linton (Ed.), New avenues for the prevention of pain, Vol. 1, Elsevier, Amsterdam, 2002, pp. 205–213.

Boersma, K., Linton, S.J., Overmeer, T., Janson, M., Vlaeyen, J.W.S. and de Jong, J., Lowering fear-avoidance and enhancing function through exposure in vivo: A multiple baseline study across six patients with back pain, Pain, 108 (2004) 8–16.

Bongers, P.M., de Winter, C.R., Kompier, M.A. and Hildebrandt, V.H., Psychosocial factors at work and musculoskeletal disease, Scandinavian Journal of Work and Environmental Health, 19 (1993) 297–312.

Bonica, J.J., The management of pain, Lea & Febiger, Philadelphia, 1990.

Boothby, J.L., Thorn, B.E., Stroud, M.W. and Jensen, M.P., Coping with pain. In: R.J. Gatchel and D.C. Turk (Eds.), Psychosocial factors in pain: Critical perspectives, Guilford Press, New York, 1999, pp. 343–359.

Borkan, J., van Tulder, M.W., Reis, S., Schoene, M.L., Croft, P.R. and Hermoni, D., Advances in the field of low back pain in primary care: A report from the Fourth International Forum, Spine, 27 (2002) E128–132.

Brekke, M., Hjortdahl, P. and Kvien, T.K., Self-efficacy and health status in rheumatoid arthritis: A two year longitudinal observational study, Rheumatology, 40 (2001) 387–392.

Buer, N. and Linton, S.J., Fear-avoidance beliefs and catastrophizing—occurrence and risk factor in back pain and ADL in the general population, Pain, 99 (2002) 485–491.

Buer, N., Linton, S.J., Samuelsson, L. and Harms-Ringdahl, K., The role of fear-avoidance beliefs and catastrophizing in patients with fractures (submitted).

Burton, A.K. and Waddell, G., Educational and informational approaches. In: S.J. Linton (Ed.), New avenues for the prevention of chronic musculoskeletal pain and disability, Elsevier, Amsterdam, 2002, pp. 245–258.

Burton, A.K., Tillotson, K.M., Main, C.J. and Hollis, S., Psychosocial predictors of outcome in acute and subchronic low back trouble, Spine, 20 (1995) 722–728.

Burton, A.K., Battié, M.C. and Main, C.J., The relative importance of biomechanical and psychosocial factors in low back injuries. In: W. Karwowski and W. Marras (Eds.), The occupational ergonomics handbook, CRC Press, Boca Raton, FL, 1999a, pp. 1127–1138.

Burton, A.K., Waddell, G., Tillotson, K.M. and Summerton, N., Information and advice to patients with back pain can have a positive effect: A randomized controlled trial of a novel educational booklet in primary care, Spine, 24 (1999b) 2484–2491.

Bushnell, M.C., Duncan, G.H., Hofbauer, R.K., Ha, B., Chen, J. and Carrier, B., Pain perception: Is there a role for primary somatosensory cortex?, Proceedings of the National Academy of Sciences, USA, 96 (1999) 7705–7709.

Bushnell, M.C., Villemure, C. and Duncan, G.H., Psychophysical and neurophysiological studies of pain modulation by attention. In: D.D Price and M.C. Bushnell (Eds.), Psychological methods of pain control: Basic science and clinical perspectives, IASP Press, Seattle, 2004, pp. 99–116.

Callister, L.C., Khalaf, I., Semenic, S., Kartchner, R., and Vehvilainen-Julkunen, K. The pain of childbirth: Perceptions of culturally diverse women. Pain Management Nursing, 4 (2003) 145–154.

Carosella, A.-M., Lackner, J.M. and Feuerstein, M., Factors associated with early discharge from a multidisciplinary work rehabilitation program for chronic low back pain, Pain, 57 (1994) 69–76.

Cherkin, E., Deyo, R.A. and Berg, A.O., Evaluation of a physician education intervention to improve primary care for low-back pain. II. Impact of patients, Spine, 16 (1991) 1173–1178.

Cherkin, D.C., Deyo, R.A., Street, J.H. and Barlow, W., Predicting poor outcome for back pain seen in primary care using patients' own criteria, Spine, 21 (1996) 2900–2907.

Chrousos, G.P. and Gold, P.W., The concept of stress and stress system disorders, Journal of the American Medical Association, 267 (1992) 1244–1252.

Ciccone, D.S. and Just, N., Pain expectancy and work disability in patients with acute and chronic pain: A test of the fear avoidance hypothesis, The Journal of Pain: Official Journal of the American Pain Society, 2 (2001) 181–194.

Cinciripini, P.M., Stimulus control and chronic behaviour: A study of low back and head/neck/face pain patients, Behavior Modification, 7 (1984) 243–254.

Clyde, Z. and Williams, A.C., Depression and mood. In: S.J. Linton (Ed.), New avenues for the prevention of chronic musculoskeletal pain and disability, Elsevier, Amsterdam, 2002, pp. 105–121.

Craig, A.D., A new view of pain as a homeostatic emotion, Trends in Neurosciences, 26 (2003) 303–307.

Craig, K.D., Emotions and psychobiology. In: P.D. Wall and R. Melzack (Eds.), Textbook of pain, Vol. 293–309, Churchill Livingstone, Edinburgh, 1999.

Craske, M.G., Anxiety disorders: Psychological approaches to theory and treatment, Westview Press, Boulder, CO, 1999.

Crombez, G., Baeyens, F. and Eelen, P., Sensory and temporal information about impending pain: The influence of predictability on pain, Behavior Research and Therapy, 32 (1994) 611–622.

Crombez, G., Vervaet, L., Lysens, R., Eelen, P. and Baeyens, F., Do pain expectancies cause pain in chronic low back patients? A clinical investigation, Behavior Research and Therapy, 34 (1996) 919–925.

Crombez, G., Eccleston, C., Baeyens, F. and Eelen, P., Attentional disruption is enhanced by the threat of pain, Behavior Research and Therapy, 36 (1998a) 195–204.

Crombez, G., Vervaet, L., Lysens, R., Baeyens, F. and Eelen, P., Avoidance and confrontation of painful, back straining movements, in chronic back pain patients, Behavior Modification, 22 (1998b) 62–77.

Crombez, G., Vlaeyen, J.W.S., Heuts, P.H. and Lysens, R., Pain-related fear is more disabling than pain itself: Evidence on the role of pain-related fear in chronic back pain disability, Pain, 80 (1999) 329–339.

Crombie, I.K. and Davies, J.T.P., Requirements for epidemiological studies. In: I.K. Crombie, P.R. Croft, S.J. Linton, L. LeResche and M. Von Korff (Eds.), Epidemiology of pain, IASP Press, Seattle, 1999, pp. 17–24.

Crombie, I.K., Croft, P.R., Linton, S.J., LeResche, L. and Von Korff, M., Epidemiology of pain, IASP Press, Seattle, Washington, 1999, 321 pp.

Cutler, R.B., Fishbain, D.A., Rosomoff, H.L., Abdel-Moty, E., Khalil, T.M. and Rosomoff, R.S., Does nonsurgical pain center treatment of chronic pain return patients to work? A review and meta-analysis of the literature, Spine, 19 (1994) 643–652.

Davis, D.A., Thomson, M.A., Oxman, A.D. and Haynes, R.B., Changing physician performance: A systematic review of the effect of continuing medical education strategies, Journal of the American Medical Association, 274 (1995) 700–705.

DeGood, D.E. and Shutty, M.S., Assessment of pain beliefs, coping and self-efficacy. In: D.C. Turk and R. Melzack (Eds.), Handbook of pain assessment, Guilford Press, New York, 1992, pp. 214–234.

DeGood, D.E. and Shutty, M.S., Assessment of pain beliefs and coping. In: D.C. Turk and R. Melzack (Eds.), Handbook of pain assessment, Guilford Press, New York, 1999, pp. 320–345.

Di Blasi, Z., Harkness, E. and Ernst, E., Influence of context on health outcomes: A systematic review, Lancet, 357 (2001) 757–762.

Dohrenwend, B.P., Raphael, K.G., Marbach, J.J. and Gallagher, R.M., Why is depression comorbid with chronic myofascial face pain? A family test of alternative hypotheses, Pain, 83 (1999) 183–192.

Drossman, D.A., Physical and sexual abuse and gastrointestinal illness: What is the link?, American Journal of Medicine, 97 (1994) 105–107.

Drossman, D.A., Leserman, J., Nachman, G., Zhiming, L., Gluck, H., Toomey, T.C. and Mitchell, C.M., Sexual and physical abuse in women with functional or organic gastrointestinal disorders, Annals of Internal Medicine, 113 (1990) 828–833.

Dworkin, R.H., Which individuals with acute pain are most likely to develop a chronic pain syndrome?, Pain Forum, 6 (1997) 127–136.

Eccleston, C. and Crombez, G., Pain demands attention: A cognitive-affective model of the interruptive function of pain, Psychological Bulletin, 125 (1999) 356–366.

Eccleston, C., Crombez, G., Aldrich, S. and Stannard, C., Attention and somatic awareness in chronic pain, Pain, 72 (1997) 209–215.

Eccleston, C., Crombez, G., Aldrich, S. and Stannard, C., Worry and chronic pain patients: A description and analysis of individual differences, European Journal of Pain, 5 (2001) 309–318.

Edwards, P.W., Zeichner, A., Kuczmierczyk, A.R. and Boczkowski, J., Familial pain models: The relationship between family history and current pain experience, Pain, 21 (1985) 379–384.

Ektor-Andersen, J., Örbaek, P., Ingvarsson, E. and Kullendorff, M., Prediction of vocational dysfunction due to musculoskeletal symptoms by screening for psychosocial factors at the social insurance office, 10th World Congress on Pain, San Diego, CA, 2002.

Estlander, A.M., Vanharanta, H., Moneta, G.B. and Kaivanto, K., The effects of anthropetric variables, self-efficacy beliefs, and pain and disability ratings on the isometric performance of low back pain patients, Spine, 19 (1994) 941–947.

Feuerstein, M., Callan-Harris, S., Hickey, P., Dyer, D., Armbruster, W. and Carosella, A.-M., Multidisciplinary rehabilitation of chronic work-related upper extremity disorders: Long-term effects, Journal of Occupational Medicine, 35 (1993) 396–403.

Fisher, K. and Johnston, M., Emotional distress as a mediator of the relationship between pain and disability: An experimental study, British Journal of Health Psychology, 1 (1996) 207–218.

Flor, H., A way out of the vicious circle: Learning to manage chronic pain through self-control, Berlin, 1997.

Flor, H., The functional organization of the brain in chronic pain, Progress in Brain Research, 129 (2000) 313–322.

Flor, H., Birnbaumer, N. and Turk, D.C., The psychobiology of chronic pain, Advances in Behavioral Research and Therapy, 12 (1990) 47–84.

Flor, H., Birnbaumer, N., Schugens, N.M. and Lutzenberger, W., Symptom-specific psychophysiological responses in chronic pain patients, Psychophysiology, 29 (1992a) 452–460.

Flor, H., Fydrich, T. and Turk, D.C., Efficacy of multidisciplinary pain treatment centers: A meta-analytic review, Pain, 49 (1992b) 221–230.

Fordyce, W.E., Behavioral methods for chronic pain and illness, C.V. Mosby, St. Louis, MO, 1976.

Fordyce, W.E., Brockway, J.A., Bergman, J.A. and Spengler, D., Acute back pain: A control-group comparison of behavioral vs. traditional management methods, Journal of Behavioral Medicine, 9 (1986) 127–140.

Fritz, J.M., George, S.Z. and Delitto, A., The role of fear-avoidance beliefs in acute low back pain: Relationships with current and future disability and work status, Pain, 94 (2001) 7–15.

Fry, R., Adult physical illness and childhood sexual abuse, Journal of Psychosomatic Research, 37 (1993) 89–103.

Gatchel, R.J., Psychological disorders and chronic pain: Cause and effect relationships. In: R.J. Gatchel and D.C. Turk (Eds.), Psychological approaches to pain management: A practitioner's handbook, Vol. 1, Guilford Press, New York, 1996, pp. 33–54.

Gatchel, R.J. and Turk, D.C., Psychological approaches to pain management: A practitioner's handbook, Guilford Press, New York, 1996, 519 pp.

Gatchel, R.J., Polatin, P.B. and Kinney, R.K., Predicting outcome of chronic back pain using clinical predictors of psychopathology: a prospective analysis, Health Psychology, 14 (1995) 415–420.

Geisser, M.E. and Roth, R.S., Knowledge of and agreement with chronic pain diagnosis: Relation to affective distress, pain beliefs and coping, pain intensity, and disability, Journal of Occupational Rehabilitation, 8 (1998) 73–88.

Geisser, M.E., Roth, R.S., Bachman, J.E. and Eckert, T.A., The relationship between symptoms of post-traumatic stress disorder and pain, affective disturbance and disability among patients with accident and non-accident related pain, Pain, 66 (1997) 207–214.

Goossens, M.E.J.B., Economic aspects of chronic musculoskeletal pain. In: S.J. Linton (Ed.), New avenues for the prevention of chronic musculoskeletal pain and disability, Vol. 1, Elsevier, Amsterdam, 2002, pp. 23–31.

Goossens, M.E.J.B. and Evers, S.M.A.A., Economic evaluation of back pain interventions, Journal of Occupational Rehabilitation, 7 (1997) 15–32.

Goubert, L., Crombez, G., and Peters, M. (2004). Pain-related fear and avoidance: A conditioning perspective. In G.J.G. Asmundson, J.W.S. Vlaeyen and G. Crombez (Eds.), Understanding and treating fear of pain (pp. 25-50). Oxford, England: Oxford University Press.

Gramling, S.E., Clawson, E.P. and McDonald, M.K., Perceptual and cognitive abnormality model of hypochondriasis: Amplification and physiological reactivity in women, Psychosomatic Medicine, 58 (1996) 423–431.

Greenwood, K.A., Thurston, R., Rumble, M., Waters, S.J. and Keefe, F.J., Anger and persistent pain: Current status and future directions, Pain, 103 (2003) 1–5.

Grimshaw, J.M., Changing provider behaviour: An overview of systematic reviews of interventions to promote implementation of research findings by health care professionals. In: A. Haines and A. Donald (Eds.), Getting research findings into practice, British Medical Journal, London, 2002.

Grisart, J.M. and Plaghki, L.H., Impaired selective attention in chronic pain patients, European Journal of Pain, 3 (1999) 325–333.

Guo, H.R., Tanaka, S. and Cameron, L.L., Back pain among workers in the United States: National estimates and workers at high risk, American Journal of Industrial Medicine, 28 (1995) 591–602.

Hadjistavropoulos, H.D., Owens, K.M.B., Hadjistavropoulos, T. and Asmundson, G.J.G., Hypochondriasis and health anxiety among pain patients. In: G.J.G. Asmundson, S. Taylor and B.J. Cox (Eds.), Health anxiety: Clinical and research perspectives on hypochondriasis and related conditions, John Wiley, New York, 2001, pp. 298–323.

Hahn, R.A., The nocebo phenomenon: Scope and foundations. In: A. Harrington (Ed.), The placebo effect: An interdisciplinary exploration, Harvard University Press, Cambridge, MA, 1997, pp. 56–76.

Hannay, D.R., The symptom iceberg: A study of community health, Routledge & Kegan Paul, London, 1979.

Headrick, L.A., Speroff, T., Pelecanos, H.I. and Cebul, R.D., Efforts to improve compliance with the National Cholesterol Education Program guidelines: Results of a randomized controlled trial, Archives of Internal Medicine, 152 (1992) 2490–2496.

Helme, R.D. and Gibson, S.J., Pain in older people. In: I.K. Crombie, P.R. Croft, S.J. Linton, L. LeResche and M. Von Korff (Eds.), Epidemiology of pain, IASP Press, Seattle, 1999, pp. 103–112.

Hoogendoorn, W.E., van Poppel, M.N.M., Bongers, P.M., Koes, B.W. and Bouter, L.M., Systematic review of psychosocial factors at work and in the personal situation as risk factors for back pain, Spine, 25 (2000) 2114–2125.

Hurley, D., Dusoir, T., McDonough, S., Moore, A., Linton, S.J. and Baxter, G., Biopsychosocial screening questionnaire for patients with low back pain: Preliminary report of utility in physiotherapy practice in Northern Ireland, Clinical Journal of Pain, 16 (2000) 214–228.

Hurley, D., Dusoir, T., McDonough, S., Moore, A. and Baxter, G., How effective is the Acute Low Back Pain Screening Questionnaire for predicting 1-year follow-up in patients with low back pain?, Clinical Journal of Pain, 17 (2001) 256–263.

Indahl, A., Velund, L. and Reikeraas, O., Good prognosis for low back pain when left untampered: A randomized clinical trial, Spine, 20 (1995) 473–477.

Jensen, I.B., Linton, S.J., Overmeer, T. and Bergström, G., Ryggboken: en bok till dig som har ont i ryggen [Back pain: What everyone should know about it], AFA, Stockholm, 2004.

Jensen, M.P., Enhancing motivation to change in pain treatment. In: D.C. Turk and R.J. Gatchel (Eds.), Psychological approaches to pain management: A practitioner's handbook, Guilford Press, New York, 2002, pp. 71–93.

Jensen, M.P., Turner, J.A., Romano, J.M. and Lawler, B.K., Relationship of pain-specific beliefs to chronic pain adjustment, Pain, 57 (1994) 301–309.

Johansson, E. and Lindberg, P., Low back pain patients in primary care: Subgroups based on the Multidimensional Pain Inventory, International Journal of Behavioral Medicine, 7 (2000) 340–352.

Jonsson, E. and Nachemson, A., Ont i ryggen, ont i nacken: en evidensbaserad kunskapssammanställning, Vol. I & II, The Swedish Council on Technology Assessment in Health Care, Stockholm, 2000.

Karasek, R. and Theorell, T., Healthy work: Stress, productivity, and the reconstruction of working life, Basic Books, New York, 1990, 381 pp.

Keefe, F.J. and Williams, D.A., Pain behavior assessment. In: D.C. Turk and R. Melzack (Eds.), Handbook of pain assessment, Guilford Press, New York, 1992, pp. 275–294.

Keefe, F.J., Caldwell, D.S. and Baucom, D., Spouse-assisted coping skills training in the management of osteoarthritis knee pain, Arthritis Care Research, 9 (1996) 279–291.

Keller, V.F. and Carroll, J.G., A new model for physician–patient communication, Patient Education and Counseling, 23 (1994) 134–140.

Kendall, N.A.S., Linton, S.J. and Main, C.J., Guide to assessing psychosocial yellow flags in acute low back pain: Risk factors for long-term disability and work loss., Accident Rehabilitation & Compensation Insurance Corporation of New Zealand and the National Health Committee, Wellington, New Zealand, 1997.

Kendall, N.A.S., Linton, S.J. and Main, C., Psychosocial yellow flags for acute low back pain: "Yellow flags" as an analogue to "red flags", European Journal of Pain, 2 (1998) 87–89.

Keogh, E., Ellery, D., Hunt, C. and Hannent, I., Selective attentional bias for pain-related stimuli amongst pain fearful individuals, Pain, 91 (2001) 91–100.

Kerns, R.D. and Payne, A., Treating families of chronic pain patients. In: R.J. Gatchel and D.C. Turk (Eds.), Psychological approaches to pain management: A practitioner's handbook, Guilford Press, New York, 1996, pp. 283–304.

Kerns, R.D., Haythornthwaite, J., Southwick, S. and Giller, E.L., The role of marital interaction in chronic pain and depressive symptom severity, Journal of Psychosomatic Research, 34 (1990) 401–408.

Kerns, R.D., Otis, J.D. and Wise, E.A., Treating families of chronic pain patients: Application of a cognitive-behavioral transactional model. In: D.C. Turk and R.J. Gatchel (Eds.), Psychological approaches to pain management: A practitioner's handbook, Guilford Press, New York, 2002, pp. 256–275.

Kettell, J., Jones, R. and Lydeard, S., Reasons for consultation in irritable bowel syndrome: Symptoms and patient characteristics, British Journal of General Practice, 42 (1992) 459–461.

Klenerman, L., Slade, P.D., Stanley, I.M., Pennie, B., Reilly, J.P., Atchison, L.E., Troup, J.D. and Rose, M.J., The prediction of chronicity in patients with an acute attack of low back pain in a general practice setting, Spine, 20 (1995) 478–484.

Koes, B.W., Bouter, L.M. and van der Heijden, G.J.M.G., Methodological quality of randomized clinical trials on treatment efficacy in low back pain, Spine, 20 (1995) 228–235.

Koes, B.W., van Tulder, M.W., Ostelo, R., Burton, A.K. and Waddell, G., Clinical guidelines for the management of low back pain in primary care, Spine, 26 (2001) 2504–2514.

Koetting O'Byrne, K., Peterson, L. and Saldana, L., Survey of pediatric hospitals' preparation programs: Evidence of the impact of health psychology research, Health Psychology, 16 (1997) 147–154.

Kores, R.C., Murphy, W.E., Rosenthal, T.L., Elias, D.B. and North, W.C., Predicting outcome of chronic pain treatment via a modified self-efficacy scale, Behavior Research and Therapy, 28 (1990) 165–169.

Landrieu, P., Said, G. and Allaire, C., Dominantly transmitted congenital indifference to pain, Annals of Neurology, 27 (1990) 574–578.

Lazarus, R.S. and Folkman, S., Stress, appraisal, and coping, Springer, New York, 1984.

Leserman, J., Li, Z., Drossman, D. and Hu, Y., Selected symptoms associated with sexual and physical abuse history among female patients with gastrointestinal disorders: The impact on subsequent health care visits, Psychological Medicine, 28 (1998) 417–425.

Leventhal, E.A., Hansell, S., Diefenbach, M., Leventhal, H. and Glass, D.C., Negative affect and self-report of physical symptoms: Two longitudinal studies of older adults, Health Psychology, 15 (1996) 193–199.

Levine, J.D. and Gordon, N.C., Influence of the method of drug administration on analgesic response, Nature, 312 (1984) 755–756.

Levine, J.D., Gordon, N.C., Smith, R. and Fields, H.L., Analgesic responses to morphine and placebo in individuals with postoperative pain, Pain, 10 (1981) 379–389.

Levine, J.D., Gordon, N.C., Smith, R. and Fields, H.L., Post-operative pain: Effect of extent of injury and attention, Brain Research, 234 (1982) 500–504.

Ley, P., Professional non-compliance: A neglected problem, British Journal of Clinical Psychology, 20 (1981) 151–154.

Lindström, I., Öhlund, C., Eek, C., Wallin, L., Peterson, L.E., Fordyce, W.E. and Nachemson, A.L., The effect of graded activity on patients with subacute low back pain: A randomized prospective clinical study with an operant-conditioning behavioral approach, Physical Therapy, 72 (1992) 279–293.

Linton, S.J., Applied relaxation as a method of coping with chronic pain: A therapist's guide, Scandinavian Journal of Behavior Therapy, 11 (1983) 161–174.

Linton, S.J., The manager's role in employees' successful return to work following back injury, Work and Stress, 5 (1991) 189–195.

Linton, S.J., Smärtans psykologi, Folksam Förlag, Stockholm, 1992.

Linton, S.J., The role of psychological factors in back pain and its remediation, Pain Reviews, 1 (1994) 231–243.

Linton, S.J., Early interventions for the secondary prevention of chronic musculoskeletal pain. In: J.N. Campbell (Ed.), Pain 1996: An updated review, IASP Press, Seattle, 1996.

Linton, S.J., Cognitive-behavioral therapy in the prevention of pain: The therapist's manual, Department of Occupational and Environmental Medicine, Örebro, Sweden, 1997a.

Linton, S.J., Overlooked and underrated? The role of acute pain intensity in the development of chronic back pain problems, Pain Forum, 6 (1997b) 145–147.

Linton, S.J., A population-based study of the relationship between sexual abuse and back pain: Establishing a link, Pain, 73 (1997c) 47–53.

Linton, S.J., Prevention of disability due to chronic musculoskeletal pain. In: R. Melzack and P.D. Wall (Eds.), The textbook of pain, Churchill Livingstone, London, 1999a, pp. 1535–1548.

Linton, S.J., Prevention with special reference to chronic musculoskeletal disorders. In: R.J. Gatchel and D.C. Turk (Eds.), Psychosocial factors in pain, Vol. 1, Guilford Press, New York, 1999b, pp. 374–389.

Linton, S.J., Cognitive-behavioral therapy in the early treatment and prevention of chronic pain: A therapist's manual for groups, Author, Örebro, 2000a, 40 pp.

Linton, S.J., Psychologic risk factors for neck and back pain. In: A. Nachemsom and E. Jonsson (Eds.), Neck and back pain: The scientific evidence of causes, diagnosis, and treatment, Lippincott Williams & Wilkins, Philadelphia, 2000b, pp. 57–78.

Linton, S.J., A review of psychological risk factors in back and neck pain, Spine, 25 (2000c) 1148–1156.

Linton, S.J., Utility of cognitive-behavioral psychological treatments. In: A. Nachemson and E. Jonsson (Eds.), Neck and back pain: The scientific evidence of causes, diagnosis, and treatment, Lippincott Williams & Wilkins, Philadelphia, 2000d, pp. 361–381.

Linton, S.J., Occupational psychological factors increase the risk for back pain: A systematic review, Journal of Occupational Rehabilitation, 11 (2001) 53–66.

Linton, S.J., A cognitive-behavioral approach to the prevention of chronic back pain. In: R.J. Gatchel and D.C. Turk (Eds.), Psychological approaches to pain management, Guilford Press, New York, 2002a, pp. 317–333.

Linton, S.J., A prospective study of the effects of self-reported physical and sexual abuse on the development of musculoskeletal pain, Pain, 96 (2002b) 347–351.

Linton, S.J., Why does chronic pain develop? A behavioral approach. In: S.J. Linton (Ed.), New avenues for the prevention of chronic musculoskeletal pain and disability, Elsevier, Amsterdam, 2002c, pp. 67–82.

Linton, S.J. and Andersson, T., Can chronic disability be prevented? A randomized trial of a cognitive-behavior intervention and two forms of information for patients with spinal pain, Spine, 25 (2000) 2825–2831.

Linton, S.J. and Boersma, K., Overcoming our fears in clinical practice: Barriers to the clinical implementation of yellow flags, Early Rehabilitation, Hoensbroek, The Netherlands, 2002.

Linton, S.J. and Boersma, K., Early identification of patients at risk of developing a persistent back problem: The predictive validity of the Örebro Musculoskeletal Pain Questionnaire, Clinical Journal of Pain (2003).

Linton, S.J. and Boersma, K., Something is broken: Patient models of back pain, Scandinavian Association for the Study of Pain, Reykjavik, Iceland, 2004.

Linton, S.J. and Boersma, K., The early identification of patients risking the development of chronic pain: The role of fear-avoidance in screening. In: G.J. Asmundson, J.W.S. Vlaeyen and G. Crombez (Eds.), Understanding and treating fear of pain, Oxford University Press, Oxford, 2004, pp. 213–235.

Linton, S.J. and Bradley, L.A., An 18-month follow-up of a secondary prevention program for back pain: Help and hindrance factors related to outcome maintenance, Clinical Journal of Pain, 8 (1992) 227–236.

Linton, S.J. and Bradley, L.A., Strategies for the prevention of chronic pain. In: R.J. Gatchel and D.C. Turk (Eds.), Psychological approaches to pain management: a practitioner's handbook, Guilford Press, New York, 1996, pp. 438–457.

Linton, S.J. and Buer, N., Working despite pain: factors associated with work attendance versus dysfunction, International Journal of Behavioral Medicine, 2 (1995) 252–262.

Linton, S.J. and Götestam, K.G., Controlling pain reports through operant conditioning: A laboratory demonstration, Perceptual and Motor Skills, 60 (1985a) 427–437.

Linton, S.J. and Götestam, K.G., Relations between pain, anxiety, mood and muscle tension in chronic pain patients, Psychotherapy and Psychosomatics, 43 (1985b) 90–95.

Linton, S.J. and Halldén, K., Risk factors and the natural course of acute and recurrent musculoskeletal pain: developing a screening instrument. In: T.S. Jensen, J.A. Turner and Z. Wiesenfeld-Hallin (Eds.), Proceedings of the 8th World Congress on Pain: Progress in pain research and management, Vol. 8, IASP Press, Seattle, 1997, pp. 527–536.

Linton, S.J. and Halldén, K., Can we screen for problematic back pain? A screening questionnaire for predicting outcome in acute and subacute back pain, Clinical Journal of Pain, 14 (1998) 209–215.

Linton, S.J. and Nordin, E. A five-year follow-up of the outcome and economic results of a randomized controlled trial of early cognitive-behavioral intervention for back pain. Submitted for publication.

Linton, S.J. and Ryberg, M., Do epidemiological results replicate? The prevalence and health-economic consequences of back and neck pain in the general public, European Journal of Pain, 4 (2000) 1–8.

Linton, S.J. and Ryberg, M., A cognitive-behavioral group intervention as prevention for persistent neck and back pain in a non-patient population: A randomized controlled trial, Pain, 90 (2001) 83–90.

Linton, S.J. and Skevington, S.M., Psychological factors and the epidemiology of pain. In: I. Crombie, P.R. Croft, S.J. Linton, L. LeResche and M. Von Korff (Eds.), The epidemiology of pain, IASP Press, Seattle, 1999, pp. 25–42.

Linton, S.J. and Warg, L.E., Attributions (beliefs) and job satisfaction associated with back pain in an industrial setting, Perceptual and Motor Skills, 76 (1993) 51–62.

Linton, S.J., Bradley, L.A., Jensen, I., Spangfort, E. and Sundell, L., The secondary prevention of low back pain: A controlled study with follow-up, Pain, 36 (1989) 197–207.

Linton, S.J., Hellsing, A.L. and Bergström, G., Exercise for workers with musculoskeletal pain: Does enhancing compliance decrease pain?, Journal of Occupational Rehabilitation, 6 (1996a) 177–190.

Linton, S.J., Lardén, M. and Gillow, Å.M., Sexual abuse and chronic musculoskeletal pain: Prevalence and psychological factors, Clinical Journal of Pain, 12 (1996b) 215–221.

Linton, S.J., Hellsing, A.L. and Halldén, K., A population based study of spinal pain among 35 to 45 year olds: Prevalence, sick leave, and health-care utilization, Spine, 23 (1998) 1457–1463.

Linton, S.J., Buer, N., Vlaeyen, J. and Hellsing, A.L., Are fear-avoidance beliefs related to a new episode of back pain? A prospective study, Psychology and Health, 14 (2000) 1051–1059.

Linton, S.J., Overmeer, T., Janson, M., Vlaeyen, J.W.S. and de Jong, J.R., Graded in-vivo exposure treatment for fear-avoidant pain patients with function disability: A case study, Cognitive Behavior Therapy, 31 (2002a) 49–58.

Linton, S.J., Vlaeyen, J.W.S. and Ostelo, R., The back pain beliefs of general practitioners and physical therapists: Are professionals fear-avoidant?, Journal of Occupational Rehabilitation, 12 (2002b) 223–232.

Linton, S.J., Boersma, K., Jansson, M., Svärd, L. and Botvalde, M., The effects of cognitive-behavioral and physical therapy preventive interventions on pain related sick leave: A randomized controlled trial, Clinical Journal of Pain (in press).

Lloyd, M.H., Gauld, S. and Soutar, C.A., Epidemiologic study of back pain in miners and office workers, Spine, 11 (1986) 136–140.

Loisel, P., Abenhaim, L., Durand, P., Esdaile, J.M., Suissa, S., Gosselin, L., Simard, R., Turcotte, J. and Lemaire, J., A population based randomized clinical trial on back pain management, Spine, 22 (1997) 2911–2918.

Lucock, M.P. and Morley, S., The health anxiety questionnaire, British Journal of Health Psychology, 1 (1996) 137–150.

Lundberg, U. and Johansson, G., Stress and health risks in repetitive work and supervisory monitoring work. In: R. Backs and W. Boucsein (Eds.), Engineering psychophysiology: Issues and application, Lawrence Erlbaum, Hillsdale, NJ, 2000, pp. 339–359.

Lundberg, U. and Melin, B., Stress in the development of musculoskeletal pain. In: S.J. Linton (Ed.), New avenues for the prevention of chronic musculoskeletal pain and disability, Elsevier, Amsterdam, 2002, pp. 165–179.

Lyons, A.C., Fanshawe, C. and Lip, G.Y.H., Knowledge, communication and expectancies of cardiac catheterization: The patient's perspective, Psychology, Health and Medicine, 7 (2002) 461–467.

Main, C.J. and Spanswick, C.C., Pain management: An interdisciplinary approach, Churchill Livingstone, Edinburgh, 2000, 438 pp.

Manning, M. and Wright, T.L., Self-efficacy expectancies, outcome expectancies and the persistence of pain control in childbirth, Journal of Personality and Social Psychology, 45 (1983) 421–431.

Mannion, A.F., Dolan, P. and Adams, M.A., Psychological questionnaires: do abnormal scores precede or follow first time low back pain?, Spine, 21 (1996) 2603–2611.

Mannion, A.F., Junge, A., Taimela, S., Müntener, M., Lorenzo, K. and Dvorak, J., Active therapy for chronic low back pain. Part 3. Factors influencing self-rated disability and its change following therapy, Spine, 26 (2001) 920–929.

Marhold, C., Linton, S.J. and Melin, L., Cognitive behavioral return-to-work program: effects on pain patients with a history of long-term versus short-term sick leave, Pain, 91 (2001) 155–163.

Marteau, T.M., Sowden, A.J. and Armstrong, D., Implementing research findings into practice: Beyond the information deficit model. In: A. Haines and A. Donald (Eds.), Getting research findings into practice, British Medical Journal, London, 2002, pp. 68–76.

Martin, L.L., Ward, D.W., Achee, J.W. and Wyer, R.S., Mood as input: People have to interpret the motivational implications of their moods, Journal of Personality and Social Psychology, 64 (1993) 317–326.

Martin, R., Lemos, K. and Leventhal, H., The psychology of physical symptoms and illness behavior. In: G.J.G. Asmundson, S. Taylor and B.J. Cox (Eds.), Health anxiety: Clinical and research perspectives on hypochondriasis and related conditions, John Wiley, New York, 2001, pp. 22–45.

Marvel, M.K., Epstein, R.M., Flowers, K. and Beckman, H.B., Soliciting the patient's agenda: Have we improved?, Journal of the American Medical Association, 281 (1999) 283–287.

McBeth, J. and Macfarlane, G.J., The prevalence of regional and widespread musculoskeletal pain symptoms. In: S.J. Linton (Ed.), New avenues for the prevention of chronic musculoskeletal pain and disability, Elsevier, Amsterdam, 2002, pp. 7–22.

McCracken, L.M., Zayfert, C. and Gross, R.T., The Pain Anxiety Symptoms Scale: Development and validation of a scale to measure fear of pain., Pain, 50 (1992) 63–67.

McGrath, P.J., There is more to pain measurement in children than "ouch", Canadian Psychology, 37 (1996) 63–75.

Meichenbaum, D. and Turk, D.C., Facilitating treatment adherence: A practitioner's guidebook, Plenum Press, New York, 1987, 310 pp.

Melin, B. and Lundberg, U., A biopsychosocial approach to work-stress and musculoskeletal disorders, Journal of Psychophysiology, 11 (1997) 238–247.

Melzack, R., Pain measurement and assessment, Raven Press, New York, 1983, 293 pp.

Melzack, R., Pain and stress: A new perspective. In: R.J. Gatchel and D.C. Turk (Eds.), Psychosocial factors in pain: Critical perspectives, Guilford Press, New York, 1999, pp. 89–106.

Melzack, R. and Wall, P.D., Pain mechanisms: A new theory, Science, 150 (1965) 971–979.

Miron, D., Duncan, G.H. and Bushnell, M.C., Effects of attention on the intensity and unpleasantness of thermal pain, Pain, 39 (1989).

Moberg, V., A time on earth, Warner Books, New York, 1984.

Moerman, D.E., Meaning, medicine and the placebo effect, Cambridge University Press, Cambridge, 2002.

Moore, J.E., Von Korff, M., Cherkin, D., Saunders, K. and Lorig, K., A randomized trial of a cognitive-behavioral program for enhancing back pain self-care in a primary care setting, Pain, 88 (2000) 145–153.

Moore, R. and Brödsgaard, I., Cross-cultural investigations of pain. In: I.K. Crombie, P.R. Croft, S.J. Linton and M. Von Korff (Eds.), Epidemiology of pain, IASP Press, Seattle, 1999, pp. 53–80.

Morley, S., Eccleston, C. and Williams, A., Systematic review and meta-analysis of randomised controlled trials of cognitive behaviour therapy and behaviour therapy for chronic pain in adults, excluding headache, Pain, 80 (1999) 1–13.

Morris, D.B., Sociocultural and religious meanings of pain. In: R.J. Gatchel and D.C. Turk (Eds.), Psychosocial factors in pain: Critical perspectives, Guilford Press, New York, 1999, pp. 118–131.

Munro, H.S., Suggestive therapeutics, applied hypnotism, psychic science: A manual of practical psychotherapy, designed for the practitioner of medicine, surgery, and dentistry, C.V. Mosby, St. Louis, MO, 1917, 481 pp.

Nachemson, A.L., Newest knowledge of low back pain, Clinical Orthopaedics, 279 (1992) 8–20.

Nachemson, A. and Jonsson, E., Neck and back pain: The scientific evidence of causes, diagnosis, and treatment, Lippincott Williams & Wilkins, Philadelphia, 2000, 495 pp.

Nagasako, E.M., Oaklander, A.L. and Dworkin, R.H., Congenital insensitivity to pain: An update, Pain, 101 (2003) 213–219.

National Research Council, Musculoskeletal disorders and the workplace, National Academy Press, Washington, DC, 2001.

Nettelbladt, childbirth pain, (1976).

Nicholas, M.K., Reducing disability in injured workers: The importance of collaborative management. In: S.J. Linton (Ed.), New avenues for the prevention of chronic musculoskeletal pain and disability, Elsevier, Amsterdam, 2002, pp. 33–46.

Nordlund, A.I. and Waddell, G., Cost of back pain in some OECD countries. In: A. Nachemson and E. Jonsson (Eds.), Neck and back pain: The scientific evidence of causes, diagnosis, and treatment, Vol. 1, Lippincott Williams & Wilkins, Philadelphia, 2000, pp. 421–425.

Ogden, J., Health psychology: A textbook, Open University Press, Buckingham, UK, 2000, 396 pp.

Ohrback, R. and McCall, W.D., The stress–hyperactivity–pain theory of myogenic pain, Pain Forum, 118 (1996) 238–247.

Ottosson, J.O., Patient–läkarrelationen: Läkekonst på vetenskaplig grund [The patient–doctor relationship: The art of healing from a scientific perspective]. In: Swedish Council on Technology Assessment in Health Care (Ed.), Natur och Kultur, Stockholm, 1999, pp. 375.

Overmeer, T., Linton, S.J. and Boersma, K., Do physical therapists recognize established risk factors? Swedish physical therapists' evaluation in comparison to guidelines, Physiotherapy, 90 (2004) 35–41.

Overmeer, T., Linton, S.J., Holmquist, L., Eriksson, M. and Engfeldt, P., Do evidence-based guidelines have an impact in primary care? A cross-sectional study of Swedish physicians and physiotherapists, Spine, 30(1) (2005), 146–151.

Papageorgiou, A.C., Croft, P.R., Thomas, E., Ferry, S., Jayson, M.I.V. and Silman, A.J., Influence of previous pain experience on the episode incidence of low back pain: Results from the South Manchester Back Pain Study, Pain, 66 (1996) 181–185.

Pennebaker, J.W., The psychology of physical symptoms, Springer, New York, 1982.

Pennebaker, J.W., Opening up: The healing power of expressing emotions, Guilford Press, New York, 1990.

Philips, H.C. and Grant, L., The evolution of chronic back pain problems: A longitudinal study, Behavior Research and Therapy, 29 (1991) 435–441.

Piasecki, M., Clinical communication handbook, Blackwell Publishing Co., Malden, MA, 2003, 107 pp.

Pincus, T. and Morely, S.J., Cognitive processing bias in chronic pain: A review and integration, Psychological Bulletin, 127 (2001) 599–617.

Pincus, T. and Morely, S.J., Cognitive appraisal. In: S.J. Linton (Ed.), New avenues for the prevention of chronic musculoskeletal pain and disability, Elsevier, Amsterdam, 2002, pp. 123–141.

Pincus, T., Burton, A.K., Vogel, S. and Field, A.P., A systematic review of psychological factors as predictors of chronicity/disability in prospective cohorts of low back pain, Spine, 27 (2002) E109–120.

Pollo, A., Amanzio, M., Arslanian, A., Casadio, C., Maggi, G., and Benedetti, F. (2001). Response expectancies in placebo analgesia and their clinical relevance. Pain, 93(1), 77–84.

Prochaska, J.O. and DiClemente, C.C., Transtheoretical therapy: Toward a more integrative model of change, Psychotherapy: Theory, Research and Practice, 19 (1982) 276–288.

Rachlin, H., Behavior and learning, W.H. Freeman, San Francisco, 1976, 613 pp.

Rachman, S., Anxiety, Psychology Press, Hove, UK, 1998, 179 pp.

Reid, S., Haugh, L.D., Hazard, R.G. and Tripathi, M., Occupational low back pain: Recovery curves and factors associated with disability, Journal of Occupational Rehabilitation, 7 (1997) 1–14.

Robinson, M.E. and Riley, J.L., The role of emotions in pain. In: R.J. Gatchel and D.C. Turk (Eds.), Psychosocial factors in pain: Critical perspectives, Guilford Press, New York, 1999, pp. 74–88.

Romano, J.M. and Turner, J.A., Chronic pain and depression: Does the evidence support a relationship, Psychological Bulletin, 97 (1985) 18–34.

Romano, J.M., Turner, J.A. and Jensen, M., The family environment in chronic pain patients: Comparison to controls and relationships to patient functioning, Journal of Clinical Psychology in Medical Settings, 4 (1997) 383–395.

Rosenstiel, A.K. and Keefe, F.J., The use of coping strategies in chronic low back pain patients: Relationships to patient characteristics and current adjustment, Pain, 17 (1983) 33–44.

Rossignol, H., Suissa, S. and Abenhaim, L., The evolution of compensated occupational spinal injuries, Spine, 17 (1992) 1043–1047.

Sackett, D.L., Richardson, W.S., Rosenberg, W. and Haynes, R.B., Evidence-based medicine: How to practice and teach EBM, Churchill Livingstone, New York, 1997.

Salkovskis, P.M. and Warwick, H.M.C., Making sense of hypochondriasis: A cognitive model of health anxiety. In: G.J.G. Asmundson, S. Taylor and B.J. Cox (Eds.), Health anxiety: Clinical and research perspectives on hypochondriasis and related conditions, John Wiley, New York, 2001, pp. 46–64.

Sanders, S.H., Operant conditioning with chronic pain: Back to basics. In: D.C. Turk and R.J. Gatchel (Eds.), Psychological approaches to pain management: A practitioner's handbook, Guilford Press, New York, 2002, pp. 128–137.

Scambler, G. and Scambler, A., The illness iceberg and aspects of consulting behavior. In: R. Fitzpatrick and J. Hinton (Eds.), The experience of illness, Tavistock, London, 1985, pp. 32–50.

Scarinci, I.C., McDonald-Haile, J., Bradley, L.A. and Richter, J.E., Altered pain perception and psychosocial features among women with gastrointestinal disorders and history of abuse: A preliminary model, American Journal of Medicine, 97 (1994) 108–118.

Schwartzer, R. and Fuchs, R., Self-efficacy and health behaviors: Theoretical approaches and a new model. In: M. Conner and P. Norman (Eds.), Predicting health behavior: Research and practice with social cognition models, Open University Press, Buckingham, UK, 1996, pp. 163–196.

Seyle, H., Stress, Acta Medical Publishers, Montreal, 1950.

Shaw, W.S., Feuerstein, M. and Huang, G.D., Secondary prevention and the workplace. In: S.J. Linton (Ed.), New avenues for the prevention of chronic musculoskeletal pain and disability, Elsevier, Amsterdam, 2002, pp. 215–235.

Sheridan, D.P. and Winogrond, I.R., The preventive approach to patient care, Elsevier, Amsterdam, 1987, 442 pp.

Shifren, K., Park, D.C., Bennett, J.M. and Morrell, R.W., Do cognitive processes predict mental health in individuals with rheumatoid arthritis?, Journal of Behavioral Medicine, 22 (1999) 529–547.

Sibley, J.C., Sackett, D.L., Neufeld, V., Gerrard, B., Rudnick, K.V. and Fraser, W., A randomized trial of continuing medical education, New England Journal of Medicine, 306 (1982) 511–515.

Sieben, J.M., Vlaeyen, J.W.S., Tuerlinckx, S. and Portegijs, P.J.M., Pain-related fear in acute low back pain: The first two weeks of a new episode, European Journal of Pain, 6 (2002) 229–237.

Siegrist, J., Adverse health effects of high-effort/low-reward conditions, Journal of Occupational Health Psychology, 1 (1996) 27–41.

Skevington, S.M., Psychology of pain, John Wiley, London, 1995.

Smith, T., Concepts and methods in the study of anger, hostility, and health. In: A. Siegmen and T. Smith (Eds.), Anger, hostility, and the heart, Lawrence Erlbaum, Hillsdale, NJ, 1994.

Snider, B.S., Asmundson, G.J. and Wiese, K.C., Automatic and strategic processing of threat cues in patients with chronic pain: A modified Stroop evaluation, Clinical Journal of Pain, 16 (2000) 144–154.

Stevens, M.J., Heise, R.A. and Pfost, K.S., Consumption of attention versus affect elicited by cognitions in modifying acute pain, Psychological Reports, 64 (1989) 284–286.

Stewart, M.S., Effective physician–patient communication and health outcomes: A review, Canadian Medical Association Journal, 152 (1995) 1423–1433.

Sullivan, M.J.L. and Neish, N., The effects of disclosure on pain during dental hygiene treatment: The moderating role of catastrophizing, Pain, 79 (1999) 155–163.

Sullivan, M.J.L. and Stanish, W.D., Psychologically based occupational rehabilitation: The Pain-Disability Prevention program, Clinical Journal of Pain, 19 (2003) 97–104.

Sullivan, M.J.L., Bishop, S.R. and Pivik, J., The Pain Catastrophizing Scale: Development and validation, Psychological Assessment, 7 (1995) 524–532.

Sullivan, M.J.L., Rouse, D., Bishop, S. and Johnston, S., Thought suppression, catastrophizing, and pain, Cognitive Therapy and Research, 21 (1997) 555–568.

Sullivan, M.J.L., Haythornthwaite, J.A., Keefe, F.J., Martin, M., Bradley, L.A. and Lefebvre, J.C., Theoretical perspectives on the relation between catastrophizing and pain, Clinical Journal of Pain, 17 (2001) 52–64.

Sullivan, M.J.L., Rodgers, W.M., Wilson, P.M., Bell, G.J., Murray, T.C. and Fraser, S.N., An experimental investigation of the relation between catastrophizing and activity intolerance, Pain, 100 (2002) 47–53.

Symonds, T.L., Burton, A.K., Tillotson, K.M. and Main, C.J., Absence resulting from low back trouble can be reduced by psychosocial intervention at the work place, Spine, 20 (1995) 2738–2745.

Symonds, T.L., Burton, A.K., L.M., T. and Main, C.J., Do attitudes and beliefs influence work loss due to low back pain?, Occupational Medicine, 48 (1996) 3–10.

Szpalski, M., Nordin, M., Skovron, M.L., Melot, C. and Cukier, D., Health care utilization for low back pain in Belgium: Influence of sociocultural factors and health beliefs, Spine, 20 (1995) 431–442.

Teasell, R.W. and Bombardier, C., Employment-related factors in chronic pain, Chronic Pain Initiative: Chronic Pain Expert Advisory Panel Report, Ontario Workplace Safety Insurance Board, Toronto, 2000.

Thomas, K.B., General practice consultations: Is there any point in being positive?, British Medical Journal, 294 (1987) 1200–1202.

Turk, D.C., Biopsychosocial perspective on chronic pain. In: R.J. Gatchel and D.C. Turk (Eds.), Psychological approaches to pain management: A practitioner's handbook, Vol. 1, Guilford Press, New York, 1996a, pp. 3–32.

Turk, D.C., Efficacy of multidisciplinary pain centers in the treatment of chronic pain. In: M.J.M. Cohen and J.N. Campbell (Eds.), Pain treatment centers at a crossroads: A practical and conceptual reappraisal, Vol. 7, IASP Press, Seattle, 1996b, pp. 257–273.

Turk, D.C., The role of demographic and psychosocial factors in transition from acute to chronic pain. In: T.S. Jensen,

J.A. Turner and Z. Wiesenfeld-Hallin (Eds.), Proceedings of the 8th World Congress on Pain, Progress in pain research and management, Vol. 8, IASP Press, Seattle, 1997, pp. 185–213.

Turk, D.C. and Flor, H., Chronic pain: A biobehavioral perspective. In: R.J. Gatchel and D.C. Turk (Eds.), Psychosocial factors in pain: Critical perspectives, Vol. 1, Guilford Press, New York, 1999, pp. 18–34.

Turk, D.C. and Rudy, T.E., Neglected topics in the treatment of chronic pain patients: Relapse, noncompliance, and adherence enhancement, Pain, 44 (1991) 5–28.

Turkat, I.D., An investigation of parental modeling in the etiology of illness behavior, Behavior Research and Therapy, 20 (1982) 547–552.

Turner, J., LeResche, L., von Korff, M. and Ehrlich, K., Primary care back pain patient characteristics, visit content, and short-term outcomes, Spine, 23 (1998) 463–469.

van den Hoogen, H.J.M., Koes, B.W., Devillé, W., van Eijk, J.T.M. and Bouter, L.M., The prognosis of low back pain in general practice, Spine, 22 (1997) 1515–1521.

van den Hoogen, H.J.M., Koes, B.W., van Eijk, T.M., Bouter, L.M. and Devillé, W., On the course of low back pain in general practice: A one year follow-up study, Annals of Rheumatic Diseases, 57 (1998) 13–19.

van Houdenhove, G., Neerinckx, W., Onghena, P., Lysens, R. and Vertommen, H., Premorbid "overactive" lifestyle in chronic fatigue syndrome and fibromyalgia: An etiological factor or proof of good citizenship?, Journal of Psychosomatic Research, 51 (2001) 571–576.

van Tulder, M.W., Disseminating and implementing the results of back pain research in primary care, Spine, 27 (2002) E121–E127.

van Tulder, M.W., Koes, B.W. and Bouter, L.M., A cost-of-illness study of back pain in The Netherlands, Pain, 62 (1995) 233–240.

van Tulder, M.W., Ostelo, R., Vlaeyen, J.W.S., Linton, S.J., Morely, S.J. and Assendelft, W.J.J., Behavioral treatment for chronic low back pain: A systematic review within the framework of the Cochrane Back Review Group, Spine, 25 (2000) 2688–2699.

Villemure, C. and Bushnell, M.C., Cognitive modulation of pain: How do attention and emotion influence pain processing?, Pain, 95 (2002) 195–199.

Vlaeyen, J.W.S. and Linton, S.J., Fear-avoidance and its consequences in chronic musculoskeletal pain: A state of the art, Pain, 85 (2000) 317–332.

Vlaeyen, J.W.S. and Linton, S.J., Pain-related fear and its consequences in chronic musculoskeletal pain. In: S.J. Linton (Ed.), New avenues for the prevention of chronic musculoskeletal pain and disability, Elsevier, Amsterdam, 2002, pp. 81–103.

Vlaeyen, J.W.S. and Morely, S.J. (2004). Active despite pain: The putative role of stop-rules and current mood. Pain, 110(3), 512–516.

Vlaeyen, J.W.S., Kole-Snijders, A.M.J., Boeren, R.G.B. and van Eek, H., Fear of movement/(re)injury in chronic low back pain and its relation to behavioral performance, Pain, 62 (1995a) 363–372.

Vlaeyen, J.W.S., Kole-Snijders, A.M.J., Rotteveel, A., Ruesink, R. and Heuts, P.H.T.G., The role of fear of movement/(re)injury in pain disability, Journal of Occupational Rehabilitation, 5 (1995b) 235–252.

Vlaeyen, J.W.S., de Jong, J., Geilen, M., Heuts, P.H.T.G. and van Breukelen, G., Graded exposure in vivo in the treatment of pain-related fear: A replicated single-case experimental design in four patients with chronic low back pain, Behavior Research and Therapy, 39 (2001) 151–166.

Von Korff, M., Perspectives on management of back pain in primary care. In: G.F. Gebhart, D.L. Hammond and T.S. Jensen (Eds.), Proceedings of the 7th World Congress on Pain: Progress in pain research and management, Vol. 2, IASP Press, Seattle, 1994, pp. 97–110.

Von Korff, M., Pain management in primary care: An individualized stepped/care approach. In: R.J. Gatchel and D.C. Turk (Eds.), Psychosocial factors in pain, Guilford Press, New York, 1999, pp. 360–373.

Von Korff, M. and Simon, G.E., The relationship between pain and depression, British Journal of Psychiatry, 168 (1996) 101–108.

Von Korff, M., Moore, J.E., Lorig, K., Cherkin, D.C., Saunders, K., González, V.M., Laurent, D., Rutter, C. and Comite, F., A randomized trial of a lay-led self-management group intervention for back pain patients in primary care, Spine, 23 (1998) 2608–2615.

Vowles, K.E. and Gross, R.T., Work-related beliefs about injury and physical capability for work in individuals with chronic pain, Pain, 101 (2003) 291–298.

Waddell, G., Low back pain: A twentieth century health care enigma, Spine, 21 (1996) 2820–2825.

Waddell, G., The back pain revolution, Churchill Livingstone, Edinburgh, 1998.

Waddell, G., Models of disability: Using low back pain as an example, Royal Society of Medicine Press, London, 2002, 26 pp.

Waddell, G. and Nordlund, A.I., Review of social security systems. In: A. Nachemson and E. Jonsson (Eds.), Neck and back pain: The scientific evidence of causes, diagnosis, and treatment, Lippincott Williams & Wilkins, Philadelphia, 2000, pp. 427–471.

Waddell, G., Newton, M., Henderson, I., Somerville, D. and Main, C.J., A Fear-Avoidance Beliefs Questionnaire (FABQ) and the role of fear-avoidance beliefs in chronic low back pain and disability, Pain, 52 (1993) 157–168.

Waddell, G., Feder, G. and Lewis, M., Systematic reviews of bed rest and advice to stay active for acute low back pain, British Journal of General Practice, 47 (1997) 647–652.

Waddell, G., Burton, A.K. and Main, C.J., Screening to identify people at risk of long-term incapacity for work: A conceptual and scientific review, London, 2003.

Waldenström, A., No pain, still gain, Department of Physiological Sciences, J. Schouenborg, Lund University, Lund, 2004, pp. 78.

Waldenstrom, U., Bergman, V., and Vasell, G. (1996). The complexity of labor pain: experiences of 278 women. Journal of Psychosomatic Obstetrics and Gynecology, 17(4), 215–228.

Walker, J., Control and the psychology of health, Open University Press, Buckingham, UK, 2001, 256 pp.

Walker, J.M. and Sofaer, B., Predictors of psychological distress in chronic pain patients, Journal of Advanced Nursing, 27 (1998) 320–326.

Wall, P.D., Pain: The science of suffering, Weidenfeld & Nicolson, London, 1999.

Wall, P.D. and Melzack, R., Textbook of pain, Churchill Livingstone, Edinburgh, 1999, 1588 pp.

Walters, E.T., Injury-related behavior and neuronal plasticity: An evolutionary perspective on sensitization, hyperalgesia, and analgesia, International Review of Neurobiology, 36 (1994) 325–427.

Weiser, S. and Cedraschi, C., Psychosocial issues in the prevention of chronic low back pain—a literature review, Bailliere's Clinical Rheumatology, 6 (1992) 657–684.

Westgaard, R.H. and Winkel, J., On occupational ergonomic risk factors for musculoskeletal disorders and related intervention practice. In: S.J. Linton (Ed.), New avenues for the prevention of chronic musculoskeletal pain and disability, Vol. 1, Elsevier, Amsterdam, 2002, pp. 143–164.

White, B. and Sanders, S.H., The influence on patients' pain intensity ratings of antecedent reinforcement of pain talk or well talk, Journal of Behavior Therapy and Experimental Psychiatry, 17 (1986) 155–159.

Williams, A.C., Facial expression of pain: An evolutionary account, Behavioral and Brain Sciences, 25 (2002) 439–488.

Williams, A.C. and Richardson, P.H., What does the BDI measure in chronic pain?, Pain, 55 (1993) 259–266.

Williams, D.A., Acute pain: with special emphasis on painful medical procedures. In: R.J. Gatchel and D.C. Turk (Eds.), Psychosocial factors in pain: Critical perspectives, Guilford Press, New York, 1999, pp. 151–163.

Worthlin, G., Communication and the physician–patient relationship: A physician and consumer communication survey, West Haven, CT, 1995.

Wurtele, S.K., Kaplan, G.M. and Keairnes, M., Childhood sexual abuse among chronic pain patients, Clinical Journal of Pain, 6 (1990) 110–113.

Zelman, D.C., Howland, E.W., Nichols, S.N. and Cleeland, C.S., The effects of induced mood on laboratory pain, Pain, 46 (1991) 105–111.

Index